D1582157

MAY 04
X-RAY

MRI MANUAL OF PELVIC CANCER

MRI MANUAL OF PELVIC CANCER

Paul Hulse and Bernadette Carrington
Consultant Radiologists
Christie Hospital, Manchester, UK

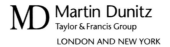

Martin Dunitz
Taylor & Francis Group
LONDON AND NEW YORK

© 2004 Martin Dunitz, an imprint of the Taylor & Francis Group

First published in the United Kingdom 2004
by Martin Dunitz, an imprint of the Taylor and Francis Group,
11 New Fetter Lane, London EC4P 4EE
Tel: +44 (0) 20 7583 9855; Fax: +44 (0) 20 7842 2298;
Email: info@dunitz.co.uk; website: http://www.dunitz.co.uk

ISBN 1 85996 069 3

Distributed in the USA by
Fulfilment Center
Taylor & Francis
10650 Toebben Drive
Independence, KY 41051, USA
Toll Free Tel.: +1 800 634 7064; E-mail: taylorandfrancis@thomsonlearning.com

Distributed in Canada by
Taylor & Francis
74 Rolark Drive
Scarborough, Ontario M1R 4G2, Canada
Toll Free Tel.: =1 877 226 2237; E-mail: tal_fran@istar.ca

Distributed in the rest of the world by
Thomson Publishing Services
Cheriton House
North Way
Andover, Hampshire SP10 5BE, UK
Tel.: +44 (0)1264 332424; E-mail:
salesorder.tandf@thomsonpublishingservices.co.uk

Typeset by Servis Filmsetting, Manchester, UK
Printed and bound in Spain by Grafos S.A.

Dedication

To Michèle and Paddy

Contents

Contributors

Rhidian Bramley
Consultant Radiologist
Christie Hospital
Manchester, UK

Suzanne Bonington
Consultant Radiologist
Christie Hospital
Manchester, UK

Bernadette M Carrington
Consultant Radiologist
Christie Hospital
Manchester, UK

Michael Dobson
Consultant Radiologist
Royal Preston Hospital
Preston, UK

Neelam Dugar
Consultant Radiologist
Doncaster Royal Infirmary
Doncaster, UK

Jane M Hawnaur
Consultant Radiologist & Honorary Senior Lecturer
Manchester Royal Infirmary
Manchester, UK

Paul A Hulse
Consultant Radiologist
Christie Hospital
Manchester, UK

Andrew Jones
Consultant Physicist
North West Medical Physics
Christie Hospital
Manchester, UK

Jeremy A L Lawrance
Consultant Radiologist
Christie Hospital
Manchester, UK

Fenella J Moulding
Specialist Registrar in Radiology
Christie Hospital
Manchester, UK

Sue Roach
Specialist Registrar in Radiology
Christie Hospital
Manchester, UK

M Ben Taylor
Consultant Radiologist
Christie Hospital
Manchester, UK

Susan M Todd
Superintendent Radiographer
Christie Hospital
Manchester, UK

Preface

Magnetic resonance imaging is now established as an invaluable imaging modality. Its marvellous contrast resolution has made it particularly useful for the evaluation of patients with cancer. This book has been compiled to provide clinical radiologists with a working knowledge and a comprehensive set of images of the various pelvic cancers.

There are introductory chapters on pelvic cancer staging, MRI technique and pelvic anatomy. Other chapters deal with cancer arising in the various locations within the pelvis. There is a short account of each disease and a set of images demonstrating the tumour, node and metastasis stages based on the most recent revision of the Union Internationale Contre le Cancer (UICC) and American Joint Committee on Cancer (AJCC) Cancer Staging Manuals published in 2002. There are also images highlighting pitfalls in the MRI diagnosis and staging of each cancer as well as illustrations of recurrent disease and appearances following chemo-radiotherapy. The two final chapters discuss and illustrate imaging before exenterative surgery and the imaging of metastatic disease within the pelvis.

Our intention is that the book should be used as a bench reference for those radiologists reporting MRI of common and rarer cancers.

Paul A Hulse
Bernadette M Carrington

Manchester, September 2003

Acknowledgments

Production of a book such as this requires a tremendous team effort from many individuals. We would particularly like to thank our secretaries, Patricia Jones and Kami Ramnarain, and the other secretaries in the Radiology Department at the Christie Hospital, for their work in the preparation of the manuscripts and images. In addition, our radiographers have been very helpful in performing searches and retrieving images from storage. They are also thanked for the high quality of their work.

Bernadette Carrington deserves a special word of gratitude for supplying supplementary images from her collection to improve many of the chapters.

Finally, we would like to acknowledge the tolerance of our contributors who have patiently revised their chapters at the editors' request as the remit of the project expanded during its evolution.

PAH
BMC

Abbreviations

APR	Abdomino-perineal resection
BPH	Benign prostatic hypertrophy
CIN	Cervical intraepithelial neoplasia
CSI	Chemical shift imaging
CT	Computed tomography
DCE	Dynamic contrast enhancement/enhanced
DRE	Digital rectal examination
DTPA	Diethylenetriaminepentaacetic acid dimeglumine
ERCs	Endorectal coils
EBRT	External beam radiotherapy
EORTC	European Organisation for Research and Treatment of Cancer
EUA	Examination under anaesthesia
5-FU	5-fluorouracil
FDG PET	^{18}-Fluorodeoxyglucose positron emission tomography
FFE	Fast field echo
FIESTA	Fast imaging employing steady state acquisition
FIGO	Federation Internationale Gynecologie et Oncologie
FISP	Fast imaging steady state precession
FOV	Field of view
FSE	Fast spin echo
Gd	Gadolinium
GE	Gradient echo
GEPDI	Gradient echo proton density image
GI	Gastrointestinal
HIV	Human immunodeficiency virus
HNPCC	Hereditary nonpolyposis colorectal cancer
HPV	Human papilloma virus
IVC	Inferior vena cava
IAF	Ischioanal fossa
JSM	Jewett-Strong-Marshall
MSAD	Maximum short axis diameter
PIN	Prostatic intraepithelial neoplasia
PSA	Prostate specific antigen
ROC	Receiver operating characteristic
SPIO	Super-paramagnetic iron oxide
STIR	Short tau inversion recovery
SV	Seminal vesicle
T1WI	T1 Weighted image(s)
T2WI	T2 Weighted image(s) (Usually fast or turbo spin echo)
TEs	Echo times
TME	Total meso-rectal excision
TNM	Tumour node metastasis
TR	Repetition time
TRUS	Transrectal ultrasound
TSE	Turbo spin echo
TURP	Transurethral resection of the prostate
UICC	Union Internationale Contre le Cancer
UKCCR	United Kingdom Coordinating Committee on Cancer Research
US	Ultrasound
VAIN	Vaginal intraepithelial neoplasia
VIN	Vulval intraepithelial neoplasia

1   Diagnosis and Staging of Pelvic Tumours: the Role of MR Imaging

Bernadette M. Carrington

INTRODUCTION

Cancer is due to an abnormal proliferation of cells which are resistant to normal regulatory mechanisms and which have the propensity to infiltrate the host organ, to invade locally and to activate mechanisms allowing more widespread dissemination through the body via blood vessels or lymphatics.

Critical initial steps in cancer management are confirmation by histological diagnosis, and determination of tumour extent by staging. This fundamental information is central to all management decisions, and provides prognostic information. Accurate stratification of patients by tumour type and stage is also a prerequisite of cancer research, enabling valid comparison of outcomes between treatment groups.

TUMOUR DIAGNOSIS

MR imaging offers exquisite detail of pelvic anatomy, but is rarely the means by which primary pelvic tumours are diagnosed. Most pelvic malignancy is diagnosed on clinical examination supplemented by findings from EUA (examination under anaesthesia), cystoscopy, colposcopy and rigid sigmoidoscopy. The initial radiological assessment will depend on the experience of the requesting clinician and the availability of local radiology services. In the investigation of a pelvic mass, transabdominal ultrasound is often the first examination performed. Transvaginal and transrectal ultrasound (US) techniques offer better image resolution. Computed tomography (CT) may be performed if disease is suspected to involve the thorax and abdomen. MR imaging is increasingly utilised in the initial assessment of pelvic tumours. This trend is expected to continue as MR imaging becomes more widely available and local radiological expertise develops.

Tissue confirmation of malignancy is required whenever possible. This may be achieved by cytological analysis of surface accessible lesions such as cervical cancer, or via fine needle aspiration biopsy of deeper lesions (e.g. enlarged lymph nodes). Core needle biopsy is used to obtain larger volume and more reliable tissue samples, when a definitive histological diagnosis is required. Some patients may require excision or incision biopsy, with resection of all or part of the tumour respectively. Excision biopsy is ideal since it allows accurate histopathological staging of the primary tumour, and offers a potential for cure. In exceptional circumstances, patients do not have histopathological confirmation of cancer, but this rarely happens in pelvic malignancy.

Image-guided biopsy can be used to target lesions, which would

otherwise require invasive procedures to obtain tissue. Ultrasound provides 'real time' imaging guidance and is the preferred modality in experienced hands. An example is transrectal ultrasound guided prostatic biopsy, which is a routine diagnostic investigation for prostatic carcinoma. CT-guided fine needle aspiration biopsy can be used to sample pelvic masses and enlarged iliac lymph nodes. Although MR-compatible biopsy equipment exists, MR-guided tumour biopsy is not widely used since most tumours are amenable to CT- or ultrasound-guided biopsy, allowing more time-efficient utilisation of MR imaging resources.

TUMOUR STAGING

Tumour extent at diagnosis may be estimated clinically by physical examination or by other means such as measurement of biochemical tumour markers. Histopathological findings on biopsy may also suggest tumour extent, high grade tumours being more likely to invade and metastasise early. Small superficial tumours of the bladder, cervix and rectum may be adequately staged by direct examination (cystoscopy, colposcopy or sigmoidoscopy) and excision biopsy. When a deeper and more extensive tumour is present, further investigation is required. The aim of imaging is to accurately determine locoregional tumour extent and to identify any metastatic spread. These findings are then described in terms of a tumour stage.

MRI is recognised as a key tool for locoregional pelvic tumour staging. It offers exquisite anatomical delineation of a tumour in multiple planes and allows identification of intra-organ tumour extent and invasion of adjacent structures. It is recommended that at least one MRI sequence be performed through the abdomen to allow evaluation of the retroperitoneal nodal stations, visualisation of more of the axial skeleton and assessment of the kidneys. Machine time constraints do not usually permit full MR imaging assessment of the liver and small volume omental and mesenteric disease may not be identified on MR imaging without increased patient scan time and the use of intravenous contrast media. The lungs are not optimally assessed by MR imaging. Therefore, thoracoabdominal CT is required in addition to pelvic MR imaging to determine tumour stage accurately. Additional need for extra-pelvic imaging to stage patients will be addressed in the chapters dealing with individual malignancies.

TUMOUR STAGING SYSTEMS

Tumour staging systems are internationally agreed graduated classifications of tumour spread.

All the tumour staging systems incorporate common principles:

- There is a graduation from 'early' confined tumours which are given low numbers in the classification systems, to 'late' more advanced and widespread tumours which are given higher numbers in the classification systems. The presence and extent of lymph node metastases are treated similarly. Visceral and bone metastases are grouped in a general metastasis category but are not quantified.

- Each primary tumour has an individual staging classification tailored to its pattern of spread. The difference between tumour extent for each stage is clearly demarcated.

- The systems must be easily applied, forming a shorthand summary of the tumour extent, which is understood within the national and international cancer community.

- The precise information supplied must be of relevance to therapeutic decision-making.

- The staging systems are an indicator of likely prognosis since each step within the system correlates with worsening outcome.

In oncology practice additional benefits accrue from cancer staging systems:

- The efficacy of new treatments can be assessed in similarly staged, and therefore, standardised populations.

- The performance of cancer treatment centres can be compared nationally and internationally.

- The exchange of information is facilitated between different cancer organisations.

The most commonly used staging system is the *Tumour Node Metastasis* (TNM) classification, which has common stratification groups for each tumour type. The TNM cancer staging classifications are reviewed regularly by the International Union against Cancer (Union Internationale Contre le Cancer, UICC) with contributions from associated national and international organisations. The American classification is the 'AJCC Cancer Staging Manual' produced by the American Joint Committee on Cancer and it correlates exactly with the TNM classification. Additional staging systems are in existence, which usually have fewer stratification groups. In gynaecological malignancy, the main alternate staging system is the *Federation Internationale Gynécologie et Obstétrique* (FIGO) classification. Bladder cancer may also be staged according to the Jewett-Strong-Marshall classification (principally in the USA). Colorectal cancer is commonly staged by the Duke's classification (principally in the UK).

STAGE MIGRATION (STAGE SHIFT)

Two factors contribute to the phenomenon of stage migration. The first is the periodic amendments all cancer staging systems undergo which may lead to tumours being up- or down-staged in the new system. The second is the impact of cross-sectional imaging, which generally up-stages more tumours than it down-stages when compared to clinical staging. This results in fewer patients categorised as having early stage disease and more patients categorised as having later stage disease, with an overall apparent improvement in survival, stage for stage, compared with non-imaged patients. This is because the patients who are radiologically up-staged usually have a smaller volume of disease than those who are clinically categorised as belonging to the same stage. The up-staged patients are likely to improve the overall survival rate for the higher stage group, and this may also result in apparent improved tumour response rates. In addition, the early stage disease group is less confounded by inaccurate clinical staging of patients with more advanced tumours, and so this group too will appear to have improved tumour response rates and survival.

The stage migration phenomenon should be remembered when interpreting modern clinical trial results and comparing them to historical controls. In this situation, stage migration may contribute to spurious increased efficacy of the new therapies.

PRINCIPLES OF ONCORADIOLOGICAL PRACTICE IN TUMOUR DIAGNOSIS AND STAGING

The aims of cancer imaging are to:

- Provide the means to obtain histological confirmation of cancer by image-guided biopsy.

- Select the optimal imaging modality for the tumour to be assessed.

- Design imaging protocols that take account of pathways of tumour spread.

- Differentiate between tumour and benign conditions which can mimic tumour.

- Allocate tumour stage on the basis of imaging findings.

- Maintain a common imaging modality and imaging protocol before and after treatment to allow assessment of response.

Each oncological staging report needs to incorporate standard information including an accurate description of tumour size, local extent, the presence of enlarged lymph nodes, which are more likely to be metastatic, together with their location and short axis diameter, and the presence of any distant metastases. This information should be summarised using an appropriate staging system, which is clearly understood by the clinicians involved in the patient's care. Where there is uncertainty about the exact stage then this should be recorded e.g. "the MR stage of this patient's prostate tumour is either T2B N0 M0 or T3a N0 M0". It is also necessary to identify important normal structures, for example unobstructed kidneys, and to mention any co-morbid conditions that may have an implication for patient treatment such as severe diverticular disease in a patient who may undergo radiotherapy.

As a general rule, staging accuracy improves through the following hierarchy: clinical, radiological, surgical, pathological, with histopathological assessment being the gold standard. Therefore, it is important to correlate radiological staging with any clinical, surgical or pathological staging. This provides an opportunity to identify the strengths and weaknesses of radiological staging and to learn on a case-by-case basis.

FURTHER READING

1. Hermanek P. (Ed.) (1997) *TNM Atlas Illustrated Guide to the TNM/pTNM Classification of Malignant Tumours*, 4th Edn. Springer-Verlag, Berlin, Heidelberg, New York.

2. Greene FL, Page DL, Fleming ID *et al.* (2002) *AJCC Cancer Staging Manual*, 6th Edn. Springer, New York.

3. International Federation of Gynecology and Obstetrics. Staging Announcement. (1995) FIGO Staging of gynaecologic cancers; cervix and vulva. *Int. J. Gynaecol. Obstet.* 5: 319.

4. Jewett H and Strong G. (1946) Infiltrating carcinoma of the bladder: relation of depth of penetration of the bladder wall to incidence of local extension in metastases. *J. Urol.* 55: 366–372.

2 MR Imaging Techniques in Pelvic Cancer

Susan M Todd and Andrew P Jones

INTRODUCTION

Pelvic cancer imaging interpretation is crucially dependent on the quality of the imaging examination performed. This in turn depends on several factors:

- Equipment available;
- Imaging protocols;
- Motivated patients;
- Expert radiographers/technologists.

MR IMAGING EQUIPMENT

Most magnetic resonance imaging scanners are superconducting magnets operating at 0.5, 1.0 or 1.5 Tesla. A surface coil, either a phased array body or pelvis coil, which wraps around the patient is ideal for pelvic imaging. The phased array coil receives the signal from the patient and has a number of individual surface coil elements (arranged above and below the patient) that feed into separate receivers. The information from all of the surface coils is combined together to form the final image. The advantages of phased array coils are (i) a high signal-to-noise ratio associated with small diameter component surface coils, and (ii) a relatively large field of view (FOV) is achieved. For example, the maximum FOV for phased array body/pelvic coils is 30–35 cm, and some systems enable additional elements to be attached to the phased array coil so that the FOV can be increased to 50 cm. This compares well with the FOV for body coils which are usually in the region of 50 cm. See *Figures 2.1a and b.*

MR IMAGING PROTOCOLS

For all pelvic cancers, a standardised imaging protocol should be agreed so as to:

- ensure imaging covers all the potential regions of tumour spread within the pelvis;
- keep scan times to the minimum necessary for patient comfort and efficient use of the MR equipment;
- allow consistent interpretation of the examination;
- ensure reproducibility of subsequent MRI examinations.

Accepted practice involves the use of orthogonal plane T1W and T2W sequences, with off-axis planes or additional sequences being used for well-defined indications. Suggested basic imaging parameters are summarised in *Table 2.1.*

T1W Sequences (spin echo or gradient echo)

T1W sequences give an overview of the abdomen and pelvis for detection of lymph node enlargement, bone marrow metastases, and hydronephrosis and hydroureter. They also allow evaluation of tumour bulk and extension into pelvic fat and provide some tissue specific information, for example, haemorrhage and water. They are most commonly performed in the coronal and transaxial planes.

Coronal plane

Following a scout planning image, a block of two-dimensional (2D) or three-dimensional (3D) generated slices in the coronal plane is obtained. The patient is positioned with the centre of the FOV at the level of the anterior superior iliac spines. A large FOV of 40–48 cm is selected and the body coil (or the phased array coil if sufficient FOV can be obtained) is used to visualise anatomy from above the renal hila to 2.5 cm below the symphysis pubis, with slices (7–10 mm thick) positioned from the sacrum forward to the symphysis pubis. See *Figure 2.2.*

Transaxial plane

Slices are obtained through the pelvis, from the iliac crests to the lower border of the symphysis pubis, either using the phased array or body coil (FOV 34–38 cm), slice thickness ranges from 5–10 mm. Ghosting artifact throughout the pelvis from anterior to posterior is caused by fat in the anterior abdominopelvic wall moving during respiration. This can be suppressed by changing the phase encoding direction so that it runs from side to side, i.e. right to left, or by selecting a breath-hold sequence. See *Figure 2.3.*

For tumours that metastasise to retroperitoneal lymph nodes (e.g. carcinoma of the cervix) a more cranially situated set of transaxial slices are necessary, again using the phased array or body coil (FOV 34–38 cm). These are positioned to cover from above the renal hila to immediately caudal to the iliac crests, so that there is overlap with the pelvic transaxial block. Artifacts from breathing are more pronounced in this area and can be overcome either by selecting a breath-hold sequence or by increasing the number of acquisitions (excitations) to average out the artifact. If choosing the latter, the phase encoding direction is selected to be in the anterior-posterior direction so that a rectangular field of view can be applied. This helps to reduce the scan time as fewer phase encoding steps are performed. Superior and inferior presaturation bands placed parallel to the block of slices reduce artifact from flowing blood in the inferior vena cava (IVC) and aorta. A reduced matrix is chosen to minimise the scan time.

T2W Sequences (fast or turbo spin echo)

These sequences give detailed information about the primary site of disease, demonstrating zonal anatomy of the cervix, uterus and prostate and the muscular layers of the pelvic floor, anal canal and rectal wall. The T2W sequences thereby aid accurate assessment of local spread and tissue specificity. The phased array body/pelvic coil is used and is positioned so that the centre of the coil is in line with the upper border of the symphysis pubis. Artifact from respiration can be limited by strapping the phased array coil across the patient to compress the pelvis. Respiratory artifact can be further reduced by swapping the phase and frequency encoding direction so that it runs from side to side (i.e. right to left) for the transaxial images and by placing a presaturation band over the fat in the anterior pelvic wall on the sagittal images. See *Figures 2.4a and b, and 2.5*. If images remain degraded by respiration-induced artifact, the patient can be positioned prone in an attempt to reduce motion in the pelvic organs.

Images can also be degraded by bowel peristalsis. Having the bladder partially full can help to lift the bowel loops out of the pelvis, however, if the bladder is too distended patient motion due to discomfort will introduce further artifact. In some instances, the only way to reduce or eliminate bowel peristalsis is to administer an anti-spasmodic agent. An intravenous injection of an anti-spasmodic agent/smooth muscle relaxant (e.g. 20 mg hyoscine butylbromide (Buscopan)) is recommended as its effect lasts approximately 20 minutes, allowing time to perform all the T2W sequences. See *Figures 2.6a and b*.

Phase over-sampling is necessary for all the T2W sequences to eliminate wrap into the image in the phase encoding direction from body parts outside the FOV. A separate scout is acquired and used to position the T2W sequences.

Transaxial plane

The transaxial plane is performed for all pelvic cancers. It is the most familiar plane to radiologists and optimally demonstrates disease spreading laterally, anteriorly and posteriorly from the primary site. A field of view of 20 cm allows coverage to the pelvic sidewalls. Ideally 3 mm (high resolution) slices with a small interslice gap (10% of slice thickness) are selected to cover the region of interest. Having phase and frequency encoding direction running from side to side (i.e. right to left) reduces respiratory artifact. Superior and inferior presaturation bands placed parallel to the block of slices reduce artifact from flowing blood.

Transaxial oblique/off-axis plane

For cancer of the cervix, transaxial oblique or off-axis images are useful for accurate assessment of disease spread into the parametrium. The slice block is positioned over the cervix uteri and perpendicular to the endocervical canal. The resultant images show the cervix and parametrium in true cross section. They are also valuable to demonstrate disease extension into the uterovesical ligament and to assess the integrity of the posterior bladder wall. See *Figures 2.7a and b*.

A second set of off-axis images can be obtained by positioning the slice block parallel to the endocervical canal and will also show lateral spread of disease. The slice angle can be altered so that the slices bisect any area of potential disease spread from the posterior cervix into the rectovaginal fascia or anterior wall of the rectum. See *Figures 2.8a and b*.

For rectal tumours, transaxial oblique images are again valuable for accurate assessment of disease spread. The slice block is positioned perpendicular to the tumour to demonstrate disease extending laterally, anteriorly or posteriorly.

Sagittal plane

The sagittal plane is particularly useful for evaluating midline structures, that is the vagina, uterus, prostate, urethra, anus and rectum. It demonstrates disease spreading anteriorly, posteriorly, superiorly and inferiorly. A field of view of 20 cm allows coverage from the sacral promontory to below the perineum. Ideally 3 mm (high resolution) slices with a small interslice gap (10% of slice thickness) are selected to cover the region of interest.

Coronal plane

The coronal plane is used for imaging the prostate, anus, pelvic floor and seminal vesicles. It demonstrates disease spreading laterally, superiorly and inferiorly. A field of view of 20 cm is positioned from the sacral promontory to below the perineum and is sufficient to include the pelvic sidewalls, again 3 mm (high resolution) slices with a small interslice gap (10%) are selected to cover the region of interest.

Coronal oblique plane

Coronal oblique slices are employed for imaging the prostate and demonstrate spread of disease laterally, superiorly and inferiorly. In particular, the plane bisects the interface between the base of the prostate and the bladder, to allow accurate evaluation of disease extent in this region. The slices are angled to run parallel to a line running from the apex of the prostate and bisecting its base and are positioned to include the seminal vesicles. See *Figures 2.9a and b*.

Table 2.1. Basic imaging parameters for staging pelvic cancers

Sequence, weighting and plane	Coil	Slice thickness (mm)	Field of view (cm)	Approx. in plane resolution phase/frequency in mm (Matrix size)	Comments
T1W 3 planes (scout)	Body	10.0	50.0	4×2 (128×256)	To plan subsequent slice positions
T1W Coronal	Body	7.0–10.0	40.0–48.0	2×1 (256×512)	
T1W Transaxial pelvis	Body or phased array	5.0–10.0	34.0–38.0	1.5×0.75 (256×512)	Phase direction right to left
T1W Transaxial abdomen	Body or phased array	5.0–10.0	34.0–38.0	2.5×1.5 (109×256 rectangular 6/8 FOV)	Inferior and superior presaturation bands parallel to slice block
T1W 3 planes (scout)	Phased array body/pelvic	10.0	35.0	2.5×1.5 (140×256)	To plan subsequent slice positions
T2W Sagittal	Phased array body/pelvic	3.0–5.0	20.0	1×0.7 (210×256)	Phase oversampling applied. Presaturation band positioned over anterior pelvic wall fat
T2W Transaxial (oblique for cervix and rectum)	Phased array body/pelvic	3.0–5.0	20.0	1×0.75 (210×256)	Phase oversampling applied. Phase direction right to left. Inferior and superior presaturation bands parallel to slice block
T2W Coronal (oblique for prostate)	Phased array body/pelvic	3.0–5.0	20.0	1×0.75 (210×256)	Phase oversampling applied

Imaging protocols for specific cancer types

All the following will require the T1W overview sequences plus the T2W / other sequences specified below.

Vulva: T2W sequences in all three orthogonal planes.

Vagina: T2W sagittal sequence to cover vagina.

T2W transaxial sequence, two blocks to include cervix uteri down to introitus.

Cervix uteri: T2W sagittal sequence to include corpus uteri down to introitus.

T2W transaxial oblique sequence, two blocks. One block positioned over cervix uteri and angled 90 degrees to the endocervical canal, the second block positioned over the cervix uteri and variably angled perpendicular to the plane that needs to be assessed e.g. posterior bladder/anterior rectum.

Corpus uteri: T2W sagittal sequence, to include all of the corpus uteri and down to introitus.

T2W transaxial oblique sequence, two blocks. One angled at 90 degrees to the endometrium and the second angled parallel to the endometrium.

Ovary: T2W transaxial sequence, one or two blocks to include all of disease. May need to increase slice thickness up to 6.0 mm to include the whole area of interest.

T2W coronal sequence. May need to increase slice thickness to encompass whole of disease.

T2W sagittal sequence may also be useful.

Prostate: T2W sagittal sequence.

T2W transaxial sequence to include seminal vesicles to apex of prostate.

T2W coronal oblique sequence to include seminal vesicles.

Bladder: T2W sequences in all three orthogonal planes. May need to increase slice thickness up to 6.0 mm depending on distension of the bladder.

Rectum and Colon: Rectum – start with T2W sagittal sequence, then transaxial oblique and coronal blocks positioned on the sagittal images.

Sigmoid – start with T2W transaxial sequence, then position coronal and sagittal blocks on transaxial images.

Pelvic Floor,
Urethra and Anus: T2W sequences in all three orthogonal planes.

Bone Metastases: Short Tau Inversion Recovery (STIR) coronal and T1W transaxial, to cover from iliac crests to below symphysis pubis.

Pelvic Lymph Node
Metastases: T2W transaxial sequence (one or two overlapping blocks) to cover from bifurcation of the aorta to below symphysis pubis.

Recurrent Tumour: Follow site specific T2W sequences as suggested above.

Pelvic Clearance: T2W sequences in all three orthogonal planes, to include pelvic sidewalls, and from sacral promontory down to symphysis pubis.

Chemical fat saturation

Chemical or frequency selective fat saturation techniques rely on the difference in resonant frequencies of water and fat (220 Hertz at 1.5 Tesla). A saturation pulse centred only over the frequency for fat can selectively remove the signal contribution of fat from the image. More recently, water and fat selective excitation methods have become available using binomial pulse techniques. All fat saturation techniques can be applied to both T1W and T2W sequences. See *Figure 2.10*. They are useful to delineate invasion from the primary tumour site into surrounding fat and to distinguish fat within lesions (e.g. ovarian masses).

Contrast enhancement

Intravenous injection of a Gadolinium (Gd)-based contrast agent is not routinely employed in imaging of the pelvis for malignancy. This is largely due to:

- the inherent high contrast within the pelvic organs on T2W images;
- the contrast differences between tumours and pelvic organs and tissues on T2W images;
- the enhancement of normal tissues and structures in the pelvis, such as the venous plexus surrounding the vagina, cervix/corpus uteri and the prostate gland, which often serves to decrease the conspicuity of tumour.

However, a contrast agent injection is valuable in certain instances:

- to delineate the extent of disease or treatment effect within muscle groups;
- to assess the depth of myometrial and bladder wall involvement when administered dynamically in patients with endometrial or bladder cancers;
- to clarify the composition of complex ovarian tumours;
- to determine the extent of sarcoma spread.

Hard copy images

To enable ease of comparison between examinations, hard copy images are printed as follows:

coronal images: posterior to anterior (back to front of patient);

transaxial images: superior to inferior (top to bottom of patient);

sagittal images: right to left with anterior of image facing to the left of the printed film;

post-contrast agent
T1W images: same window width and window centre as pre-contrast agent images. This ensures correct visual identification of contrast enhancement.

PATIENT MOTIVATION AND SUPPORT

The interaction between the patient and the radiographic/technological staff is vital to ensure a successful examination. Most patients with cancer are motivated to cooperate but may have difficulty due to pain, claustrophobia or psychological stress. With careful explanation and sympathetic handling, patients are often able to cooperate fully. Time spent in making them as comfortable as possible before the examination, assisting them during the examination and praising their efforts afterwards may ensure that the current examination is satisfactory and, importantly, that the patient is happy to undergo follow-up MR examinations.

When patients are distressed and images inadequate it is helpful to have additional time built into the imaging schedule to allow for repeating some sequences.

Strategies for claustrophobic and distressed patients include:

- sending written information to the patient prior to the MR examination date, including a contact telephone number to use for any queries;
- explaining the procedure simply to the patient prior to the MR examination;
- keeping in contact with the patient during the examination (i.e. speaking encouragingly to them between sequences);
- playing music (of the patient's choice) or video if available to help soothe the patient;
- the use of prismatic glasses, so that the patient can see out of the scanner bore;
- scanning the patient feet first so that the head has not travelled far into the scanner bore;
- scanning the patient feet first and in the prone position, the patient's chin tilted and resting on folded arms, again so that he or she can see out of the scanner;
- having the patient's friend or relative stay in the magnet room during the examination to alleviate the sense of isolation. The companion needs to comply with magnetic and radiofrequency field safety checks before entering the magnet room.

EXPERT RADIOGRAPHERS / TECHNOLOGISTS

As with all MRI examinations, radiographers require training and experience to become competent and efficient in scanning pelvic cancers. A good radiographer/technologist will be:

- quick;
- calm, assured and caring;
- familiar with the aims of pelvic cancer imaging;
- adaptable, that is able to alter sequence parameters dependent on the patient;
- able to prioritise sequences where the patient is unlikely to last a full examination;
- meticulous in attention to detail;
- able to optimise the quality of images when producing hard copy images.

NEW TECHNIQUES

Acquisition strategies

Recently a number of new sequence variants and acquisition strategies have become available on standard MR systems, which may find important applications within pelvic imaging. Potential problems with motion artifacts in non breath-hold techniques can be minimised using free-breathing approaches. The minimisation of motion blurring can improve the image quality for example at the liver lung interface. These new data acquisition strategies are generally either continuous with retrospective selection and re-ordering of phase encoding steps, or prospective, using navigator echo techniques to selectively gate the acquisition according to respiratory motion. Navigator echo methods in their simplest form, acquire effectively a one-dimensional column of data across the boundary of the liver/diaphragm and the lung for each repetition time (TR) of the sequence. The high contrast boundary is clearly demonstrated and its position can be monitored automatically and an acceptance window set to trigger data acquisition as shown in *Figure 2.11*. Navigator techniques are also used to monitor the diaphragm position during multiple breath-hold studies to ensure correct coverage of the liver, for example, in situations where a patient's breath-hold positions are not reproducible. Necessarily, nearly all such acquisition techniques which involve the selective acquisition of data can result in slight increases in scan time, however the advantages of improved image quality outweigh any disadvantage.

New sequences

A series of new sequence developments, initially primarily aimed at neurological or cardiac applications, have started to find favour in body imaging for the abdomen and pelvis. An extension to the fat saturation techniques referred to above now permits fat only or water only images to be obtained, using either narrow bandwidth frequency selective excitations or using a variety of types of binomial pulses. Optimisation of steady state gradient echo sequences, with ultra short echo times (TEs) and TRs, have enabled multi-slice acquisitions in a single breath-hold. Particular variants such as True FISP (fast imaging with steady state precession, also known as Balanced fast field echo (FFE) and fast imaging employing steady state acquisition (FIESTA)) demonstrate a unique tissue contrast (high signal is produced for tissues with a large value of T2/T1). While special versions of these sequences have specific strengths for cardiac imaging, the inherent contrast has interesting applications within general body imaging as shown in *Figure 2.12*.

Dynamic contrast enhancement (DCE)

In addition to the conventional application of DCE sequences to visualise vasculature, DCE techniques are also being actively investigated as a method of assessing tumour perfusion, oxygenation and angiogenesis. Studies in the brain, using T2* based methods, monitoring the signal decrease in brain parenchyma via a series of dynamic T2* weighted images following a bolus injection of contrast, are well established for assessing perfusion and cerebral blood volume. Similar methods based on dynamic T1 contrast enhancement following a bolus contrast injection are being used to investigate the permeability of tissue and the oxygenation state of malignant lesions in the brain and throughout the body. The signal enhancement curves obtained can be mathematically fitted using a variety of pharmacokinetic models in terms of factors linked directly to tissue permeability, angiogenesis and hypoxia. Promising results have been published, for example, in the study of carcinoma of the cervix and carcinoma of the prostate.

^{1}H Spectroscopy of the prostate

Multi-voxel ^{1}H spectroscopy or Chemical Shift Imaging (CSI) has been applied to the brain for some time. Recently, CSI techniques have been used for examination of cancer of the prostate. ^{1}H spectra show changes in creatine and choline signals in the presence of tumour and a reduction in the metabolite signal from citrate, which is present only in normal healthy tissue. In prostate cancer, spectral changes have been reported as being present, despite normal imaging appearances (*Figure 2.13*). The spectroscopy provides important information on disease spread in the peripheral zone and into the neurovascular bundle and can be used to guide biopsies, monitor response to treatment and for the assessment of possible recurrence. Recently, reductions in CSI voxel size have improved the resolution of the CSI data, although best results are reported for endo-cavity coils rather than pelvic phased array coils.

FURTHER READING

1. Elster AD and Burdette JH. (2001) *Questions and Answers in Magnetic Resonance Imaging,* 2nd Edn. Mosby, St Louis, Missouri. *Thorough but easy to read physics text providing practical answers of benefit to all involved in MRI.*

2. Husband JES, Johnson RJ and Reznek RH. (1999) *A Guide to the Practical Use of MRI in Oncology.* The Royal College of Radiologists, London, UK. *General guidelines for oncological MRI examinations.*

3. Lomas DJ. (1997) Review: Optimization of sequences for MRI of the abdomen and pelvis. *Clin. Radiol.* 52(6): 412–428. *Physics based review of MR sequences and artifacts encountered in abdomen and pelvic MR imaging.*

4. Loncaster JA, Carrington BM, Sykes JR *et al.* (2002) Prediction of radiotherapy outcome using dynamic contrast-enhanced MRI of carcinoma of the cervix. *Int. J. Radiat. Oncol. Biol. and Phys.* 54(3): 759–767. *Paper describing method and correlation between clinical outcome and dynamic contrast-enhanced MRI.*

5. Padhani AR and Husband JES. (2001) Dynamic contrast-enhanced MRI studies in oncology with an emphasis on quantification, validation and human studies. *Clin. Radiol.* 56(8): 607–620. *Reviews quantification analysis of oncological studies using dynamic contrast-enhanced MRI.*

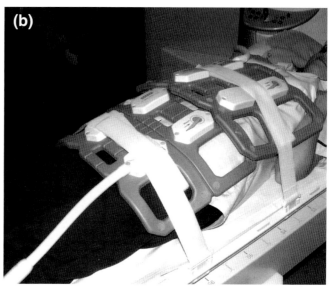

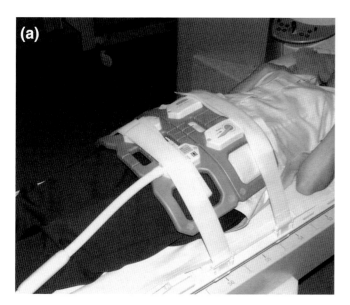

Figure 2.1.

(a) Anterior aspect of a flexible phased array body coil positioned over the lower abdomen and pelvic region. The patient is lying over posterior phased array coil elements. The maximum FOV using this coil arrangement is 35 cm. **(b)** Flexible phased array body coil with additional elements positioned over the abdomen. The maximum FOV using all the elements is now 50 cm.

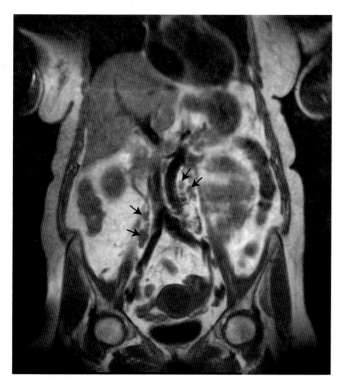

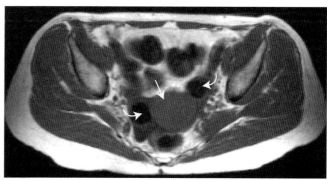

Figure 2.3.

Transaxial T1WI of the pelvis showing the intermediate signal intensity corpus uteri (straight arrow) and low signal intensity adnexal cysts (curved arrows).

Figure 2.2.

Coronal T1WI of the abdomen and pelvis demonstrating lymph node metastases (arrows).

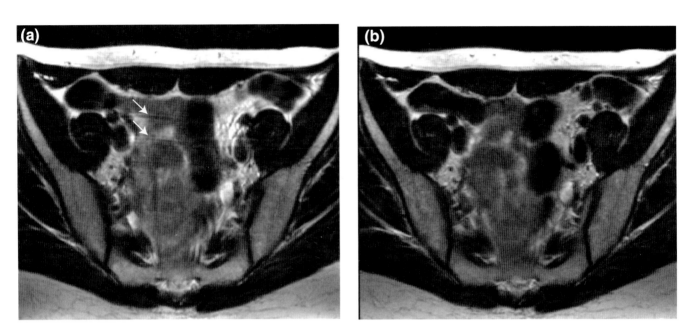

Figure 2.4.

(a) Transaxial T2WI with phase encoding direction anterior to posterior with ghosting artifact (arrows). (b) Transaxial T2WI with phase encoding direction left to right showing greatly reduced ghosting artifact.

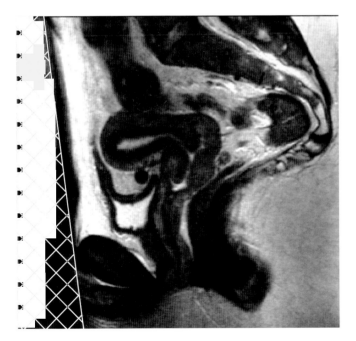

Figure 2.5.

Sagittal T2WI of the female pelvis showing the position of presaturation band (cross-hatched area).

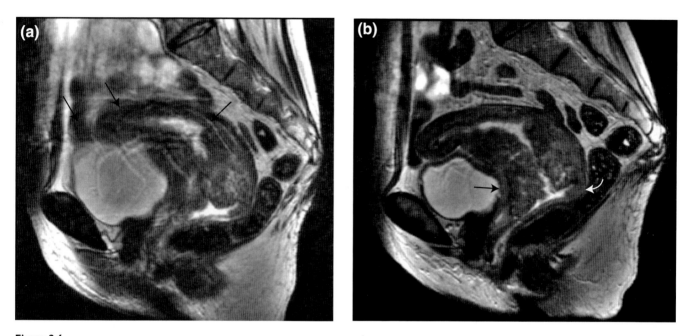

Figure 2.6.

(a) Sagittal T2WI of the female pelvis showing image degradation as a result of peristalsis (arrows). **(b)** Sagittal T2WI of the female pelvis post administration of anti-spasmodic agent. The cervical tumour and its relationship with the bladder wall (straight arrow) and rectum (curved arrow) are more clearly visualised.

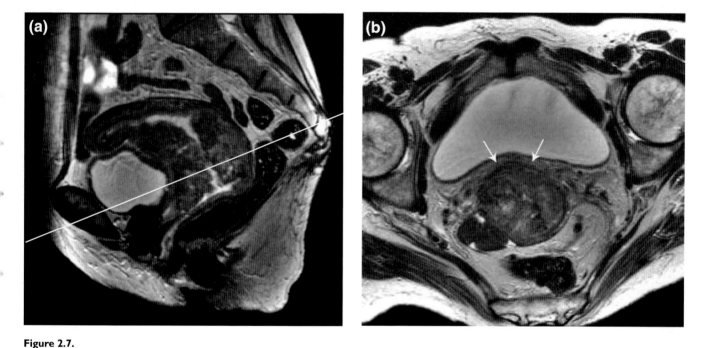

Figure 2.7.

(a) Sagittal T2WI of the female pelvis showing plane of transaxial oblique slices perpendicular to the endocervical canal (white line). **(b)** Transaxial oblique T2WI of the female pelvis from plane illustrated in (a). The intact fat plane between the cervix uteri and the bladder is clearly visualised (arrows).

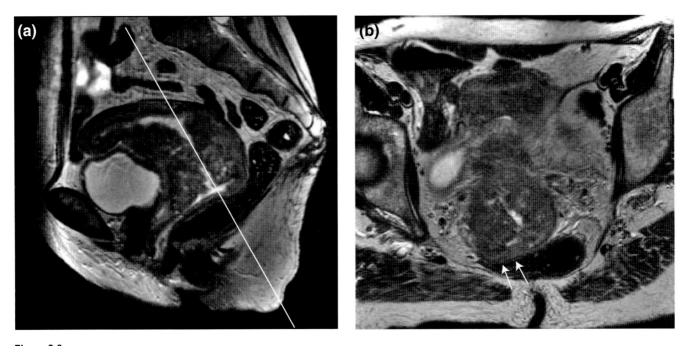

Figure 2.8.

(a) Sagittal T2WI showing plane of transaxial oblique slices parallel to the endocervical canal (white line). (b) Transaxial oblique T2WI of the female pelvis from plane illustrated in (a), showing infiltration of cervical tumour into the rectal wall (arrows).

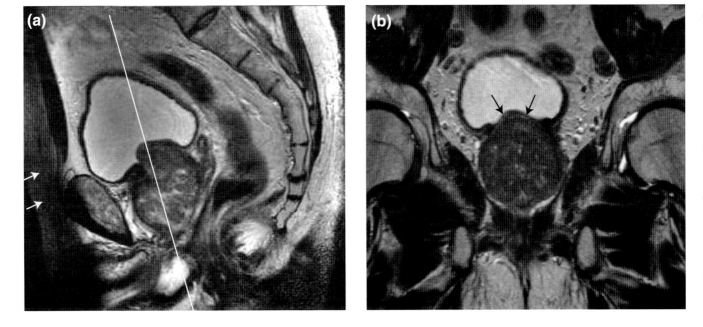

Figure 2.9.

(a) Sagittal T2WI showing plane of coronal oblique slices through the prostate (white line). Note the reduced signal from fat in the abdominopelvic wall due to positioning of presaturation band (arrows). (b) Coronal oblique T2WI of the male pelvis from plane illustrated in (a), showing disease extending into the bladder from the base of the prostate (arrows), and the lateral extent of the lesion.

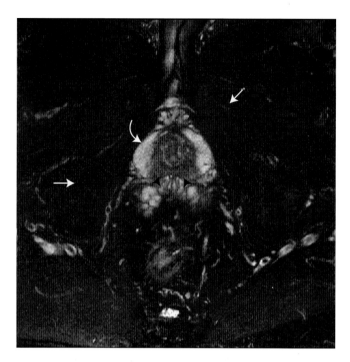

Figure 2.10.

Example of a small field of view transaxial T2WI of the male pelvis with fat saturation. Note the loss of signal from fat (arrows) which allows clear visualisation of the prostate (curved arrow) and abnormal low signal in the peripheral zone posteriorly (arrowheads) consistent with prostatic cancer.

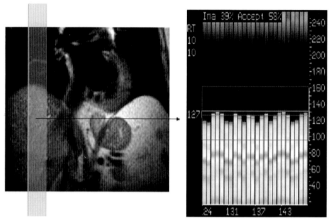

Figure 2.11.

Illustration of the use of a navigator echo for monitoring respiratory motion and triggering data acquisition. A column of data is collected for each TR of the sequence over the boundary of the liver and lung as shown on the left. The right image demonstrates a real-time display of the signal from this column, the narrow dashed box indicating acceptable positions of the diaphragm and the large dashed box extreme positions of the diaphragm. The acquisition can be triggered or retrospectively corrected by setting allowed limits on the position of the diaphragm.

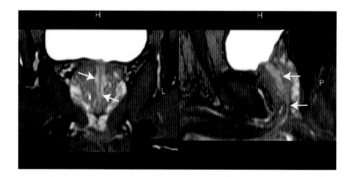

Figure 2.12.

Example images of the application of TrueFISP in the pelvis. Despite the low spatial resolution of these images there is excellent tissue contrast within the prostate such that the urethra (arrows) can be clearly visualised.

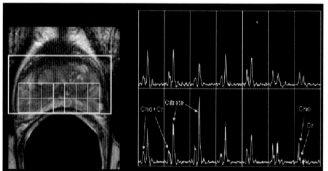

Figure 2.13.

^{1}H spectroscopic chemical shift imaging of the prostate. The position of the voxels is shown in the left image and the measured spectra for each voxel is demonstrated on the right. Citrate occurs only within normal healthy tissue. Areas of malignant tissue are characterised by a decrease in citrate signal and an increase in the choline (cho) signal. (Cr – Creatine.)

3　Anatomy of the Pelvis

Paul A Hulse

MUSCULOSKELETAL MORPHOLOGY

The **pelvic cavity** is divided into the **false** (greater) pelvis above, and the **true** (lesser) pelvis below, by an imaginary plane passing from the sacral promontory posteriorly around the arcuate lines laterally and anteriorly onto the symphysis pubis.

The bony pelvis forms an articulated ring consisting of the paired hip bones (composed of the fused iliac, ischial and pubic bones), the sacrum and the coccyx.

The pelvic sidewalls are composed of a horseshoe shaped muscular sling covered with pelvic fascia. The iliopsoas muscles form the walls of the false pelvis while the obturator internus and piriformis muscles form the walls of the true pelvis. The pelvic floor is a fibromuscular diaphragm formed from the paired levator ani muscles anteriorly and the paired coccygeal muscles posteriorly. The levator ani muscle arises from the superior and posterior aspects of the pubis, the pelvic fascia covering the obturator internus muscle and the inner surface of the ischial bone and ischial spine. It inserts into the perineal body, coccyx and the anococcygeal body. The levator ani is divided into three groups of muscles. The anterior group (levator prostate or sphincter vaginae) forms a sling around the prostate and vagina and inserts into the perineal body. The middle group (puborectalis) forms a sling around the junction of the rectum and anal canal and blends with the external anal sphincter. The posterior group (pubococcygeus and iliococcygeus) inserts into the anococcygeal body. The paired coccygei muscles form the posterior part of the pelvic floor. These arise from the ischial spines and attach to the coccyx posterior to the levator ani muscles. The groups of muscles are not resolved separately on MR imaging.

Lying centrally in the pelvic floor is the perineal body, a fibromuscular mass that gives attachment to the anal sphincter, bulbospongiosus, transverse perineal and levator ani muscles. Lying posteriorly between the anus and coccyx is the anococcygeal body a fibromuscular mass that gives attachment to levator ani and fibres from the anal sphincter. The pelvic floor divides the pelvic cavity above from the perineum and ischiorectal fossae below.

PELVIC FASCIA, VISCERAL LIGAMENTS AND PERITONEAL REFLECTIONS

The pelvis has a two-layered covering of fascia. The parietal fascia covers the walls and floor and is continuous superiorly with the iliacus and transversalis fascia. It is thickened over the obturator internus. The visceral fascia covers the bladder, uterus and rectum. Fascial condensations form a bilateral band running from pubis to sacrum. Around the urethra and at the bases of the prostate, bladder, rectum and uterus, these form supporting ligaments, which attach to the pelvic wall. The urethropelvic and parapelvic ligaments support the urethra. The pubovesical and puboprostatic ligaments support the bladder and prostate. The posterior ligaments support the rectum. The lateral cervical (cardinal) and pubocervical ligaments support the cervix and uterus. The sacrogenital ligaments pass around the side of the rectum to attach to the prostate in the male and the vagina in the female. A fascial condensation anterior to the sacrum forms the pre-sacral fascia. The sacrogenital ligaments and pre-sacral fascia are normally demonstrated on MR imaging although the other visceral ligaments are not seen unless pathologically thickened.

The pelvic cavity can be divided into intra- and extra-peritoneal compartments. The peritoneum forms a sack, which, in the pelvis, is draped over the pelvic organs to form a number of intra-peritoneal recesses. The largest is the rectovesical space. Within the male rectovesical space the opposing layers of peritoneum between the prostate and rectum fuse to form Denonvilliers fascia. In the female, the rectovesical space is divided by the uterus into the small vesicouterine recess anteriorly and the larger recto-uterine space (Pouch of Douglas) posteriorly. The opposing peritoneal layers between the vagina and rectum fuse to form the rectovaginal septum. The rectovesical space is continuous laterally with the pararectal fossae. The sigmoid colon usually indents the left pararectal fossa so that it is smaller than the right. The pararectal fossae are continuous anteriorly with the paravesical and supravesical spaces. The paravesical spaces are indented by the lateral and medial umbilical ligaments formed from the peritoneal coverings of the inferior epigastric vessels and obliterated umbilical arteries respectively.

Lying between the transversalis fascia of the anterior abdominal wall anteriorly, and the umbilicovesical fascia posteriorly, is the extra-peritoneal prevesical space. This is limited inferiorly in the male by the puboprostatic ligament and in the female by the pubovesical ligament, and laterally by the paravesical connective tissues. It extends superiorly to the level of the umbilicus. It is indented anteriorly in the mid line by the median umbilical ligament, which contains the urachus; this runs from the apex of the bladder to the umbilicus.

The peritoneal reflection and umbilical ligaments are consistently demonstrated on MR imaging.

PELVIC VISCERA

Bladder

The bladder is a muscular organ, which lies below the peritoneal reflection and rests on the pelvic floor. It is separated from the pubic bones anteriorly by the retropubic space. The vagina in the female and the seminal vesicles and vasa deferentia in the male lie posteriorly. The bladder has an apex, body, base (fundus) and neck. The apex lies anteriorly and points to the symphysis pubis. The base forms the posterior wall. The body lies between the apex and base and is formed from the inferolateral surfaces. These converge with the base at the bladder neck. The trigone is a smooth triangular area of internal mucous membrane lying between the ureteric and internal urethral orifices. When fully distended the bladder wall thickness should not exceed 5.0 mm.

MR appearance

On T1WI the bladder wall has intermediate signal intensity slightly higher than urine in the adjacent lumen. The wall is best demonstrated on T2WI because of contrast between its low signal, high signal urine and high/intermediate signal perivesical fat. The individual layers of the bladder wall cannot be consistently defined on MR imaging. Occasionally the inner mucosal layer can be identified particularly following intravenous Gd-DTPA, which results in delayed enhancement of the wall (*Figure 3.6b*).

Ureters

The ureters are retroperitoneal structures, which enter the pelvis passing over the pelvic brim close to the bifurcation of the common iliac artery. They pass postero-inferiorly onto the lateral pelvic walls, anterior to the internal iliac arteries. Subsequently, they curve anteromedially superior to the levator ani to enter the bladder where they describe an oblique course through the bladder wall. In the male, the ureter lies postero-lateral to the ductus deferens and enters the bladder just superior to the seminal vesicles. In the female, the ureter passes medial to the origin of the uterine artery from the anterior division of the internal iliac artery to the level of the ischial spine. It runs in the broad ligament of the uterus and parametrium lateral to the cervix and just above the lateral fornices of the vagina and is crossed superiorly by the uterine artery.

MR appearance

The ureters can be identified on high resolution T1WI and T2WI in the pelvis, they have thin low signal intensity walls. They are most easily identified on T2WI when they are obstructed in their distal course so that they become distended with high signal intensity urine.

Urethra

The **male urethra** is divided into four parts. The preprostatic urethra is 1.0–1.5 cm long and extends from the neck of the bladder to the superior aspect of the prostate. The prostatic urethra is 3.0–4.0 cm long; on its posterior wall it has a median ridge, the urethral crest. In the middle of the crest is the seminal colliculus (verumontanum), which has a slit-like orifice, which opens into a small cul-de-sac, the prostatic utricle. The ejaculatory ducts open onto the orifice of the prostatic utricle. On either side of the urethral crest is the prostatic sinus into which the prostatic ductules open. The membranous urethra is 1.5 cm long and continuous with the prostatic urethra. It is the portion that passes through the external urethral sphincter within the urogenital diaphragm. Consequently, it is the narrowest and least distensible part of the urethra. The spongy urethra is 15.0–16.0 cm long and extends from the membranous urethra to the external urethral orifice. It is divided into bulbous and penile portions. The bulbous urethra lies in the bulb of the penis where it is expanded to form the intrabulbar fossa. This contains the orifices of the bulbo-urethral glands (Cowper's glands). The penile urethra is dilated within the glans penis to form the navicular fossa. Multiple minute openings of the mucus-secreting urethral glands open along the length of the spongy urethra.

MR appearance

The proximal prostatic urethra and the spongy urethra are not demonstrated on MR imaging unless a Foley catheter is *in-situ*. On T2WI axial images, the membranous urethra appears as a low signal intensity ring surrounded by high signal intensity epithelium.

The **female urethra** is 4.0 cm long and passes from the bladder neck to the vaginal vestibule, opening directly anterior to the vaginal orifice and behind the clitoris. It lies anterior to, and describes a course parallel to the axis of the vagina. It passes with the vagina through the urogenital diaphragm. The ducts of multiple para-urethral glands open onto the vestibule on each side of the external urethral orifice.

MR appearance

On T2WI the female urethra appears as four concentric rings of alternating signal intensity. An outer low signal ring corresponds to the striated muscle layer, a middle high signal ring corresponds to the smooth muscle layer and submucosa, and the inner two rings correspond to mucosa lined by stratified squamous epithelium and the lumen (*Figures 3.7b, 3.9b and 3.17*).

Prostate

The prostate is a pyramidal structure approximately 3.0–4.5 cm long composed of glandular and fibromuscular tissue. It is enclosed by a 2.0–3.0 mm band of concentrically orientated fibromuscular stromal tissue, inseparable from the prostate gland that forms a false capsule. This is deficient at the apex allowing a route of extracapsular tumour spread. A fibrous prostatic sheath that is continuous with the pubo-prostatic ligaments surrounds the capsule. Between the prostatic capsule and sheath is the prostatic venous plexus. The prostate is broader superiorly with a base closely related to bladder neck. Inferiorly, the apex rests on the urogenital diaphragm in contact with fascia of the urethral sphincter and deep perineal muscles. Its anterior surface is separated from the symphysis pubis by loose areolar tissue in the retropubic space, which contains the puboprostatic ligament and part of the prostatic venous plexus. Infero-laterally the prostate rests on the levator ani muscles. Postero-superiorly, lie the seminal vesicles and ejaculatory ducts and posteriorly the surface is separated from the adjacent rectum by Denonvillier's fascia. The nonglandular anterior fibromuscular band extends over the antero-lateral surface of the prostate. Above the level of the ejaculatory ducts the small transitional zone surrounds the urethra. This is covered postero-laterally by the horseshoe-shaped central zone through which the ejaculatory ducts pass. This in turn is surrounded on its posterior, inferior and lateral surfaces by the peripheral zone.

MR appearance
On T1WI, the prostate, seminal vesicles and periprostatic veins are of uniform intermediate to low signal. On T2WI, the zonal anatomy is clearly demonstrated. The central zone and transitional zone, commonly termed the central gland, have low signal compared to the high signal intensity peripheral zone. The anterior fibromuscular band has low signal on T1WI and T2WI, and is contrasted with the relatively high signal from fat in the retropubic space. The verumontanum is often visualised on T2WI as a high signal intensity structure. The prostatic capsule is consistently identified as a low signal intensity structure on T1WI. Following intravenous Gd-DTPA enhancement is variable. The periurethral region enhances during the early phase and subsequently the whole gland enhances homogeneously (*Figures 3.8 and 3.26*).

Zonal anatomy changes with increasing age. The central zone shrinks as the transitional zone enlarges due to benign prostatic hypertrophy. This causes compression of the peripheral zone and creates a low signal intensity band (surgical pseudo-capsule) between it and the hypertrophied transitional zone (*Figures 3.22 and 3.25*).

Seminal vesicles, vas deferens and ejaculatory ducts

The seminal vesicles are lobulated sacks 5.0 cm long with a terminal duct positioned inferiorly. They lie obliquely behind the bladder and converge towards the mid line. The superior parts of the seminal vesi-cles lie posterior to the ureters and above the level of the peritoneal reflection within the rectovesical space. They are therefore separated from the rectum by a double layer of peritoneum. The inferior part of each seminal vesicle lies below the peritoneal reflection and is separated from the rectum by Denonvilliers' fascia. The duct of the seminal vesicle joins the vas deferens to form the ejaculatory ducts.

The vas deferens originates in the tail of the epididymis, ascends in the spermatic cord and passes through the inguinal canal to enter the pelvis crossing the external iliac vessels. It traverses the pelvic sidewall lying external to the peritoneum and then passes medially behind the bladder anterior to and above the ureter and medial to the seminal vesicles where it is dilated to form an ampulla.

The paired ejaculatory ducts arise adjacent to the neck of the bladder and run in close proximity passing antero-inferiorly through the prostate where they converge and open onto the prostatic utricles.

MR appearance
On T1WI, the seminal vesicles are of intermediate signal intensity similar to muscle contrasted with the pelvic fat. On T2WI the walls appear of low signal intensity and the contents of high signal intensity. A clear fat plane should be present in the angle between the anterior surface of the seminal vesicle and the posterior surface of the bladder (*Figures 3.22, 3.23 and 3.24*).

Vagina

This is a musculo-membranous tube, which extends from the vulva postero-superiorly to surround the cervix of the uterus. It is normally collapsed, with its anterior and posterior walls apposed. It broadens superiorly to form a continuous recess around the cervix divided into the shallow anterior fornix and the deeper posterior and lateral fornices. The anterior wall is approximately 1.5 cm shorter than the posterior wall. The vagina is arbitrarily divided into thirds, the important division being between the upper two-thirds and the lower third, demarcated anteriorly by the junction of the bladder and urethra at the bladder neck. Anteriorly the vagina is closely related to the base of the bladder and the urethra. Posteriorly the upper third of the vagina at the level of the vaginal fornices is related to the peritoneal reflection in the pouch of Douglas, the middle third is related to the ampulla of the rectum and the lower third to the perineal body and anal canal. In postmenopausal women the vagina shrinks and the cervix is less prominent so that the vaginal fornices are virtually effaced.

MR appearance
Layered anatomy of the vagina can be recognised on MR imaging. Mucous secretions within the lumen and the inner mucosal layer may be seen as low signal on T1WI and high signal on T2WI. The surrounding layer of submucosa, collagen, and longitudinal and circular smooth muscle have low signal on T1WI and T2WI. The surrounding adventitia that contains the vaginal venous plexus appears of high

signal intensity on T2WI *(Figures 3.17 and 3.18)*.

Following intravenous Gd-DTPA the vaginal muscle wall and sub-mucosa enhance. A central low signal intensity line, which probably represents the vaginal lumen, is occasionally identified *(Figures 3.6 and 3.7)*. The vaginal appearances vary with the phase of the menstrual cycle. The wall thickness is thicker in the proliferative phase than the secretory phase. Vaginal secretions are most prominent in the late proliferative and early to mid secretory phase. In the postmenopausal woman, the vaginal wall is thin and of low signal intensity on T1 and T2WI.

Uterus and uterine tubes

The uterus is a pear-shaped muscular organ lying centrally in the pelvis between the bladder anteriorly and the rectum posteriorly. It is divided into the fundus, which lies above the level of the uterine tube orifices, the body and the isthmus, which constricts inferiorly to form the cervix. The cervix is divided into supra-vaginal and infra-vaginal parts. The fundus, body and isthmus of the uterus are pre-dominantly muscular whereas the cervix is predominantly fibrous in composition. The uterine cavity communicates supero-laterally with the uterine (Fallopian) tubes and inferiorly with the cervical canal at the internal os. The cervical canal communicates with the vagina via the external os.

Anterior and posterior reflections of the peritoneum pass over the uterine tubes to form the broad ligaments. These also enclose the round ligaments of the uterus, the ovarian ligament and the uterine vessels. The round ligament arises antero-inferiorly to the origin of the uterine tube from the body of the uterus and passes through the inguinal canal to insert into the labia majora. The ovarian ligament arises postero-inferior to the origin of the uterine tubes, and passes in the mesovarium to attach to the ovary.

The uterine tubes extend from the uterine cornua to open into the peritoneal cavity close to the ovaries. They run in the mesosalpinx formed by the free edges of the broad ligament. They have an infundibulum, a funnel-shaped distal end, which extends beyond the broad ligament to overhang the ovary with its fimbriae; an ampulla forming the widest and longest parts of the uterine tube and an isthmus that is continuous with the interstitial portion lying within the uterine wall.

MR appearance

On MRI the demarcation between the uterine body and cervix is denoted by a waist in the uterine contour and the entrance of the uterine blood vessels at the level of the internal os.

On T1WI, the uterus appears of low to intermediate signal inten-sity. On T2WI, three separate layers are distinguished – the endometrium, junctional zone and myometrium. The endometrium lies centrally and appears of high signal. Its thickness varies with the phase of the menstrual cycle, being thinnest after menstruation and thickest during the mid-secretory phase. The outer layer of myometrium is of intermediate signal intensity that increases through

the menstrual cycle to a maximum intensity in the mid-secretory phase. Between the endometrium and myometrium is the junctional zone that appears of low signal intensity. Uterine appearances also vary under the influence of oral contraceptives with the myometrium appearing of high signal intensity on T1 and T2WI.

The cervix is of variable composition consisting of an outer zone of smooth muscle, which appears of intermediate signal on T2WI, an inner zone of fibrous stroma, which appears low signal on T2WI, and a central area of high signal intensity due to epithelium and mucus in the cervical canal.

In the shrunken uterus of the postmenopausal woman, the zonal anatomy is not well distinguished, the endometrium is thin and the myometrium is of lower signal intensity.

Following intravenous Gd-DTPA zonal anatomy can be displayed on T1WI. The myometrium and endometrium enhance but the junc-tional zone remains of low signal intensity. The paracervical tissues and inner cervical epithelium enhance but the cervical stroma remains of low signal intensity.

Parametrium

The parametrium is the extra-peritoneal connective tissue that lies adjacent to the uterine body (parametrium), the cervix (paracervix), and vagina (paracolpos), which together are termed the parametrium clinically. The parametrium is rich in vascular and lymphatic tissue and contains the ureters, which pass lateral to the supra-vaginal part of the cervix. The floor of the parametrium is formed from the lateral cervical (cardinal) ligaments and divides the paracervical parametria from the paracolpos. The uterovesical ligaments demarcate the lateral margin of the parametrial tissues.

MR appearance

The parametrium appears of intermediate to high signal intensity on T1WI and heterogeneously high signal intensity on T2WI *(Figure 3.16)*. The parametrial tissues enhance following intravenous Gd-DTPA.

Ovary

The ovaries are almond-shaped structures usually located in the ovarian fossae close to the lateral pelvic sidewall. Their size varies with age. In the adult, the ovary measures up to 3.0 cm in its longest dimension, but atrophies following the menopause reducing to a dimension of less than 2.0 cm.

The ovary is attached to the posterior surface of the broad liga-ment by a double fold of peritoneum, the mesovarium. Further support is given by the ovarian ligament proper and the suspensory ligament of the ovary that is continuous with the broad ligament attaching to the pelvic sidewall and in which the ovarian vessels and lymphatics run.

Each adult ovary contains approximately 70000 follicles. With each menstrual cycle some of these develop into Graafian follicles, one of which matures and releases an ovum at ovulation, leaving the corpus luteum. Therefore, the ovarian cortex contains immature follicles, Graafian follicles and corpora lutea.

MR appearance

The adult ovary appears of intermediate signal intensity on T1WI. On T2WI the central stroma is of low signal intensity with hyper-intense follicles identified in the high signal intensity peripheral cortex *(Figure 3.16)*. Following intravenous Gd-DTPA, the central ovarian stroma enhances and contrasts with the low signal ovarian follicles.

Sometimes the ovaries can be difficult to locate on MR imaging. If the round ligament is identified and traced posteriorly, the ovaries lie in close proximity to it attached to it by the ovarian ligament. Peripherally located follicular cysts and surrounding small vessels help to differentiate the ovaries from adjacent bowel. Occasionally the ovaries are transposed from the pelvis using the ovarian vessels as a pedicle to an intraperitoneal paracolic or retrocaecal location in order to remove them from a pelvic radiation field. Knowledge of this is important to avoid confusion with metastatic disease.

Rectum

The rectum describes an S-shape in the sagittal plane formed by the recto-sigmoid junction superiorly and the indentation of the pubo-rectalis muscle of the pelvic floor (the anorectal flexure) inferiorly. In the coronal plane, there are three lateral flexures caused by internal mucosal folds, which overlie thickenings of the circular muscle layer of the rectal wall (valves of Houston). The terminal part of the rectum is dilated to form an ampulla that is supported by the pelvic floor and anococcygeal ligaments.

The rectum has no mesentery and is only partially invested by peritoneum. In its upper third, peritoneum covers the anterior and lateral surfaces; in the middle third, only the anterior surface; and in the lower third there is no peritoneal covering.

Above the level of the levator ani and below the peritoneal reflection, a loose layer of connective tissue comprising the perirectal fat, blood vessels, nerves and lymphatics encloses the rectum. The visceral and parietal layers of perirectal fascia surround this. The rectum and tissues enclosed by the visceral layer of perirectal fascia, also termed the mesorectal fascia, form a distinct anatomical entity, the mesorectum. This is important because radical removal of the rectum is achieved at total mesorectal excision surgery by dissecting along the plane that separates the visceral (mesorectal) from the parietal layers of perirectal pelvic fascia.

MR appearance

The bowel wall appears of low signal on T1WI and intermediate signal on T2WI. When distended, the wall thickness of the recto-sigmoid and anal canal should not exceed 5 mm and 10 mm, respectively. As the bowel wall thickens in the lower rectum, four concentric layers can be discerned. An outside low signal intensity ring represents the outer muscular layer *(muscularis propria)*, within this a layer of higher signal intensity represents the submucosa, this encloses a layer of low

signal intensity corresponding to the muscularis mucosa and lamina propria, and centrally lies a high signal intensity layer representing the mucosa. On post-contrast T1WI, the submucosal and mucosal layers enhance but the intervening layer of muscularis mucosa and outer muscular layer do not, permitting differentiation between the layers.

Anal canal

The anal canal begins at the narrowing of the rectal ampulla formed by the indentation of the puborectalis portion of the levator ani and ends at the anal verge. The upper part of the anal canal is lined with transitional (urothelial type) or rectal glandular mucosa. The lower part of the anal canal is lined with squamous mucosa. The line of demarcation (pectinate line, dentate line) between the two parts lies 2.5–3.0 cm proximal to the anal verge and is visible macroscopically but not on MR imaging. It forms a transitional area of squamous and non-squamous mucosa and indicates the watershed for arterial supply, venous and lymphatic drainage. Above the pectinate line the anal canal is supplied by the superior rectal artery with blood from the inferior mesenteric artery and drained by the superior rectal vein into the portal venous system. Below the pectinate line, blood supply is from the inferior rectal artery, a branch of the internal iliac artery, and venous drainage is via the inferior rectal veins to the systemic venous system. At the level of the pectinate line arterial supply and venous drainage passes in both directions via anastomoses formed by the middle rectal arteries and veins. Lymphatic drainage above the level of the pectinate line is to the internal iliac lymph nodes and below the level of the pectinate line to the superficial inguinal lymph nodes.

The anal canal has a large voluntary external sphincter formed from striated muscle, which blends superiorly with the puborectalis muscle. The internal anal sphincter is involuntary and is formed from a thickening of the circular smooth muscle layer, which invests the upper two-thirds of the anal canal. Between the internal and external sphincters lies a continuation of the longitudinal muscle layer of the rectum, which inserts via a fascial extension into the pectinate line.

MR appearance

On MRI the upper and lower parts of the anal canal are identified and appear different. The upper part contains the internal anal sphincter, the longitudinal muscle layer and the puborectalis muscle. The lower part contains the internal anal sphincter, the longitudinal muscle layer and the external anal sphincter. The longitudinal muscle layer lies in a slit like space between the internal anal sphincter and the external anal sphincter and puborectalis muscle, the intersphincteric space. On T2WI all the muscles except the internal sphincter, which has intermediate signal intensity, have low signal intensity *(Figure 3.28)*.

PERINEUM

The perineum lies below the pelvic diaphragm. It is a diamond-shaped space, which is bounded antero-laterally by the ischiopubic rami, laterally by the ischial tuberosities and postero-laterally by the lower borders of the sacrotuberous ligaments. A line drawn between the ischial tuberosities passes just anterior to the anus and divides the perineum into the urogenital triangle anteriorly and the anal triangle posteriorly.

Urogenital triangle

This compartment contains the urogenital diaphragm, which is a triangular double-layer of fascia, which spans the pubic arch and attaches to the ischiopubic rami. The inferior fascial layer of the urogenital diaphragm forms the perineal membrane, which gives attachment to the bulb and crura of the penis or clitoris. It is pierced by the urethra in both sexes and the vagina in the female.

Below the urogenital diaphragm lies the superficial perineal pouch. The muscles of the superficial perineal pouch are analogous in both sexes but smaller in the female.

In the male, the bulbospongiosus muscles cover the corpus spongiosum, which encloses the urethra, to form the bulb of the penis. The ischiocavernosus muscles arise from the ischial rami, cover the corpora cavernosa and fuse anteriorly together and with the bulb of the penis to form the body of the penis.

In the female, the bulbospongiosus muscles cover the vestibular bulbs. The bulbs arise from the perineal membrane, are united anteriorly by a median commissure and lie each side of the vestibule. The vestibule contains the openings of the vagina, urethra and ducts of the greater vestibular (Bartholins) glands, which lie at the posterior border of each vestibular bulb. The ischiocavernosus muscles fuse with the paired corpora cavernosa to form the crura of the clitoris.

The superficial transverse perineal muscle is a slender muscle that runs along the posterior border of the perineal membrane and attaches to the perineal body and ischial rami.

Deep to the perineal membrane lies the deep perineal pouch, bounded superiorly by the superior layer of the urogenital diaphragm. This principally consists of the deep transverse perineal muscles and the sphincter urethrae. In the male, it contains the bulbourethral (Cowper's) glands and ducts, and in the female, is pierced by the vagina.

Anal triangle

This contains the anus, anal sphincters, levator ani, and wedge-shaped ischiorectal and ischioanal fossae. The ischiorectal and ischioanal fossae lie between the ischium and rectum and anal canal respectively. They are bounded superiorly by the posterior fibres of levator ani and inferiorly by the perineal skin. The fossae communicate with each other around the anal canal but are separated by the anococcygeal body, the anal canal and the perineal body.

ARTERIES

The abdominal aorta bifurcates at the L4 level to form the common iliac arteries. These pass infero-laterally to divide at the level of the pelvic brim into the external and internal iliac arteries. They lie anterior to the common iliac veins. The external iliac artery follows the iliopsoas muscle to pass under the inguinal ligament. It gives origin to the deep circumflex iliac and inferior epigastric arteries, which supply the anterior abdominal wall. It lies antero-lateral to the external iliac vein. The internal iliac artery supplies the pelvic viscera, buttocks, medial thighs and perineum. It passes postero-medially into the pelvis dividing into anterior and posterior divisions at the superior edge of the greater sciatic foramen. The anterior division gives rise to the umbilical, obturator, vesical, middle rectal, vaginal, uterine, internal pudendal and inferior gluteal arteries. The posterior division gives rise to the superior gluteal, iliolumbar and lateral sacral arteries.

VEINS

The venous drainage of the pelvic viscera is mainly via a network of interconnecting veins, which form the pelvic venous plexuses (rectal, vesical, prostatic, uterine, vaginal). These principally drain to the internal iliac veins but also drain via the superior rectal vein to the inferior mesenteric vein and through the lateral sacral veins to the internal vertebral venous plexus.

The internal and external iliac veins join to form the common iliac veins, which unite to form the inferior vena cava at the level of the L5 vertebra. The left common iliac vein describes a more horizontal course than the right so that it may appear quite large and elongated on transverse axial cross-sectional imaging.

MR appearance
Blood vessels can be distinguished from lymph nodes on MRI because of their different signal characteristics. Patent vessels usually appear as low signal on spin echo images because of flow voids.

LYMPH NODES

The pelvic lymph nodes are arranged in chains and usually named according to the artery, which they accompany. Unlike the abdominal organs, the pelvic viscera do not possess a hilum. Lymphatic drainage, therefore, occurs to the nodal chains on both sides of the pelvis and not to organs' hilar nodes.

Inguinal lymph nodes

These lie outside of the pelvis below the inguinal ligament but drain to the external iliac lymph nodes within the pelvis. They are divided into superficial and deep groups. The superficial inguinal nodes receive lymphatic drainage from the lower limb, the anterior abdominal wall below the umbilicus, the gluteal region, the anus and perianal skin, the perianal genitalia, the vagina below the hymen, the uterine fundus and the round ligaments of the uterus.

The deep inguinal lymph nodes are located medial to the femoral vein and receive lymphatic drainage from the superficial inguinal nodes, the glans penis and the clitoris.

External iliac nodes

These receive lymphatic drainage from the bladder, the membranous urethra, the prostate, the cervix and the upper part of the vagina. They drain to the common iliac nodes.

Internal iliac nodes

These receive lymphatic drainage from the rectum, anal canal, bladder, lower ureter, body and cervix of the uterus, upper part of the vagina, seminal vesicles, prostate and vas deferens. They drain to the common iliac nodes and the surgical obturator nodes.

Obturator nodes

These are divided into the proximal (surgical) obturator nodes and the distal (anatomical) obturator node. The surgical obturator nodes receive lymphatic drainage from the internal iliac nodes and drain to the external iliac nodes. They are located adjacent to the obturator nerve and vessel seen posterior to the iliopsoas muscle on transaxial imaging. The anatomical obturator node is part of the internal iliac group and lies within the obturator canal.

Sacral lymph nodes

These are part of the internal iliac group and receive a similar lymphatic drainage. They drain to the lateral aortic lymph nodes. They are located along the medial and lateral sacral vessels.

Common iliac lymph nodes

These receive lymphatic drainage from the internal and external iliac nodes and drain to the lumbar nodes.

Lumbar nodes

These are composed of right and left lateral aortic chains, pre-aortic and retro-aortic chains. The lateral aortic chains receive lymphatic drainage from the legs, pelvic viscera and lower abdominal wall via the common iliac and sacral nodes. They also receive direct drainage from the ovary and testis. The pre-aortic nodes receive drainage from the rectum, anal canal, colon and anterior abdominal wall. The retro-aortic nodes receive drainage from the posterior abdominal wall.

MR appearance

Lymph nodes appear of intermediate signal intensity on T1WI and variable signal intensity on T2WI, although usually greater than the signal intensity of muscle. Lymph nodes enhance to a variable degree following intravenous Gd-DTPA but this does not help to differentiate malignant from hyperplastic lymph nodes. Pelvic lymph nodes greater than 1.0 cm in short axis diameter and inguinal nodes greater than 1.5 cm in short axis diameter are considered enlarged (Table 3.1). Lymph nodes in the perirectal, paracervical and pre-sacral spaces are not normally seen, so that their identification on MRI is a good indicator that they are abnormal.

Table 3.1. Upper limit of normal sized pelvic lymph nodes

Location	Short axis diameter (mm)
Inguinal	15.0
Common iliac	9.0
Internal iliac	7.0
Obturator	8.0
Pre-sacral, paracervical, perirectal	Not normally identified

NERVES

The pelvis is innervated by the sacral and coccygeal plexi. The sacral plexus lies on the anterior surface of the piriformis muscle just beneath the sacroiliac joint. It gives rise to the sciatic and pudendal nerves. The sciatic nerve leaves the pelvis through the greater sciatic foramen and enters the posterior thigh lateral to the ischial tuberosity. The pudendal nerve also leaves the pelvis through the greater sciatic foramen between the piriformis and coccygeus muscles, hooks around the ischial spine and sacrospinous ligament and enters the perineum via the lesser sciatic foramen.

Passing through the pelvis are the femoral and obturator nerves which originate from the lumbar plexus. The femoral nerve lies in the groove between the iliacus and psoas muscles. The obturator nerve runs along the medial border of the psoas, across the pelvic sidewall, to exit through the obturator foramen.

MR appearance

Nerves appear as low / intermediate signal on T1WI and have a speckled appearance on T2WI, with low signal axons and high signal myelin and other supporting connective tissue. Only the sacral plexus, sciatic and femoral nerves are usually identified on MRI.

FURTHER READING

1. Hricak H and Carrington BM. (1991) *MRI of the pelvis: a text atlas.* Martin Dunitz, London. *Definitive text atlas of pelvic pathology.*

2. Vinnicombe SJ and Husband JE. (1999) In: *Applied radiological anatomy* (Eds. Butler P, Mitchell AMW, and Ellis H). Cambridge University Press, Cambridge. *Valuable overview of radiological anatomy.*

3. Moore KL and Dalley AF. (1999) *Clinically oriented anatomy,* 4th Edn. Lippincott, Williams and Wilkins, Baltimore, Maryland. *Well-illustrated clinical anatomy text.*

4. Netter FH. (1989) *Atlas of human anatomy.* Ciba-Geigy, Summit, New Jersey. *Invaluable bench reference.*

5. Ryu J and Kim B. (2001) MR imaging of the male and female urethra. *Radiographics* 21: 1169–1185. *Useful review.*

6. Siegelman ES, Outwater EK, Banner MP, *et al.* (1997) High resolution MR imaging of the vagina. *Radiographics* 17: 1183–1203. *Useful review.*

7. Hussain SM, Stoker J, Laméris, JS. (1995) Anal sphincter complex: Endoanal MR imaging of normal anatomy. *Radiology* 197: 671–677.

8. Debatin JF and Patak MA. (1999) MRI of the small and large bowel. *Eur. Radiol.* 9(8): 1523–1534. *Useful review.*

9. Coakley F and Hricak H. (2000) Radiologic anatomy of the prostate gland: a clinical approach. *Radiol. Clin. North Am.* 38(1): 15–30. *Useful review.*

10. Barentsz JO, Sager GJ and Witjes JA. (2000) MR imaging of the urinary bladder. *Magn. Reson. Imaging Clin. N. Am.* 8(4): 853–867. *Useful review.*

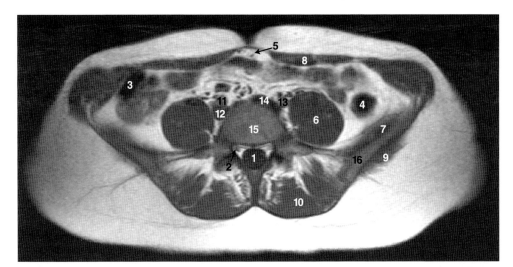

Figure 3.1.

Transaxial T1WI at level of L5 vertebra.
(1) Thecal sac
(2) L5 nerve root
(3) Caecum
(4) Descending colon
(5) Urachus
(6) Psoas muscle
(7) Iliacus muscle
(8) Rectus abdominis muscle
(9) Gluteus maximus muscle
(10) Erector spinae muscle
(11) Right common iliac artery
(12) Right common iliac vein
(13) Left common iliac artery
(14) Left common iliac vein
(15) L5 vertebral body
(16) Iliac blade

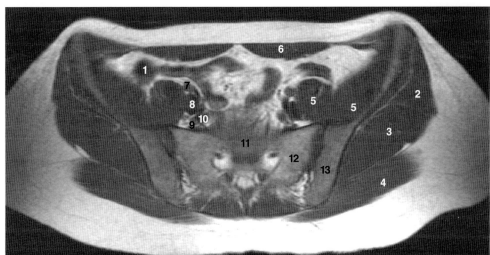

Figure 3.2.

Transaxial T1WI at level of S1 vertebra.
(1) Caecum
(2) Gluteus minimus muscle
(3) Gluteus medius muscle
(4) Gluteus maximus muscle
(5) Iliopsoas muscle
(6) Rectus abdominis muscle
(7) External iliac artery
(8) External iliac vein
(9) Internal iliac artery
(10) Internal iliac vein
(11) Body of sacrum
(12) Sacral ala
(13) Body of ilium

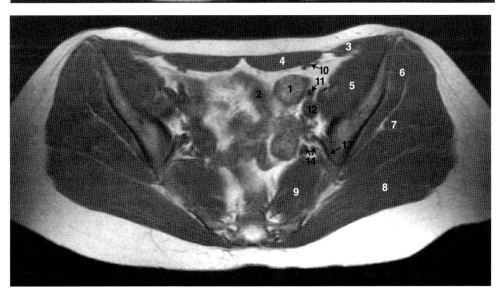

Figure 3.3.

Transaxial T1WI at level of mid sacrum.
(1) Sigmoid colon
(2) Small intestine
(3) Internal oblique muscle
(4) Rectus abdominis muscle
(5) Iliopsoas muscle
(6) Gluteus minimus muscle
(7) Gluteus medius muscle
(8) Gluteus maximus muscle
(9) Piriformis muscle
(10) Inferior epigastric vessels
(11) External iliac artery
(12) External iliac vein
(13) Superior gluteal artery
(14) Branches of internal iliac artery and vein

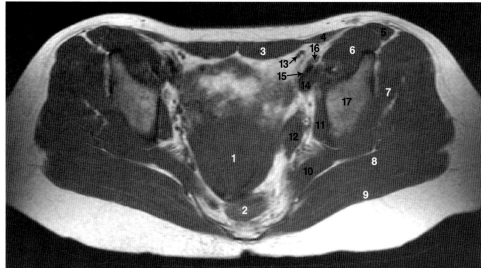

Figure 3.4.

Transaxial T1WI at level of acetabular roof.

(1) Uterus (retroverted)
(2) Rectum
(3) Rectus abdominis muscle
(4) Internal oblique muscle
(5) Sartorius muscle
(6) Iliopsoas muscle
(7) Gluteus minimus muscle
(8) Gluteus medius muscle
(9) Gluteus maximus muscle
(10) Piriformis muscle
(11) Obturator internus muscle
(12) Left ovary
(13) Inferior epigastric vessels
(14) External iliac vein
(15) External iliac artery
(16) Deep circumflex iliac vessels
(17) Acetabular roof

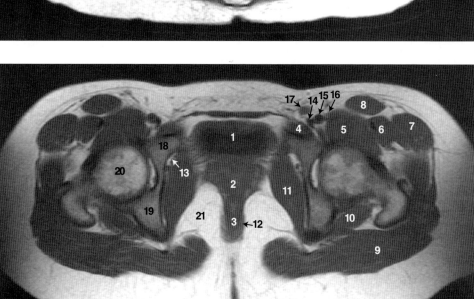

Figure 3.5.

Transaxial T1WI at level of femoral head.

(1) Urinary bladder
(2) Vagina
(3) Rectum
(4) Obturator externus muscle
(5) Iliopsoas muscle
(6) Rectus femoris muscle
(7) Tensor fascia lata muscle
(8) Sartorius muscle
(9) Gluteus maximus muscle
(10) Piriformis muscle
(11) Obturator internus muscle
(12) Levator ani muscle
(13) Obturator vessels and nerve
(14) Common femoral vein
(15) Common femoral artery
(16) Femoral nerve
(17) Deep inguinal lymph node
(18) Superior pubic ramus
(19) Ischium
(20) Head of femur
(21) Ischiorectal/anal fossa

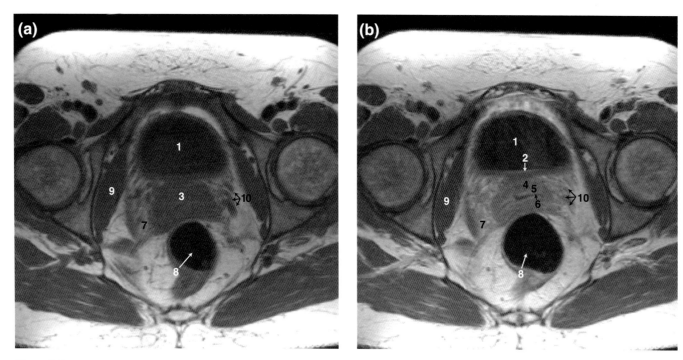

Figure 3.6.

Transaxial TIWI of female pelvis at level of femoral heads **(a)** before and **(b)** after intravenous Gadolinium-DTPA.
- (1) Bladder
- (2) Bladder mucosa
- (3) Vagina
- (4) Vagina-muscle wall
- (5) Vagina-submucosa
- (6) Vagina-lumen
- (7) Paracolpos
- (8) Rectum
- (9) Obturator internus muscle
- (10) Blood vessels in paracolpos

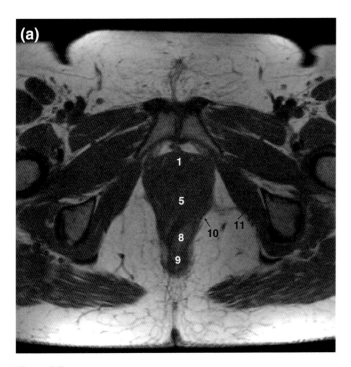
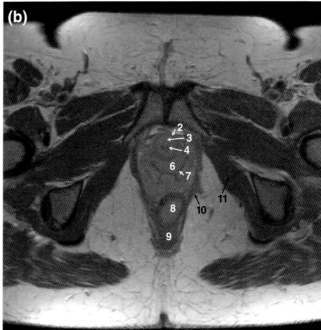

Figure 3.7.

Transaxial T1WI of female pelvis at level of symphysis pubis **(a)** before and **(b)** after intravenous Gadolinium-DTPA.

(1) Urethra
(2) Urethra-striated muscle layer
(3) Urethra-smooth muscle layer and submucosa
(4) Urethra-lumen
(5) Vagina
(6) Vagina-muscle wall
(7) Vagina-lumen
(8) Anal canal
(9) Anococcygeal body
(10) Levator ani muscle
(11) Obturator internus muscle

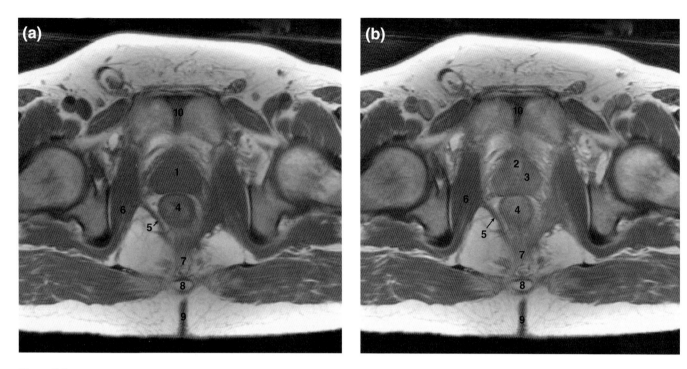

Figure 3.8.

Transaxial T1WI of male pelvis at level of symphysis pubis **(a)** before and **(b)** after intravenous Gadolinium-DTPA

  (1) Prostate
  (2) Prostate – periurethral region
  (3) Prostate – central and peripheral zone
  (4) Anal canal
  (5) Levator ani muscle
  (6) Obturator internus muscle
  (7) Anococcygeal raphe
  (8) Coccyx
  (9) Natal cleft
(10) Symphysis pubis

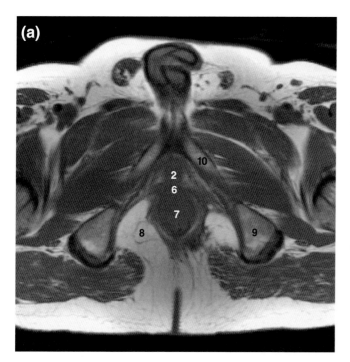
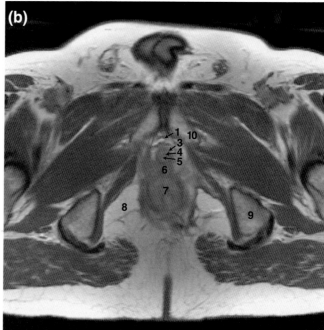

Figure 3.9.

Transaxial T1WI of male pelvis at level of perineum **(a)** before and **(b)** after intravenous Gadolinium-DTPA.
- (1) Deep dorsal vein of penis
- (2) Urethra
- (3) Urethra-striated muscle layer
- (4) Urethra-smooth muscle layer and submucosa
- (5) Urethra-lumen
- (6) Perineal body
- (7) Anal canal
- (8) Ischioanal fossa
- (9) Ischial tuberosity
- (10) Inferior pubic ramus

Figure 3.10.

Transaxial T1WI at level of symphysis pubis.
- (1) Anal canal
- (2) Ischioanal fossa
- (3) Pectineus muscle
- (4) Obturator externus muscle
- (5) Obturator internus muscle
- (6) Sartorius muscle
- (7) Rectus femoris muscle
- (8) Tensor fascia lata muscle
- (9) Iliopsoas muscle
- (10) Vastus lateralis muscle
- (11) Gluteus maximus muscle
- (12) Gemellus muscle
- (13) Body of pubis
- (14) Neck of femur
- (15) Greater trochanter of femur
- (16) Ischial tuberosity

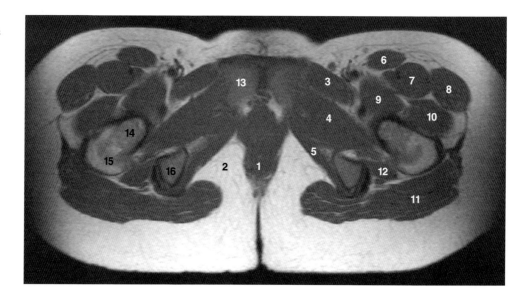

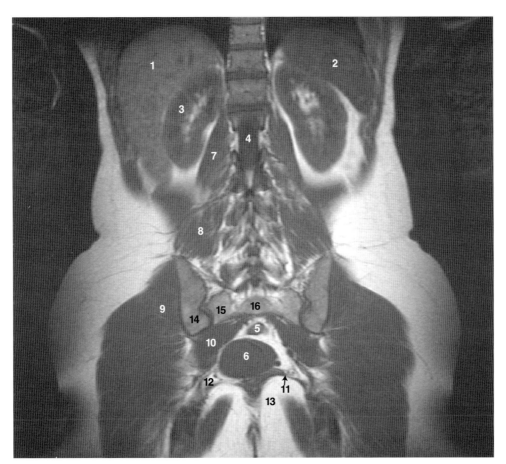

Figure 3.11.

Coronal T1WI of female posterior abdomen and pelvis.
- (1) Liver
- (2) Spleen
- (3) Right kidney
- (4) Thecal sac
- (5) Rectum
- (6) Retroverted uterus
- (7) Psoas muscle
- (8) Quadratus lumborum muscle
- (9) Gluteus maximus muscle
- (10) Piriformis muscle
- (11) Levator ani muscle
- (12) Inferior gluteal artery and vein
- (13) Ischioanal fossa
- (14) Ilium
- (15) Sacral alum
- (16) Body of sacrum

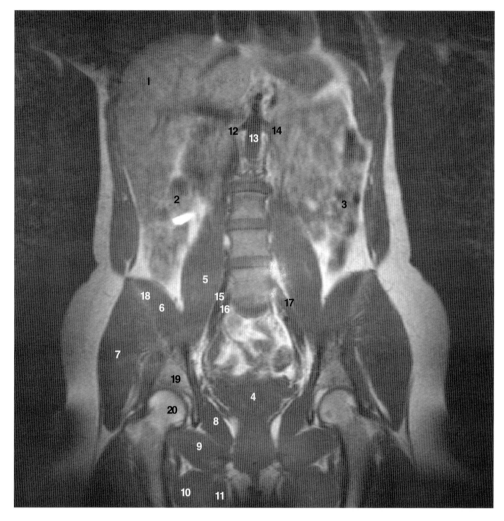

Figure 3.12.

Coronal T1WI of female mid-abdomen and pelvis.
 (1) Liver
 (2) Ascending colon
 (3) Descending colon
 (4) Uterus
 (5) Psoas muscle
 (6) Iliacus muscle
 (7) Gluteus maximus muscle
 (8) Obturator internus muscle
 (9) Obturator externus muscle
(10) Adductor brevis muscle
(11) Adductor longus muscle
(12) Right renal artery
(13) Abdominal aorta
(14) Left renal artery
(15) Right common iliac vein
(16) Right common iliac artery
(17) Left common iliac artery
(18) Iliac blade
(19) Acetabulum
(20) Head of femur

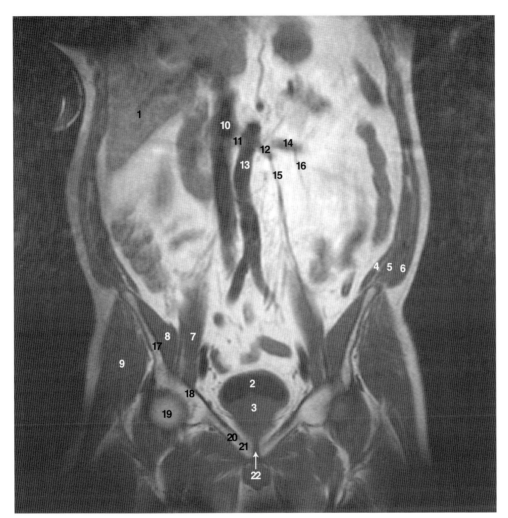

Figure 3.13.

Coronal T1WI of male mid abdomen and pelvis.
(1) Liver
(2) Urinary bladder
(3) Prostate
(4) Transversus abdominis muscle
(5) Internal oblique muscle
(6) External oblique muscle
(7) Psoas muscle
(8) Iliacus muscle
(9) Gluteus medius muscle
(10) Inferior vena cava
(11) Right renal artery
(12) Left renal artery
(13) Abdominal aorta
(14) Left renal vein
(15) Left testicular artery
(16) Left testicular vein
(17) Ilium
(18) Acetabulum
(19) Head of femur
(20) Superior pubic ramus
(21) Body of pubis
(22) Symphysis pubis

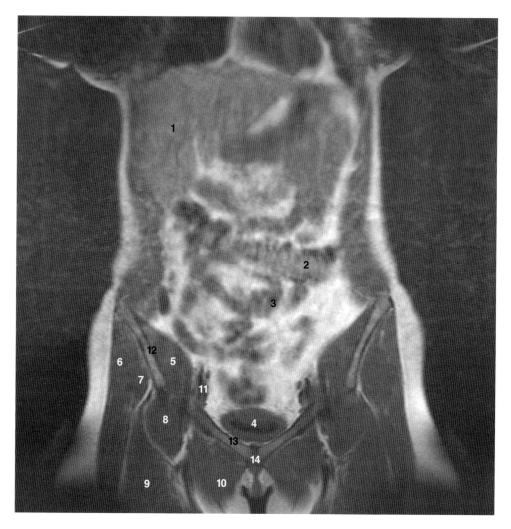

Figure 3.14.

Coronal T1WI of female anterior abdomen and pelvis.
 (1) Liver
 (2) Transverse colon
 (3) Small intestine
 (4) Urinary bladder
 (5) Iliopsoas muscle
 (6) Gluteus medius muscle
 (7) Gluteus minimus muscle
 (8) Psoas muscle
 (9) Rectus femoris muscle
(10) Adductor longus muscle
(11) External iliac vessels
(12) Ilium
(13) Superior pubic ramus
(14) Symphysis pubis

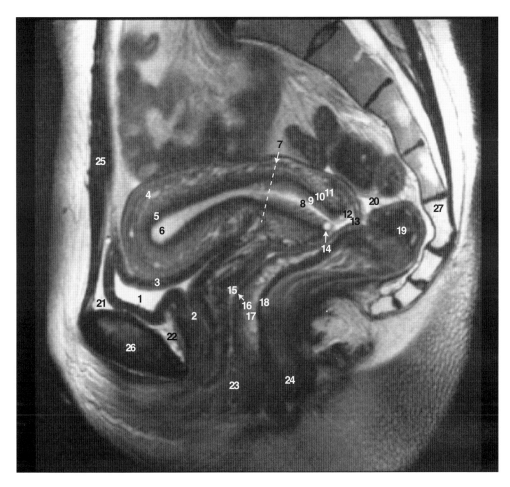

Figure 3.15.

Sagittal T2WI of female pelvis.
(1) Urinary bladder
(2) Urethra
(3) Muscular layer of bladder wall
(4) Outer myometrium
(5) Junctional zone
(6) Endometrium
(7) Plane of uterocervical junction
(8) Cervical lumen
(9) Cervical mucosa
(10) Cervix (fibromuscular layer)
(11) Cervix (outer layer)
(12) Ectocervical mucosa
(13) Posterior vaginal fornix
(14) Nabothian cyst
(15) Vaginal lumen containing secretions
(16) Vaginal wall (submucosal and muscle layers)
(17) Vaginal adventitia and venous plexus
(18) Rectovaginal septum
(19) Rectum
(20) Recto-uterine space (Pouch of Douglas) containing small volume of fluid.
(21) Prevesical space
(22) Retropubic space
(23) Introitus
(24) Anal canal
(25) Rectus abdominis muscle
(26) Pubic bone and symphysis
(27) Sacrum

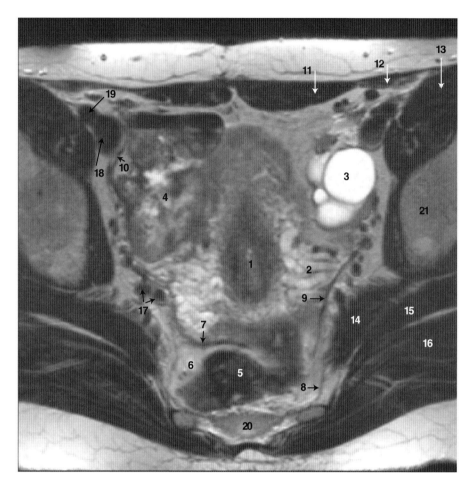

Figure 3.16.

Transaxial T2WI of female pelvis at level of acetabular roof.

(1) Uterus
(2) Parametrium
(3) Right ovarian follicular cyst
(4) Caecum
(5) Rectum
(6) Perirectal fat
(7) Perirectal fascia
(8) Perirectal fascia
(9) Peritoneum
(10) Round ligament of ovary
(11) Rectus abdominis muscle
(12) External oblique muscle
(13) Iliopsoas muscle
(14) Piriformis muscle
(15) Gluteus medius muscle
(16) Gluteus maximus muscle
(17) Internal iliac vessels
(18) External iliac vein
(19) External iliac artery
(20) Sacrum
(21) Acetabular roof

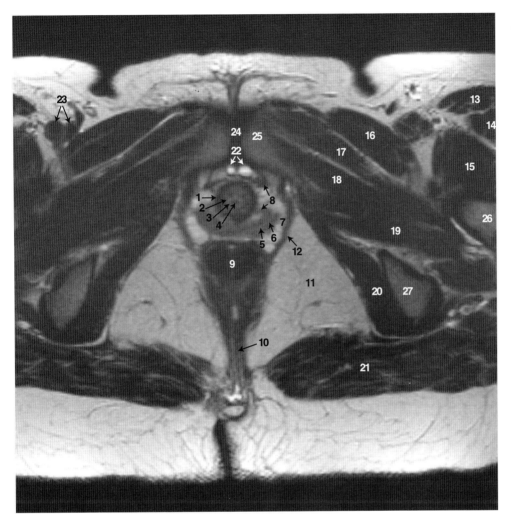

Figure 3.17.

Transaxial T2WI of female pelvis at level of symphysis pubis.
  (1) Urethra-striated muscle layer
  (2) Urethra-smooth muscle layer and submucosa
  (3) Urethra-mucosal layer
  (4) Urethra – lumen
  (5) Vagina – mucus secretions and inner mucosal layer
  (6) Vagina – submucosa and smooth muscle layer
  (7) Vagina – adventitia and venous plexus
  (8) Pubourethral and periurethral ligaments
  (9) Rectum
  (10) Anococcygeal ligament
  (11) Ischiorectal/anal fossa
  (12) Levator ani muscle
  (13) Sartorius muscle
  (14) Rectus femoris muscle
  (15) Iliopsoas muscle
  (16) Pectineus muscle
  (17) Adductor longus muscle
  (18) Adductor brevis muscle
  (19) Obturator externus muscle
  (20) Obturator internus muscle
  (21) Gluteus maximus muscle
  (22) Deep dorsal vein of clitoris
  (23) Common femoral vessels
  (24) Symphysis pubis
  (25) Body of pubis
  (26) Femur
  (27) Ischium

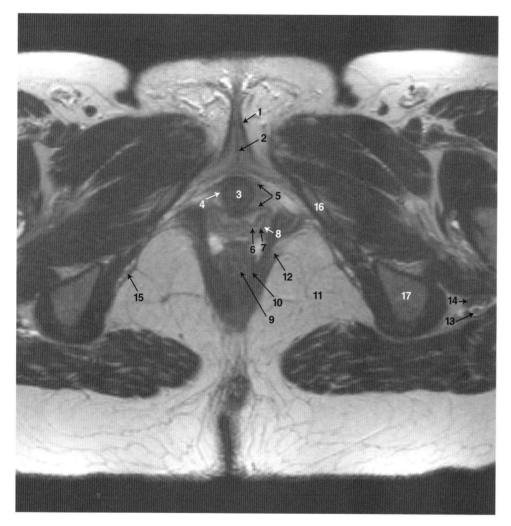

Figure 3.18.

Transaxial T2WI of female pelvis below symphysis pubis.

(1) Clitoris
(2) Corpus cavernosum
(3) Urethra
(4) Urethropelvic (parapelvic) ligament
(5) Paraurethral ligament
(6) Vagina – mucus secretions and inner mucosal layer
(7) Vagina – submucosa and smooth muscle layer
(8) Vagina – adventitia and venous plexus
(9) Anal canal – internal sphincter
(10) Anal canal – external sphincter and longitudinal muscle layer
(11) Ischioanal fossa
(12) Levator ani muscle – puborectalis portion
(13) Sciatic nerve
(14) Inferior gluteal vessels
(15) Pudendal vessels
(16) Inferior pubic ramus
(17) Ischium

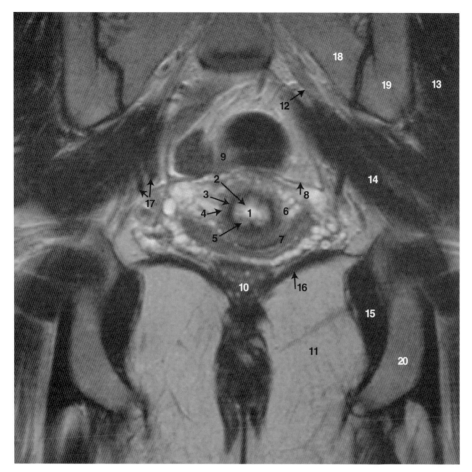

Figure 3.19.

Coronal T2WI of female mid-pelvis.
(1) Cervical lumen
(2) Cervical mucosa
(3) Cervix (fibromuscular layer)
(4) Cervix (outer layer)
(5) Nabothian cyst
(6) Paracervix containing venous plexus
(7) Bladder
(8) Peritoneum
(9) Recto-sigmoid junction
(10) Posterior wall of vagina and vaginal adventitia
(11) Ischioanal fossa
(12) Sacral nerve root component of sciatic nerve
(13) Gluteus medius muscle
(14) Piriformis muscle
(15) Obturator internus muscle
(16) Levator ani muscle
(17) Internal iliac vessels
(18) Sacral ala
(19) Ilium
(20) Ischium

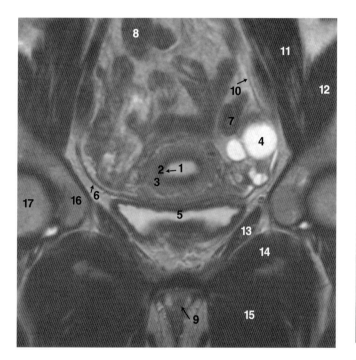

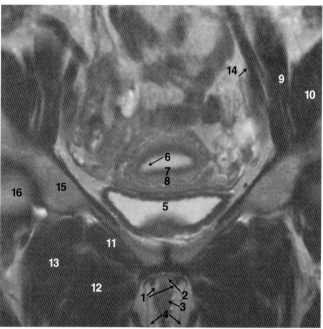

Figure 3.20.

Coronal T2WI of female anterior pelvis.
 (1) Endometrium
 (2) Uterus – junctional zone
 (3) Outer myometrium
 (4) Ovarian follicular cyst
 (5) Bladder
 (6) Broad ligament of uterus
 (7) Sigmoid colon
 (8) Small intestine
 (9) Urethra
(10) Peritoneum
(11) Psoas muscle
(12) Iliacus muscle
(13) Obturator internus muscle
(14) Obturator externus muscle
(15) Adductor magnus muscle
(16) Acetabulum
(17) Head of femur

Figure 3.21.

Coronal T2WI of female pelvis through symphysis pubis.
 (1) Crura of clitoris
 (2) Body of clitoris
 (3) Vestibule
 (4) Labia majora
 (5) Bladder
 (6) Endometrium
 (7) Uterus – junctional zone
 (8) Outer myometrium
 (9) Psoas muscle
(10) Iliacus muscle
(11) Obturator externus muscle
(12) Adductor brevis muscle
(13) Pectineus muscle
(14) External iliac vessels
(15) Acetabulum
(16) Femoral head

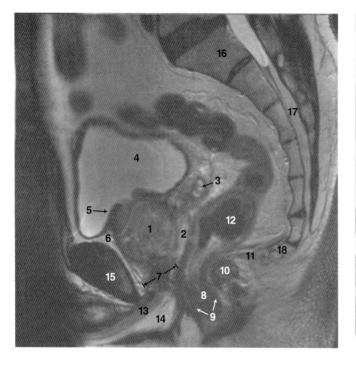

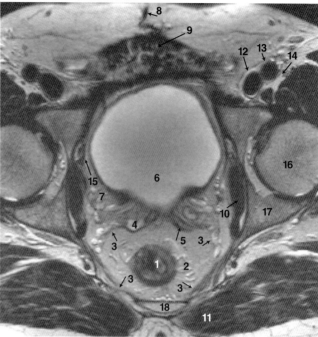

Figure 3.22.

Sagittal T2WI image of male pelvis.
 (1) Prostate with benign prostatic hypertrophy in central zone
 (2) Peripheral zone
 (3) Seminal vesicle
 (4) Bladder
 (5) Bladder trigone
 (6) Retropubic space
 (7) Urogenital diaphragm
 (8) Anal canal
 (9) External sphincter
 (10) Anococcygeal body
 (11) Anococcygeal ligament
 (12) Rectum
 (13) Corpus cavernosum
 (14) Corpus spongiosum
 (15) Symphysis pubis
 (16) Sacrum
 (17) Sacral canal
 (18) Coccyx

Figure 3.23.

Transaxial T2WI of male pelvis.
 (1) Rectum
 (2) Fat in perirectal space
 (3) Perirectal fascia enclosing mesorectum
 (4) Seminal vesicle
 (5) Vas deferens
 (6) Urinary bladder
 (7) Perivesical venous plexus
 (8) Wound scar
 (9) Rectus abdominis muscle
 (10) Obturator internus muscle
 (11) Gluteus maximus muscle
 (12) Common femoral vein
 (13) Common femoral artery
 (14) Femoral nerve
 (15) Obturator vessels and nerve in obturator foramen
 (16) Head of femur
 (17) Acetabulum
 (18) Sacrum

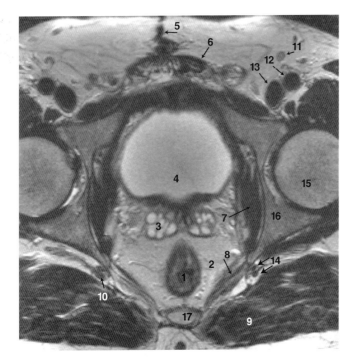

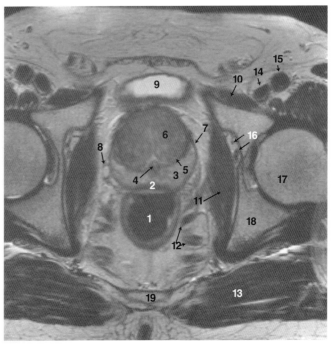

Figure 3.24.

Transaxial T2WI of male pelvis.
 (1) Rectum
 (2) Fat in perirectal space
 (3) Seminal vesicle
 (4) Bladder
 (5) Scar
 (6) Rectus abdominis muscle
 (7) Obturator internus muscle
 (8) Levator ani muscle
 (9) Gluteus maximus muscle
(10) Sciatic nerve
(11) Superficial inguinal lymph node
(12) Common femoral artery
(13) Common femoral vein
(14) Inferior gluteal vessels
(15) Head of femur
(16) Acetabulum
(17) Sacrum

Figure 3.25.

Transaxial T2WI of male pelvis at level of prostate gland showing benign prostatic hypertrophy (BPH).
 (1) Rectum
 (2) Denonvilliers fascia
 (3) Prostate – peripheral zone
 (4) Urethra
 (5) Surgical pseudo-capsule
 (6) Prostate – transitional zone with benign prostatic hypertrophy
 (7) Prostatic capsule (see text)
 (8) Vesicoprostatic venous plexus
 (9) Bladder
(10) Pectineus muscle
(11) Obturator internus muscle
(12) Muscular slips of levator ani muscle
(13) Gluteus maximus muscle
(14) Common femoral vein
(15) Common femoral artery
(16) Obturator vessels and nerve in obturator foramen
(17) Head of femur
(18) Acetabulum
(19) Sacrum

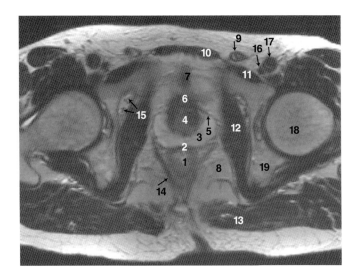

Figure 3.26.

Transaxial T2WI of male pelvis at level of prostate gland.
(1) Ano-rectum
(2) Denonvilliers fascia
(3) Prostate – peripheral zone
(4) Prostate – central gland
(5) Prostatic capsule (see text)
(6) Prostate – fibromuscular band
(7) Bladder base
(8) Ischioanal fossa
(9) Spermatic cord
(10) Rectus abdominis muscle
(11) Pectineus muscle
(12) Obturator internus muscle
(13) Gluteus maximus muscle
(14) Levator ani – puborectalis portion
(15) Obturator nerve and vessels
(16) Common femoral vein
(17) Common femoral artery
(18) Head of femur
(19) Acetabulum

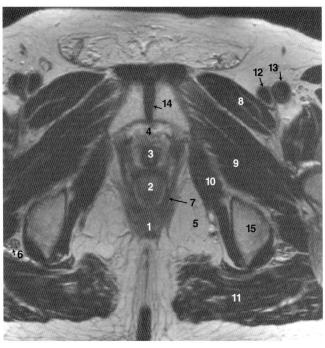

Figure 3.27.

Transaxial T2WI of male pelvis at level of symphysis pubis.
(1) Anococcygeal body
(2) Anal canal
(3) Urethra
(4) Retropubic space
(5) Ischioanal fossa
(6) Sciatic nerve
(7) Levator ani – puborectalis portion
(8) Pectineus muscle
(9) Obturator externus muscle
(10) Obturator internus muscle
(11) Gluteus maximus muscle
(12) Common femoral vein
(13) Common femoral artery
(14) Pubic symphysis
(15) Ischial tuberosity

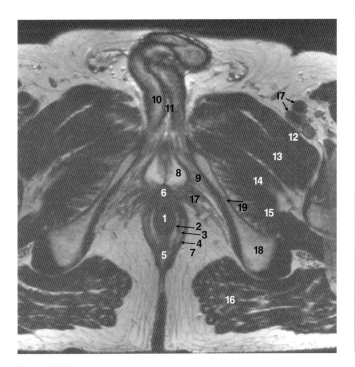

Figure 3.28.

Transaxial T2WI of male pelvis at level of perineal body.
 (1) Anal canal
 (2) Internal sphincter
 (3) Longitudinal muscle layer in intersphincteric space
 (4) External sphincter
 (5) Anococcygeal body
 (6) Perineal body
 (7) Ischioanal fossa
 (8) Bulb of penis
 (9) Crus of penis
(10) Corpus cavernosum
(11) Urethra
(12) Pectineus muscle
(13) Adductor longus muscle
(14) Adductor brevis muscle
(15) Obturator externus muscle
(16) Gluteus maximus muscle
(17) Common femoral vessels
(18) Ischial tuberosity
(19) Inferior pubic ramus

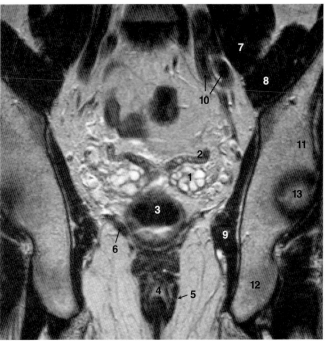

Figure 3.29.

Coronal T2WI of posterior male pelvis.
 (1) Seminal vesicle
 (2) Ductus deferens
 (3) Ampulla of rectum
 (4) Anal canal
 (5) External anal sphincter
 (6) Levator ani muscle
 (7) Psoas muscle
 (8) Iliacus muscle
 (9) Obturator internus muscle
(10) Common iliac vessels
(11) Ilium
(12) Ischium
(13) Head of femur

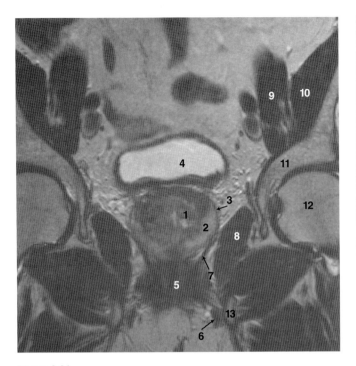

Figure 3.30.

Coronal T2WI of male pelvis.
  (1) Prostate – central gland (transitional zone with benign prostatic hypertrophy – see text)
  (2) Prostate – peripheral zone
  (3) Prostatic capsule (see text)
  (4) Urinary bladder
  (5) Perineal body
  (6) Ischiocavernosus muscle
  (7) Levator ani muscle
  (8) Obturator internus muscle
  (9) Psoas muscle
 (10) Iliacus muscle
 (11) Acetabulum
 (12) Head of femur
 (13) Ischium

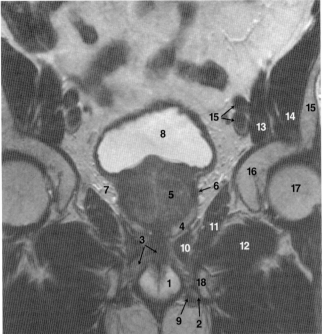

Figure 3.31.

Coronal T2WI of anterior male pelvis.
  (1) Bulb of penis
  (2) Crus of penis
  (3) Urogenital diaphragm
  (4) Prostate – peripheral zone
  (5) Prostate – central gland
  (6) Prostatic capsule (see text)
  (7) Prostatic venous plexus
  (8) Urinary bladder
  (9) Ischiocavernosus muscle
 (10) Levator ani muscle – levator prostate portion
 (11) Obturator internus muscle
 (12) Obturator externus muscle
 (13) Psoas muscle
 (14) Iliacus muscle
 (15) Ilium
 (16) Acetabulum
 (17) Head of femur
 (18) Ischium

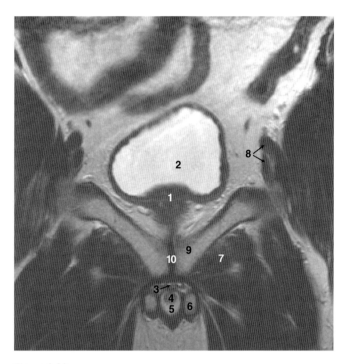

Figure 3.32.

Coronal T2WI of male pelvis through symphysis pubis.
 (1) Prostate – Fibromuscular band
 (2) Bladder
 (3) Suspensory ligament of penis
 (4) Urethra
 (5) Corpus spongiosum
 (6) Corpus cavernosum
 (7) Obturator externus
 (8) External iliac vessels
 (9) Body of pubis
(10) Symphysis pubis

4 Cervical Cancer

Bernadette M. Carrington and Rhidian Bramley

BACKGROUND INFORMATION

Epidemiology

Worldwide, cervical cancer is the third most common cancer among women after breast and colorectal cancer, with a greater incidence in developing countries and in lower socioeconomic groups. In developed countries it is the third most common gynaecological malignancy with an estimated annual incidence of 10.4 per 100 000 women in the UK and 8 per 100 000 women in the USA. The peak incidence is between 35 and 50 years. In the last 10 years, there has been a decreasing incidence due to national screening programmes for cervical cancer and for cervical intraepithelial neoplasia (CIN), its precursor. Aetiological factors implicated in the pathogenesis of CIN and cervical cancers are multiple and include smoking, immunosuppression, and sexual activity with exposure to certain types of human papilloma virus.

Histopathology

Approximately 90% of cervical carcinomas are of squamous cell origin, the remainder being adenocarcinomas or adenosquamous carcinomas. There is some evidence that adenocarcinoma is increasing in frequency. Other cervical malignancies include malignant melanoma, sarcoma, lymphoma and small cell carcinoma.

Squamous carcinomas usually arise from the squamo-columnar junction whose position varies with age. Before puberty and after the menopause it is situated inside the endocervical canal. At puberty, oestrogen influenced cervical eversion occurs, followed by squamous cell metaplasia, which has the potential to de-differentiate into squamous cell carcinoma. Adenocarcinomas arise within the endocervical canal and are more likely to remain occult, delaying clinical presentation.

Patterns of tumour spread

Cervical cancer spreads through the cervical stroma and into the parametrium. With increasing infiltration of the pericervical connective tissue and ligaments, disease may reach the pelvic sidewall. As a consequence of lateral tumour extension the patient's ureters may be engulfed and obstructed. Craniocaudal extension is to the body of the uterus, upper vagina and eventually to the lower third of the vagina. Finally, the tumour may extend into adjacent organs, particularly the bladder and rectum, but also occasionally to involve the pelvic floor or transgress the peritoneum to invade sigmoid colon or small bowel.

Lymphatic spread occurs first to the paracervical and parametrial nodes. The obturator nodes are frequently the earliest pelvic sidewall lymph nodes to be involved and pre-sacral or perirectal nodes can be infiltrated in the posterior pelvis. Nodal disease may extend along the internal and external iliac chains, the common iliac chains or the upper retroperitoneal nodal stations, and there may be non-contiguous involvement of lymph node groups. Rarely, involved supraclavicular nodes are detected on clinical examination at presentation.

Metastatic disease, with the exception of extra-pelvic nodal disease, is rare at presentation and usually manifests as pulmonary, liver or bone metastases.

Clarification of cervical cancer TNM and FIGO staging using MR imaging

It should be remembered that the FIGO staging system is clinically based, principally upon surgical and pathological findings, but also upon the results of physical examination and examination under anaesthesia in patients with advanced tumours unsuitable for surgery. It is designed to be applicable worldwide, irrespective of imaging resources. The TNM system takes into account nodal and visceral metastases, often identified by imaging.

When such systems are applied to imaging findings, areas of uncertainty arise. For example, MR evidence of bladder muscle layer invasion without involvement of the overlying mucosa might suggest stage TNM T4 or FIGO IVA disease but this stage requires tumour infiltration of the mucosa as well as the muscle layer (*Table 4.1*). When patients have tumours which infiltrate through the pelvic wall then they have tumour extension beyond the true pelvis and are stage TNM T4 or FIGO IVA. The N stage in cervical cancer only applies to pelvic lymph nodes. If there is upper retroperitoneal lymph node metastases, then the patient has TNM M1 or FIGO IVB disease and inguinal lymph node metastases are treated similarly.

Prognostic indicators

The features that have been shown to correlate with an adverse prognosis include:

- Tumour volume. For example, in early stage disease (IB and IIA), when tumour diameter exceeds 3.0 cm then there is a 40% chance of lymph node involvement.

Table 4.1. Cervical cancer: TNM (2002) and FIGO staging classification

TNM categories	FIGO stages	
TX		Primary tumour cannot be assessed
T0		No evidence of primary tumour
Tis	0	Carcinoma *in situ* (preinvasive carcinoma)
T1	I	Cervical carcinoma confined to uterus (extension to corpus should be disregarded)
T1a	IA	Invasive carcinoma diagnosed only by microscopy. All macroscopically visible lesions – even with superficial invasion – are T1b/Stage IB
T1a1	IA1	Stromal invasion no greater than 3.0 mm in depth and 7.0 mm or less in horizontal spread
T1a2	IA2	Stromal invasion more than 3.0 mm and not more than 5.0 mm with a horizontal spread 7.0 mm or less
T1b	IB	Clinically visible lesion confined to the cervix or microscopic lesion greater than T1a2/IA2
T1b1	IB1	Clinically visible lesion 4.0 cm or less in greatest dimension
T1b2	IB2	Clinically visible lesion more than 4.0 cm in greatest dimension
T2	II	Tumour invades beyond uterus but not to pelvic wall or to lower third of the vagina
T2a	IIA	Without parametrial invasion
T2b	IIB	With parametrial invasion
T3	III	Tumour extends to pelvic wall and/or involves the lower third of vagina and/or causes hydronephrosis or non-functioning kidney
T3a	IIIA	Tumour involves lower third of vagina, no extension to pelvic wall
T3b	IIIB	Tumour extends to pelvic wall and/or causes hydronephrosis or non-functioning kidney
T4	IVA	Tumour invades mucosa of bladder or rectum and/or extends beyond true pelvis
M1	IVB	Distant metastasis
N – Regional Lymph Nodes		
NX		Regional lymph nodes cannot be assessed
N0		No regional lymph node metastasis
N1		Regional lymph node metastasis

- Tumour stage. The 5-year survival rate for stage I is 91%, dropping to 15% for stage IV disease. Particularly important is the presence of lymph node metastases. For example a patient with stage Ib node negative disease has a >90% 5-year survival but stage Ib node positive disease has a 5-year survival of 50%.

- Poor tumour differentiation.

- Histological features, for example tumour vascularity and lymphatic permeation, deep cervical invasion, tumour extension into the body of the uterus and mixed adenosquamous tumour histological type.

- Diagnosis during pregnancy or at a young age.

Treatment

Surgery

Patients are eligible for surgery only if their tumour is less than T2b and if they have no known nodal metastases. Radical hysterectomy involves resection of the upper third of the vagina, the body and cervix of the uterus, the pericervical tissues including all ligaments (i.e. the cardinal, uterosacral and round ligaments), with bilateral salpingo-oophorectomy and pelvic lymph node resection. Not all patients undergo a standard radical hysterectomy, for example one ovary may be retained and either left *in situ* or transposed out of the true pelvis into the iliac fossa. Also, lymph node dissection can be extended to include upper retroperitoneal lymph nodes, or alternatively no lymph node dissection may be performed. Exceptionally, in some young patients with early stage disease, local resection of the cervix (trachelectomy) can be contemplated to preserve the patient's fertility. Patients who have positive surgical margins at the time of hysterectomy or who are lymph node positive may be referred for adjuvant radiotherapy.

Radiotherapy

Radiotherapy can be used to treat all stages of cervical cancer, although it is palliative in advanced disease (T4). External beam radiotherapy, brachytherapy (internal placement of radioactive sources), conformal radiotherapy and chemoradiotherapy are possible treatment methods. In advanced disease (T2 or greater) and in all node positive patients, the pelvic nodal stations are treated in addition to the primary tumour. Gynaecological complications of radiotherapy include cervical or vaginal stenosis, hydrosalpinx and fistula formation.

Chemotherapy

Chemotherapy may be used in the neo-adjuvant setting in patients with advanced disease before and during radiotherapy, or preoperatively in an attempt to downstage the tumour.

MR IMAGING OF CERVICAL CANCER

Technique

When imaging the pelvis, turbo spin echo sequences and phased array coil imaging offer advantages over conventional spin echo sequences and body coil imaging in terms of an improved signal-to-noise ratio. This allows thinner sections with better spatial resolution and reduced movement artifacts because of faster scan times. In addition to orthogonal plane imaging, off-axis imaging may be useful to transect the cervical tumour at 90° and/or to scan perpendicular to the interface between the cervix and rectum, or cervix and bladder. Fat suppressed imaging can be used but offers no staging advantage over conventional T1- and T2-weighted turbo spin echo sequences in cervical cancer. Body coil imaging of the upper pelvis and retroperitoneum are advised to assess for noncontiguous lymph node involvement.

Conventionally administered intravenous contrast enhancement has not been shown to improve the staging of cervical cancer but dynamic contrast-enhanced imaging may improve the detection of small tumours, the determination of extent of stromal and parametrial invasion and the detection or confirmation of invasion of adjacent organs. Dynamic contrast-enhanced imaging can be used to assess tumour perfusion and is thus an indirect method of assessing tumour hypoxia, which inversely correlates with tumour radiosensitivity and prognosis.

Endoluminal coils may be used and have been shown to improve the detection of small tumours but do not lead to a significant change in overall staging accuracy or accuracy in identifying parametrial invasion.

Current indications

Magnetic resonance imaging is the optimal method for locally staging cervical cancer because it is better than clinical staging for: overall tumour staging (including detection of lymph node metastases); tumour volume assessment; the identification of deep cervical extension and uterine body involvement. It has also been shown to have a significant impact on management in up to 50% of patients undergoing MRI examinations.

In recurrent cervical cancer, the aims of imaging are to accurately document local tumour extent and involvement of adjacent viscera in any patient for whom salvage surgery or radical radiotherapy is contemplated, and to identify nodal and metastatic tumour. MR imaging is better than CT for the diagnosis of local recurrence and for the determination of local extent. When patients are ineligible for curative therapy, imaging serves to document local and metastatic tumour burden as a baseline before chemotherapy, and can be used to monitor chemotherapy response.

Imaging features

Primary tumour

Usually, cervical cancer is of intermediate signal intensity on T1WI and higher signal intensity on T2 weighted turbo spin echo images, compared to the normal cervical stroma. Tumours may be solid or demonstrate central necrosis with or without cavitation.

Nodal disease

Local lymphatic spread to the paracervical and parametrial nodes is often not identified separate from the tumour proper.

While the size of normal lymph nodes varies in different anatomical sites, the most robust measurement for normal nodal size is a short axis diameter less than 1.0 cm. Other features suggestive of nodal involvement are: round shape, an asymmetrical cluster of nodes on the pelvic sidewall, and nodal T2-weighted signal intensity similar to the primary tumour.

In patients with squamous cell tumours, central nodal necrosis is an accurate positive predictor of metastasis even in normal sized lymph nodes.

Post treatment: surgery

During radical hysterectomy, the vagina is oversewn, may appear bow-tie shaped in the transaxial plane, and may become of low signal intensity on T2WI due to fibrotic change. The bladder and bowel may adhere to its margins. The position of retained ovaries should be documented. The site of the surgical approach may be visible and lymph node resection clips may be identified as small areas of signal void on the pelvic sidewalls adjacent to the iliac vessels and in the upper retroperitoneum.

Post treatment: radiotherapy

Marker seeds placed in the cervix to provide a landmark for external beam therapy may be visualised on MR imaging. The cervix reconstitutes after radiotherapy with resolution of the tumour mass, which is often rapid, so that within weeks there is restoration of T2WI low signal intensity fibrous stroma, whose signal intensity is often very low due to a profound fibrous reaction.

The uterus of a post-menopausal woman may decrease in size following radiotherapy. A patient of reproductive age will demonstrate more profound changes with decrease in size of the uterus, loss of the junctional zone anatomy, low signal intensity of the uterine body, marked thinning of the endometrium and low signal intensity of the cervix as it reconstitutes. The ovaries will decrease in size often demonstrating low signal intensity and will no longer have physiological cysts evident on MR imaging. The vagina also demonstrates a decrease in signal intensity.

Residual/recurrent disease

Residual disease should be considered when the cervix retains areas of high signal intensity more than 6 months after radiotherapy, but the finding is non-specific since inflammatory change or, occasionally, radiotherapy induced telangiectasia can produce similar appearances. Dynamic contrast enhancement may help differentiate residual or recurrent disease from treatment effect.

Up to one third of patients develop recurrent tumour in the pelvis by three years after treatment of their primary tumour. Central recurrence after hysterectomy manifests as a tumour mass arising from the vault of the vagina. All patients require assessment of loco-regional nodal stations and the upper retroperitoneum. CT is necessary to assess the lungs.

MRI staging accuracy

In cervical cancer, local staging accuracy ranges from 81% to 91%. This is better than conventional CT assessment, transrectal ultrasound imaging or clinical evaluation. MRI is better than CT for evaluation of tumour size, stromal invasion, and local and regional disease extension. Nodal status is assessed by MRI with an 85% to 93% accuracy, which compares well with dynamic helical CT. With high resolution MR imaging more lymph nodes are seen than on helical CT at standard slice thickness.

Pitfalls of MRI

Early stage disease

- The identification of small tumours and differentiation from post biopsy and inflammatory change may be difficult. The biopsy may leave an ill-defined area of high signal intensity on T2WI and if a cone biopsy has been performed there may be a tissue defect present.

- Nabothian cysts are mucous retention cysts which may be misinterpreted as tumour. However their site, spherical shape, fluid content and thin wall differentiate them from a cancer.

- Early parametrial extension is sometimes difficult to identify. Preservation of hypointense fibrous stroma outwith the tumour has a high negative predictive value for parametrial invasion but, conversely, complete loss of the low signal intensity fibrous stromal ring does not always indicate definite parametrial extension.

- Displacement and compression of the vaginal vault by a large exophytic cervical mass may mimic vaginal infiltration, or be misinterpreted as preservation of the outer cervical stroma. It is important to review the images in multiple planes to determine whether the tumour is truly invading the vagina.

Late stage disease

- In Stage T3a disease lower one third vaginal infiltration may be difficult to identify because of uncertainty about the demarcation between the upper two thirds and the lower one third of the vagina (arbitrarily the vagina distal to the bladder base). Laxity of the pelvic floor may alter vaginal position and large exophytic tumours may compress the vaginal wall and mimic vaginal involvement.

- Extension along the uterosacral ligaments may be difficult to define. The radiological signs of uterosacral ligament extension are thickening or lobularity of the uretosacral ligaments in continuity with the primary tumour, and signal intensity similar to that of the primary tumour on T2WI.

- Extension to the pelvic sidewall (stage T3b) is problematic because of differences in radiological interpretation. Some authorities consider tumour extending to within 0.5–1.0 cm of the sidewall to indicate stage T3b tumour, others only consider tumour actually making contact with the sidewall as stage T3b.

- Bladder involvement (stage T4) may be difficult to decide upon. While tumour can alter the signal intensity of the bladder muscle outer layer, it is only when the innermost portion of the muscle layer is of tumour signal intensity and/or there are tumour masses within the bladder lumen that Stage T4 disease can be diagnosed. Motion artifact due to bowel peristalsis can make assessment of the bladder wall difficult, particularly the bladder dome.

- Pelvic floor invasion can be difficult to distinguish from tumour tethering or adherence. If there is no plane between the tumour and the levator ani but the signal intensity of the muscle differs from that of the tumour then adherence is likely. If the tumour extends into or through the levator ani muscle then the levator has a T2-weighted signal intensity similar to the tumour proper.

FURTHER READING

1. Hawnaur J. (1998) Uterine and cervical tumours. In: *Imaging in Oncology* (eds Janet ES Husband and Rodney Reznek). Isis Medical Media Ltd, Oxford, pp. 309–328. *Considers cross-sectional imaging of these tumours and puts MRI in context.*

2. Boss EA, Barentsz JO, Massuger LFAG and Boonstra H. (2000) The Role of MR imaging in invasive cervical carcinoma. *Eur. Radiol.* 10: 256–270. *Sound review article.*

3. Nicolet V, Carignan L, Bourdon F and Prosmanne O. (2000) MR Imaging of cervical carcinoma: A practical staging approach. *Radiographics* 20:1539–1549. *Well-illustrated summary of FIGO staging.*

4. Lien HH. (1999) MR imaging of invasive carcinoma of the uterine cervix. *Acta Radiologica* 40: 236–245. *Good review article.*

5. Wagenaar HC, Trimbos JBMZ, Postema S, Anastasopoulou A *et al.* (2001) Tumour diameter and volume assessed by magnetic resonance imaging in the prediction of outcome for invasive cervical cancer. *Gynecol. Oncol.* 82: 474–482. *Highlights the relationship between tumour size and volume and patient outcome.*

6. Seki H, Azumi R, Kimura M and Sakai K. (1997) Stromal invasion by carcinoma of the cervix: Assessment with dynamic MR imaging. *AJR* 168:1579–1585. *Demonstrates the ability of dynamic MR imaging to improve detection of stromal invasion.*

7. Yang WT, Lam WWM, Yu MY, Cheung TH and Metreweli C. (2000) Comparison of dynamic helical CT and dynamic MR imaging in the evaluation of pelvic lymph nodes in cervical carcinoma. *AJR* 175: 759–766. *Identifies cystic nodal necrosis as a useful parameter in node assessment.*

8. Postema S, Pattynama PMT, Broker S *et al.* (1998) Fast dynamic contrast-enhanced colour-coded MRI in uterine cervix carcinoma: Useful for tumour staging? *Clin. Radiol.* 53: 729–734. *This study draws attention to possible overstaging with dynamic contrast enhancement.*

9. Van Vierzen PBJ, Massuger LFAG, Ruys SHJ and Barentsz JO. (1998) Fast dynamic contrast enhanced MR imaging of cervical carcinoma. *Clin. Radiol.* 53: 183–192. *This article demonstrates improved staging of cervical cancer using dynamic contrast enhanced MR imaging.*

10. Boss EA, Massuger LFAG, Pop LAM, Verhoef LCG *et al.* (2001) Post-radiotherapy contrast enhancement changes in fast dynamic MRI of the cervical carcinoma. *J. Magn. Reson. Imaging* 13: 600–606. *Explores the role of fast dynamic MRI in a small number of treated patients as a predictor of survival.*

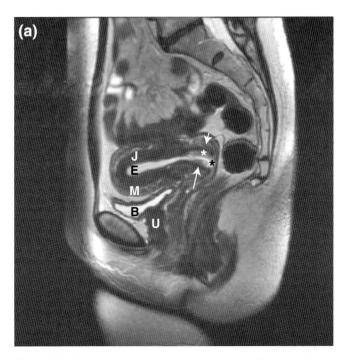

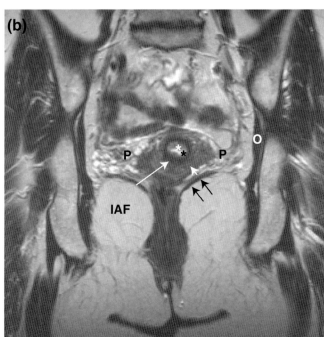

Figure 4.1. Normal cervical anatomy in a woman of reproductive age.

T2WI in **(a)** the sagittal plane and **(b)** the coronal plane, the latter providing a true transaxial image through the cervix. The endocervical lumen can be seen as a high signal intensity structure (black asterisk) surrounded by the cervical mucosa (white asterisk). The predominantly fibrous portion of the cervical stroma returns a low signal intensity and is discerned as a low signal intensity ring (long white arrow) immediately adjacent to the mucosa, while the outer cervix has an increased proportion of smooth muscle resulting in intermediate signal intensity (short white arrow). The cervix is surrounded by parametrium laterally and anteriorly (P in (b)) which is composed of fat, connective tissue, numerous blood vessels and lymphatics. The intra-organ anatomy of the uterus is well seen in (a) with the endometrial cavity (E), the junctional zone of the inner myometrium (J) and the outer myometrium (M). The pelvic floor formed by the levator ani muscular plate is well illustrated in (b) (black arrows). Bladder (B); urethra (U); ischioanal fossa; (IAF) obturator internus muscle (O).

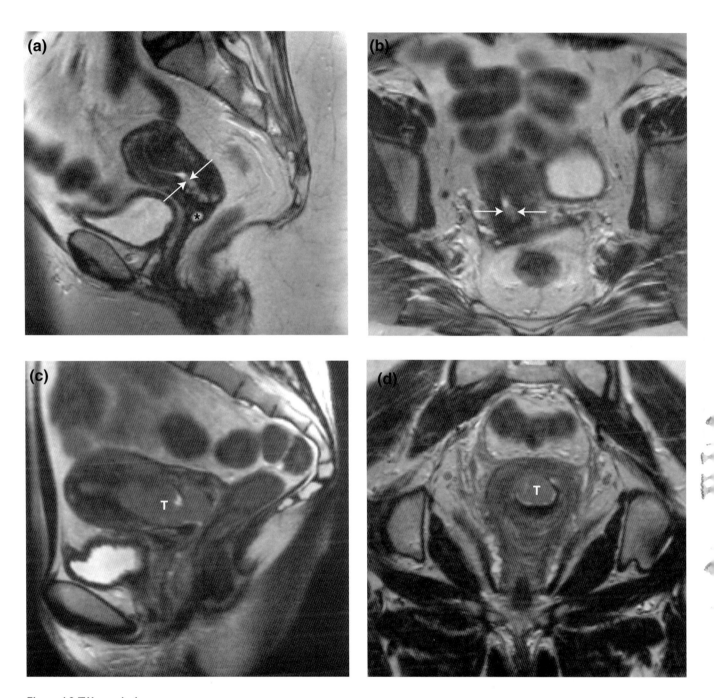

Figure 4.2. T1b cervical cancer.

T2W **(a)** sagittal and **(b)** transaxial images demonstrating a small predominantly endocervical tumour in a post-menopausal patient. The mass is of high signal intensity (arrows) but is of lower signal intensity than the endocervical secretions seen cranial to the lesion. There is slight distension of the endocervical canal. Note the preservation of normal cervical tissue around the tumour indicating that it is confined. After the menopause the junctional anatomy of the uterus is lost and the cervix is often of low signal intensity throughout. The patient has a small Nabothian cyst (asterisk in (a)). **(c)**, **(d)** Sagittal and off-axis coronal T2-weighted images in a different patient demonstrating a larger T1b endocervical tumour (T) which is confined. The tumour exceeds 4 cm in its longest diameter (craniocaudal) making it a radiological T1b2 tumour.

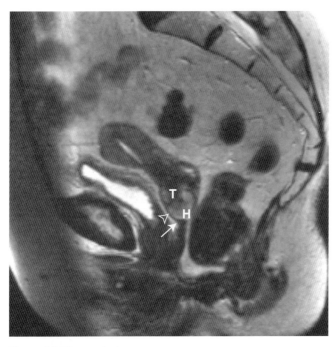

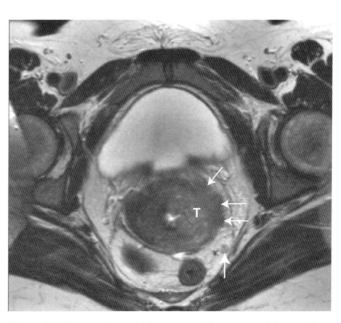

Figure 4.3. T2a cervical cancer.

Sagittal T2WI in which the tumour (T) can be seen extending to the anterior vaginal fornix (open arrowhead) with altered high signal intensity in the adjacent vaginal wall; contrast this with the uninvolved vagina more caudally (arrow). There is haemorrhage (H) within the vagina which is distended superiorly.

Figure 4.4 T2b N0/N1 cervical tumour with parametrial extension.

Off-axis transaxial T2WI demonstrating a high signal intensity tumour mass (T) involving the left cervix and extending from the endocervical canal throughout the entire cervical stroma with lobulated tumour extending beyond the lateral cervical margin and bulging into the parametrium (short arrows). There is also one left-sided posterior pelvic lymph node (long arrow) which, while small, has the same signal intensity as the tumour proper and both by its position and signal intensity is highly suspicious for an involved node.

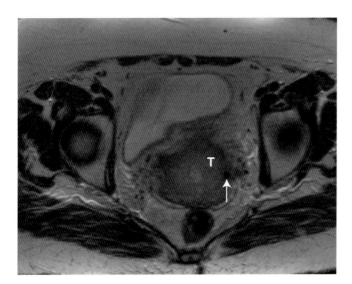

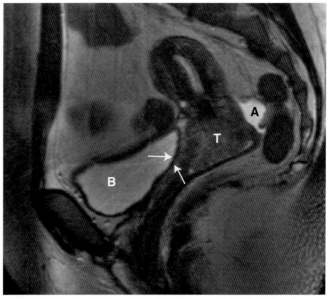

Figure 4.5. T2b cervical cancer with parametrial vascular engulfment.

Transaxial T2WI in which the cervix is entirely replaced by high signal intensity tumour (T) which engulfs a parametrial vessel (arrow), identified as an area of signal void due to flowing blood.

Figure 4.6. T2b cervical cancer with involvement of the uterovesical ligament, the anterior parametrium.

Sagittal T2WI with tumour (T) arising from the anterior lip and involving the upper third of the vagina. The tumour extends anteriorly into the uterovesical ligament, normally of high signal intensity due to its fat content. Disease abuts the posterior wall of the bladder (B) – (arrows). A small volume of ascites (A) is present in the Pouch of Douglas.

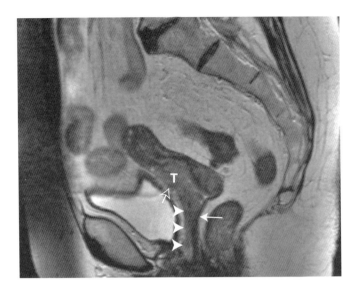

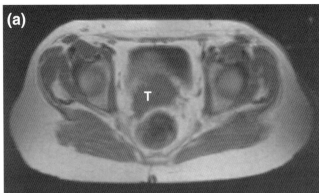

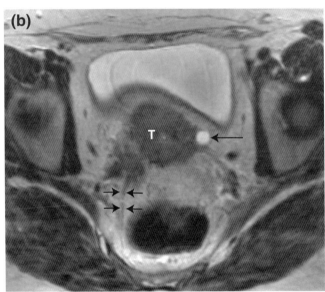

Figure 4.7. T3a cervical cancer.

Sagittal T2WI demonstrating tumour (T) extending down the anterior wall of the vagina (arrowheads) whose abnormal increased signal intensity contrasts with the normal low signal intensity of the submucosa and muscularis layers of the posterior vagina (arrow). There is also a small nodule of tumour extending into the uterovesical ligament, which is the anterior parametrium (open arrow).

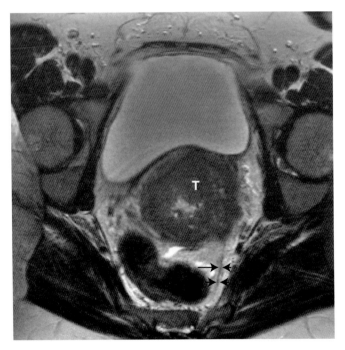

Figure 4.8. T3b cervical tumour with hydronephrosis.

Transaxial **(a)** T1WI and **(b)** high resolution T2WI showing a tumour (T) completely replacing the cervix and demonstrating spiculated extension into the parametrium. The left ureter (long arrow) is dilated and partially surrounded by tumour. Disease has extended into the proximal portion of the right uterosacral ligament (short arrows) but has not reached the pelvic sidewall. The T1WI often provide good soft tissue contrast between the tumour margin and adjacent parametrial fat.

Figure 4.9. T3b cervical tumour with uterosacral extension to the pelvic sidewall.

Transaxial T2WI demonstrating tumour (T) involving the entire cervix, infiltrating the left uterosacral ligament (arrows) which is thickened, and extending to within a centimetre of the pelvic sidewall. Clinically this tumour was fixed to the sidewall.

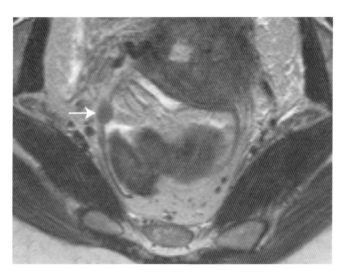

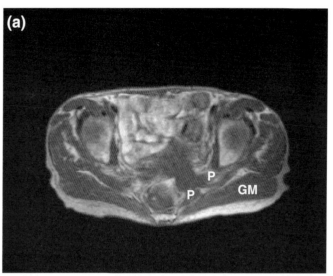

Figure 4.10.T3b cervical tumour with uterosacral extension.

Transaxial T2WI showing tumour extending along both uterosacral ligaments, to within 0.5 cm of the sidewall on the right and to within a centimetre of the sidewall on the left. Note the lobular uterosacral tumour infiltration on the right side (arrow). Tumour extension to the pelvic sidewall is diagnosed differently by various authorities. Criteria include tumour extending to within 1 cm, tumour extending to within 0.5 cm and tumour actually contacting the sidewall. Overall, however, early pelvic sidewall extension may be under-identified.

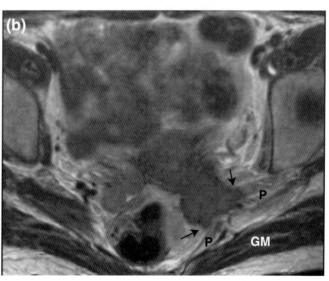

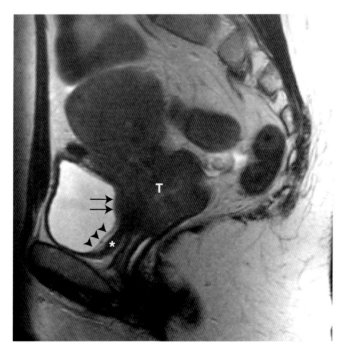

Figure 4.11.T3b cervical cancer with large volume uterosacral extension.

Transaxial **(a)** T1WI and **(b)** T2WI of a patient with substantial uterosacral tumour extending to the left pelvic sidewall (arrows) and infiltrating into the left piriformis muscle (P). The piriformis is tethered by the tumour at the site of infiltration and retracted away from the underlying gluteus maximus muscle (GM). However the tumour has not extended through the piriformis muscle. In (b) note increased T2-weighted signal intensity of the uninfiltrated portions of the piriformis muscle most likely due to reactive oedema.

Figure 4.12.T4a cervical cancer invading the bladder.

Sagittal T2WI showing a large tumour (T) infiltrating the whole uterus and extending through the bladder into the mucosa (arrows). The mucosa should demonstrate the same signal intensity as the tumour proper to allow diagnosis of bladder infiltration. Note the normal low signal intensity muscle layer of the bladder inferiorly (asterisk) and the presence of overlying mucosal bullous oedema producing high signal intensity change within the mucosa (arrowheads) which should not be diagnosed as tumour infiltration.

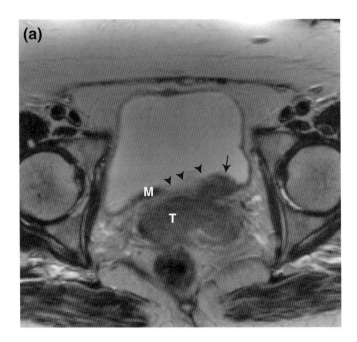

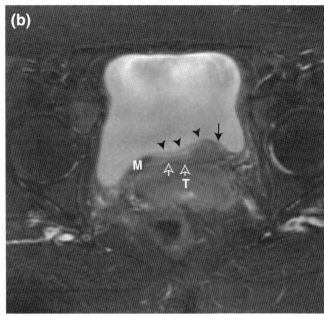

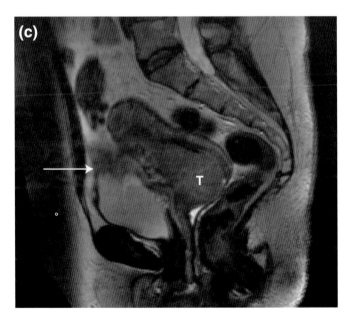

Figure 4.13. T4a cervical cancer invading the bladder.

Transaxial **(a)** T2WI, **(b)** T2W fat suppressed and **(c)** sagittal T2WI. There is a large cervical tumour (T) invading the bladder in a left posterior location with a mass of similar signal intensity to the tumour proper (arrow) seen within the bladder lumen. Note that there is bladder mucosal oedema (arrowheads) in (b) partially overlying the intravesical tumour but also extending over the posterior bladder wall. The central portion of the bladder wall in (a) and (b) is also abnormal but signal intensity is higher than the tumour proper and represents oedema. In (b) a portion of the bladder wall is shown to be partially infiltrated but to retain an intact though oedematous inner muscle layer (small open arrows), bladder muscle layer (M). In (c) the abnormal signal intensity of the posterior bladder muscle layer and its retraction towards the tumour can be appreciated. Note the apparent abnormal signal intensity at the dome of the bladder in (c) (long arrow). This was due to artifact from adjacent peristalsing small bowel. To overcome this, hyoscine butylbromide (Buscopan) could be administered if necessary.

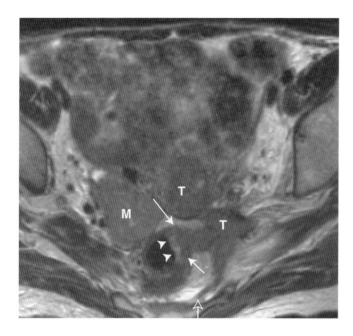

Figure 4.14. T3b cervical tumour with partial thickness rectal involvement.

Transaxial T2WI showing a cervical tumour (T) extending through the perirectal fat to infiltrate the outer rectum on the left side (arrows). Disease extends around the left uterosacral ligament to the pelvic sidewall (open arrow). The overlying rectal mucosa (arrowheads) is intact but of high signal intensity indicating oedema or haemorrhage and, because of this, although tumour is obviously invading the rectal wall, the stage is T3b by clinical criteria. Note a right adnexal mass (M) of similar signal intensity to the tumour proper, due to involvement by the primary cervical tumour.

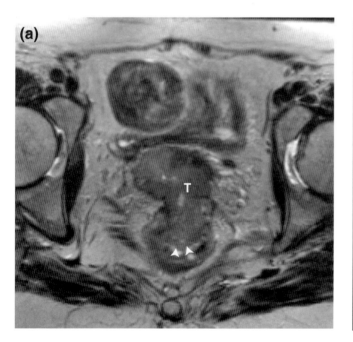

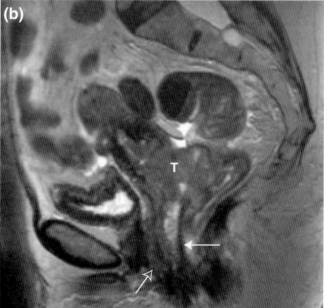

Figure 4.15. T4 cervical cancer with full thickness rectal involvement.

Transaxial **(a)** and sagittal **(b)** T2WI showing a large cervical tumour (T) extending through the posterior vaginal wall and breaching the recto-vaginal septum (arrow in (b)) to invade the rectum. There is transmural extension of tumour to the rectal lumen (arrowheads). The tumour also extends along the entire vagina to the lower third (open arrow).

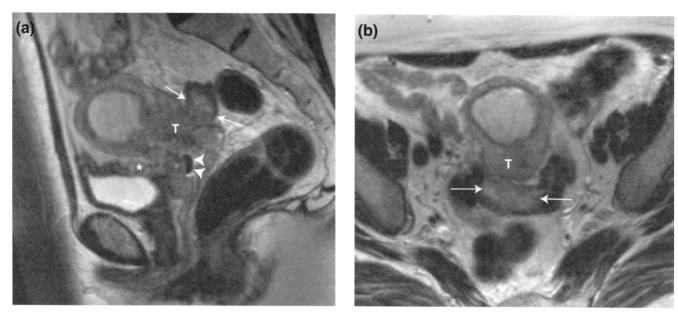

Figure 4.16. T4 cervical cancer involving the sigmoid colon.

Sagittal **(a)** and transaxial **(b)** T2WI demonstrating a cervical tumour extending postero-superiorly into the sigmoid colon (arrows). The tumour extends through the uterovesical ligament to involve the supero-posterior bladder wall (asterisk). There is an air/fluid level in this centrally necrotic tumour (arrowheads).

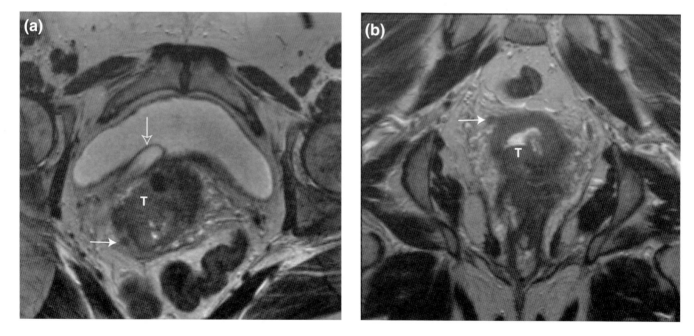

Figure 4.17. Paracervical/parametrial lymph node metastases.

Off-axis transaxial **(a)** and off-axis coronal **(b)** T2WI in two different patients illustrating paracervical / parametrial lymph node metastases (arrows) adjacent to the cervical tumour (T). These nodes are often small, but of similar signal intensity to the tumour proper, and appear separate from the primary tumour on all planes. They are infrequently seen because parametrial extension of the primary tumour often engulfs them. Note the right-sided ureterocoele (open arrow) in (a).

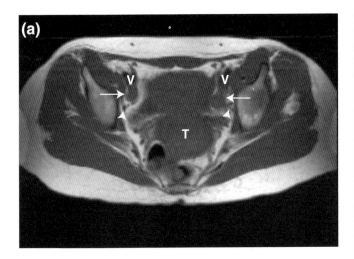

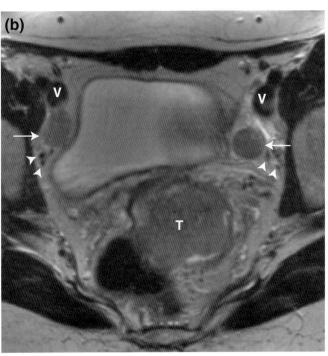

Figure 4.18. Bilateral obturator lymph node metastases.

Transaxial T1WI **(a)** and T2WI **(b)** demonstrating bilateral obturator lymph nodes (arrows) in a patient with a large cervical primary tumour (T). The nodes are situated adjacent to the obturator vessels (arrowheads) and positioned posterior to the external iliac vein (V), typically adjacent to the pelvic sidewall. These lymph nodes are highly likely to contain metastatic tumour because they are enlarged, rounded and of similar signal intensity to the primary tumour mass. Obturator nodes are the most frequently involved by metastatic tumour. It is important to evaluate both the T1WI and T2WI for nodal disease since node:fat contrast is optimal on T1WI and lymph nodes may be overlooked occasionally on T2WI if their signal intensity rises to approximate the signal intensity of fat.

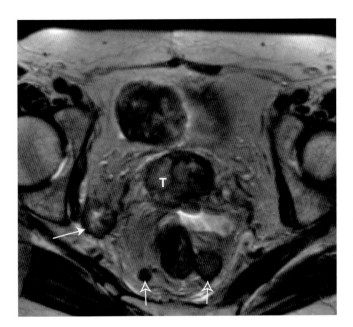

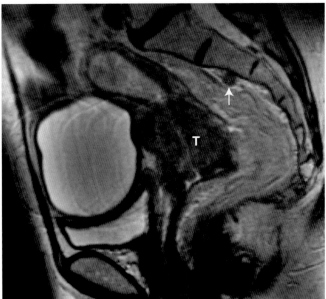

Figure 4.19. Internal iliac and perirectal lymph node metastases.

Transaxial T2WI demonstrating a high signal intensity primary cervical tumour (T) with metastatic spread to a right internal iliac (arrow) and two perirectal lymph nodes (open arrows). The right internal iliac lymph node has undergone central nodal necrosis as shown by irregular very high signal intensity within its centre.

Figure 4.20. Pre-sacral lymph node metastasis in cervical cancer.

Sagittal T2WI demonstrating a pre-sacral node at S2 level (arrow) which has the same signal intensity as the tumour proper (T). It is likely to be involved by tumour. Pre-sacral lymph nodes may be excluded from the radiotherapy field if they are located below S2 level, since the posterior margin of the field is normally vertically aligned at the S2/3 junction.

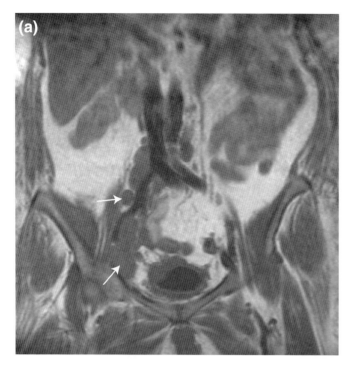

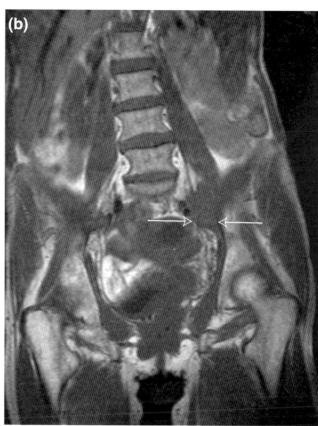

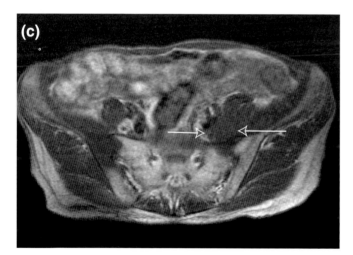

Figure 4.21. Common iliac and external iliac metastatic lymph nodes in cervical cancer.

(a) Coronal T1WI showing multiple enlarged right pelvic sidewall lymph nodes (arrows). (b) Coronal and (c) transaxial T1WI in a different patient. There are left common iliac lymph node metastases (open arrows) producing the filled in fat sign compared to the contralateral side. This site for lymph node metastases can be overlooked easily. In (c) malignant bone infiltration can be seen within the right medial ilium and in the left sacrum directly underlying the metastatic lymph node mass. Bone infiltration can be due to haematogeneous spread or direct bone erosion by the lymph node disease. Note the asymmetry of the iliopsoas muscles with increase in size on the left side. This is most likely to be due to oedema arising from impaired lymphatic drainage.

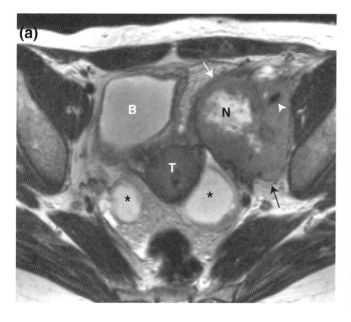

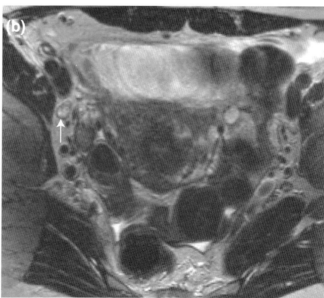

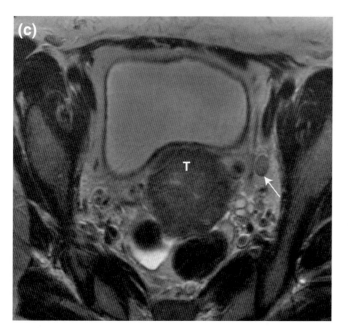

Figure 4.22. Pelvic metastatic lymph nodes.

(a) Transaxial T2WI demonstrating a primary tumour (T) with a huge left external iliac lymph node mass showing central necrosis (N) and encasing the left external iliac artery (arrowhead). The bladder (B) is displaced to the right. The patient also has bilateral adnexal cysts (asterisks). It is unusual to have such a large lymph node metastasis at presentation. (b) Transaxial T2WI showing a small right obturator lymph node (arrow) with central nodal necrosis exhibiting high signal intensity greater than pelvic fat. Histopathological analysis confirmed metastatic tumour in this node. In squamous cell carcinoma, T2-weighted central nodal necrosis is a highly accurate predictor of metastatic nodal infiltration even if the lymph node is not enlarged by size criteria. If there is uncertainty whether T2-weighted high signal intensity in a node is fat or central nodal necrosis, then fat suppressed imaging (fat saturation or STIR sequences) may help. (c) Off-axis transaxial T2WI demonstrating a large cervical primary tumour (T) with parametrial extension and a left obturator lymph node (arrow) which is of normal size but of similar signal intensity to the tumour proper. This finding indicates likely metastatic infiltration.

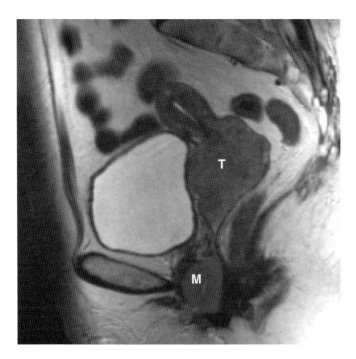

Figure 4.23. T2b M1 cervical cancer with metastasis to the lower vagina.

Sagittal T2WI showing a bulky cervical tumour (T) and a metastasis to the lower third of the vagina (M). The two lesions were separate on all imaging planes.

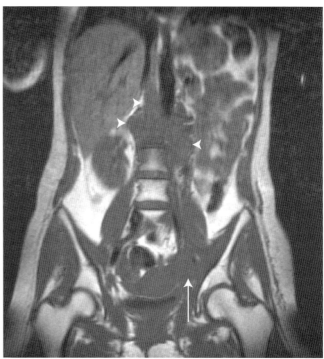

Figure 4.24. Upper retroperitoneal lymph node metastases.

Coronal T1WI demonstrating left pelvic sidewall lymph node metastases (arrow) and upper retroperitoneal lymph node metastases (arrowheads).

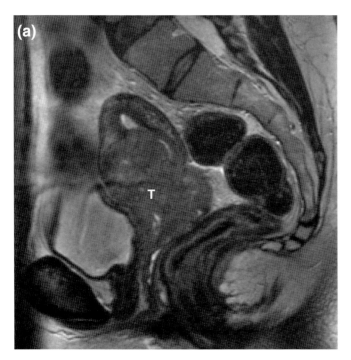

Figure 4.25. Liver metastases in cervical cancer.

(a) Sagittal T2WI demonstrating a large cervical tumour (T) extending into the parametrium, body of uterus and upper two thirds of the vagina. (b) Off axis coronal dynamic enhanced gradient recalled echo image of the liver demonstrating a large necrotic metastasis (M) with a satellite lesion (arrow).

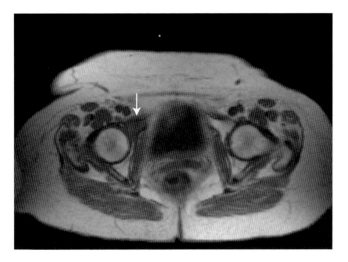

Figure 4.26. Bone metastasis in cervical cancer.

Transaxial T1WI showing an intermediate signal intensity metastasis (arrow) in the right superior pubic ramus and acetabulum. The lesion has breached the cortex anteriorly. Bone metastases contrast best with marrow fat on T1WI. (See also *Figures 4.21(b)* and *(c)*).

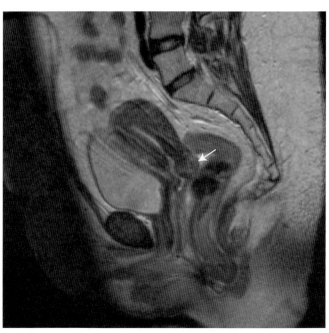

Figure 4.27. Small tumours and post biopsy change.

Sagittal T2WI demonstrating subtly altered signal intensity in and slight expansion of the posterior lip of the cervix (arrows) after biopsy. Pathological examination of the hysterectomy specimen revealed inflammatory change after biopsy but no residual tumour.

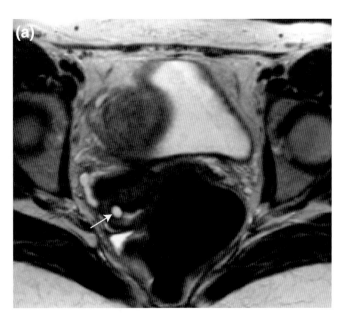

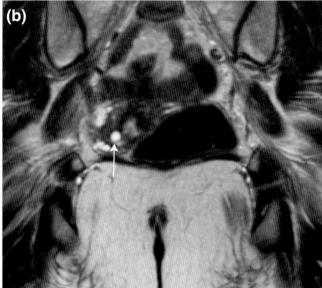

Figure 4.28. Nabothian cysts.

(a) Transaxial and **(b)** coronal T2WI demonstrating a well demarcated thin-walled high signal intensity lesion in the cervix (arrows). Nabothian cysts are mucus retention cysts formed by occlusion of the endocervical crypts by squamous metaplasia.

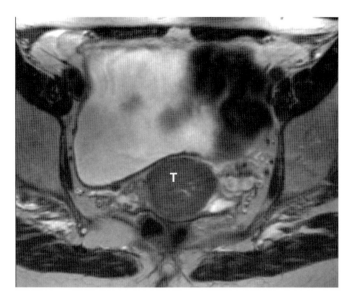

Figure 4.29. Loss of cervical fibrous stroma.

Transaxial T2WI demonstrating a tumour (T) with complete loss of the low signal intensity fibrous stroma but a smooth margin with the parametrial fat. Absence of the low signal intensity fibrous stromal ring is not an absolute indicator of tumour extension into the parametrium (see text).

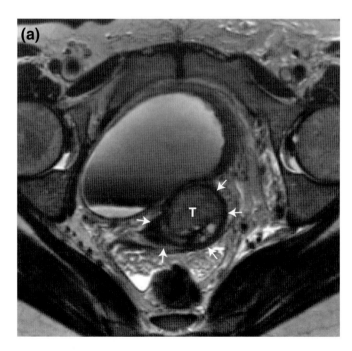
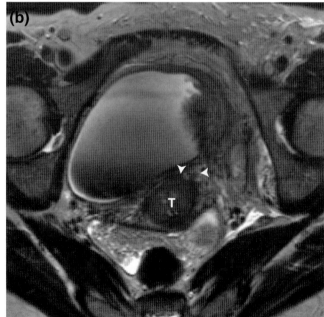

Figure 4.30. The upper vagina mimicking the outer cervical stroma.

(a), (b) Off-axis transaxial T2WI with a cervical tumour (T) seen in (a) surrounded by a low signal intensity rim (arrows) which was the vagina. More cranially in (b) the tumour can be seen to extend into the parametrium (arrowheads). The left bladder wall is irregularly thickened and of altered signal intensity due to infiltration by a large left pelvic sidewall lymph node metastasis (out of plane on this image).

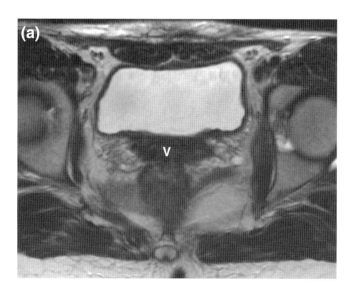

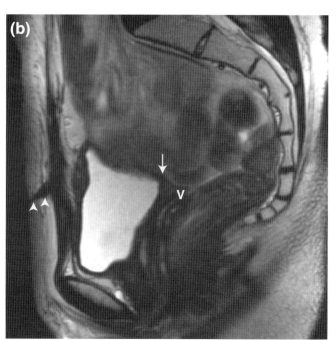

Figure 4.31. Appearances post radical hysterectomy.

Transaxial **(a)** and sagittal **(b)** T2WI demonstrating the oversewn vaginal vault (V), of low signal intensity due to fibrous change, with spread of fibrous tissue to the posterior wall of the bladder (arrow in (b)). The surgical scar is well seen in (b) (arrowheads).

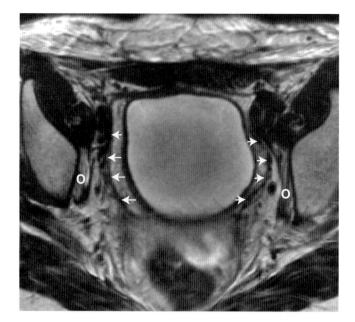

Figure 4.32. Appearances after bilateral pelvic sidewall lymph node dissection.

Transaxial T2WI showing low signal intensity linear scarring (arrows) extending anteroposteriorly along the pelvic sidewalls. There is also high signal intensity of both obturator internus muscles (O) due to post-surgical inflammatory change. There is abnormality of the anterior abdominal wall due to oedema at the laparotomy site.

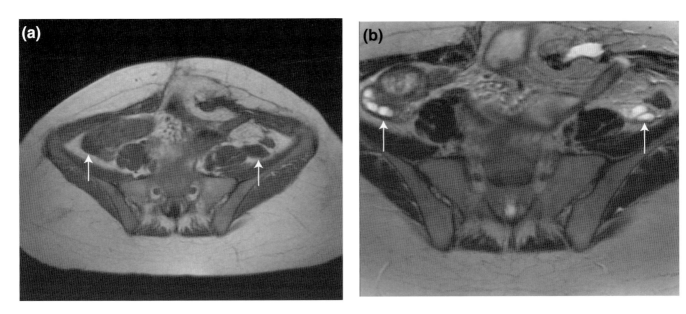

Figure 4.33. Appearances after bilateral ovarian transposition.

Transaxial **(a)** T1WI and **(b)** T2WI in a patient who underwent ovarian transposition at the time of radical hysterectomy. The ovaries (arrows) have been relocated to the iliac fossae. This procedure is performed to prevent the ovaries being included in a post-operative radiation field and thereby preserve ovarian function. The ovaries should not be confused with tumour masses.

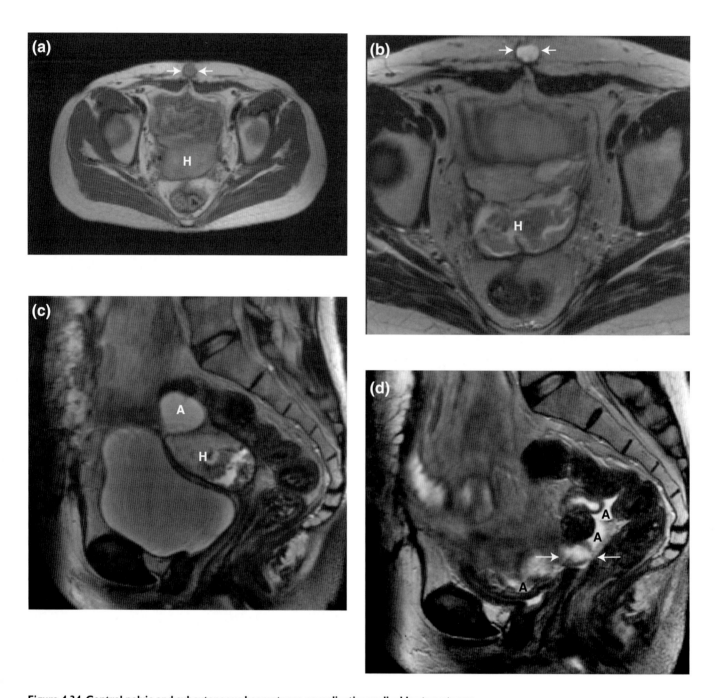

Figure 4.34. Central pelvic and subcutaneous haematoma complicating radical hysterectomy.

(a) Transaxial T1WI, (b) transaxial T2WI and (c) sagittal T2WI in which a central haematoma (H) is seen with characteristic high signal intensity on the T1WI, and T2-weighted heterogeneous appearance with a low signal intensity rim and mixed high and intermediate signal intensity content. Compared to the central pelvic haematoma, the small subcutaneous haematoma (arrows) is of similar signal intensity. There is loculated ascites (A) above the haematoma in (c). (d) Sagittal T2WI performed three months later demonstrates the small residuum of the haematoma (arrow) but persistent ascites (A). The appearance of haematomata varies with their age.

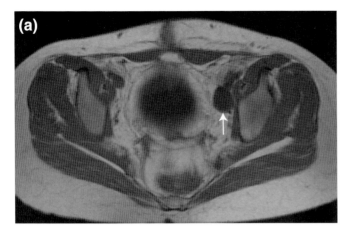

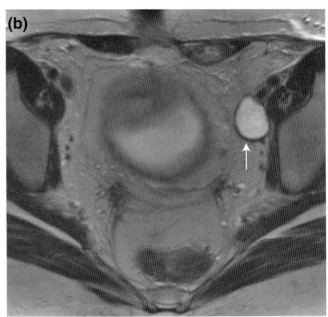

Figure 4.35. Unilocular lymphocoele after radical hysterectomy.

Transaxial **(a)** T1WI and **(b)** T2WI showing a small left-sided unilocular lymphocoele (arrow) in a common position adjacent to the external iliac vessels. Lymphocoeles are retroperitoneal collections of lymph fluid caused by surgical disruption of lymphatic trunks. They demonstrate signal intensity characteristics similar to water on T1WI and T2WI, are usually unilocular and thin-walled and often resorb spontaneously. Occasionally septations may be seen within larger lymphocoeles.

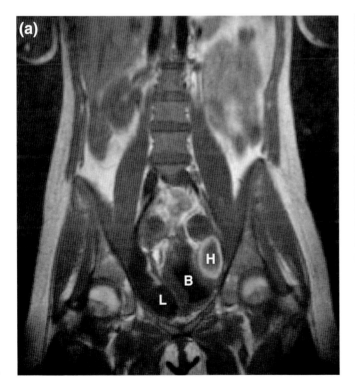

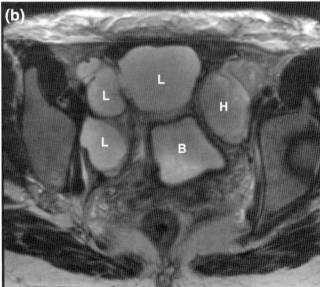

Figure 4.36. Post-surgical left pelvic sidewall haematoma and multiloculated right lymphocoele.

(a) Coronal T1WI and **(b)** transaxial T2WI demonstrating a left pelvic sidewall haematoma (H), whose nature is best elucidated on the T1WI, where there is a characteristic ring-within-ring appearance of a low to intermediate signal intensity thin margin, an inner high signal intensity ring and an inner intermediate signal intensity core. The bladder (B) is thick-walled and displaced to the left of the midline by a multiloculated lymphocoele (L) extending along the right pelvic sidewall and across the midline anteriorly. Lymphocoele are typically unilocular and thin-walled but may occasionally be multilocular.

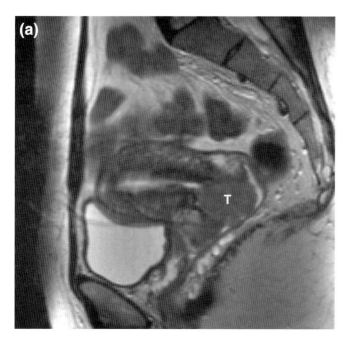

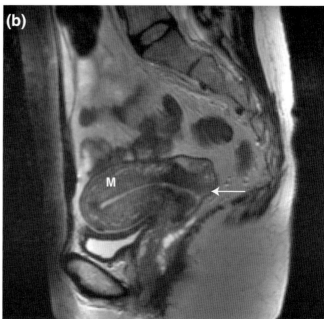

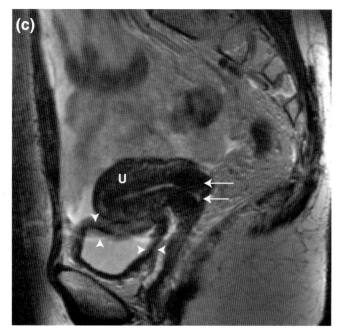

Figure 4.37. Response of cervical tumour to radiotherapy.

Sagittal T2WI **(a)** at presentation, **(b)** 2 months and **(c)** 10 months after radiotherapy. The intermediate signal intensity cervical tumour (T) can be readily identified in (a). By 2 months there is only a small area of residual abnormal signal intensity (arrow in (b)) in the posterior lip of the cervix. The anterior lip of the cervix has reconstituted. The uterine body has lost its zonal differentiation but the outer myometrium (M) is still of normal signal intensity. Rapid tumour response to radiotherapy can often occur. By 10 months post radiotherapy the cervix and vagina are of intense low signal intensity indicating a good treatment response (arrows in (c)). The uterus has atrophied and the uterine body (U) is of low signal intensity with loss of zonal anatomy. There is now treatment-induced mural thickening of the posterior and superior bladder (arrowheads).

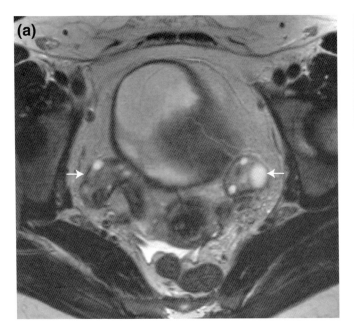 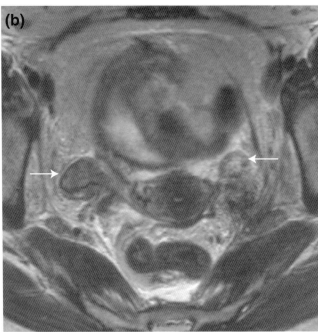

Figure 4.38. Response of the ovaries to radiotherapy.

Off-axis transaxial T2WI **(a)** before and **(b)** 4 months after radiotherapy. In (a) the ovaries (arrows) have multiple follicular cysts present with high signal intensity central stroma. In (b) 4 months after radiotherapy the ovaries (arrows) have shrunk, lost their follicular cysts and the signal intensity of the central stroma has started to decrease.

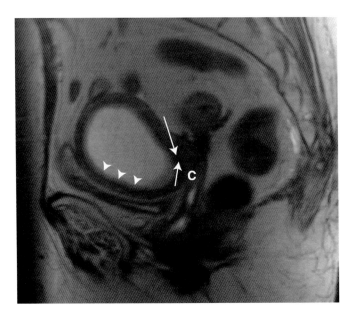

Figure 4.39. Post-radiotherapy cervical stenosis with hydrometria.

Sagittal T2WI demonstrating a distended high signal intensity endometrial cavity with visualisation of the endometrium (arrowheads) and a stenotic internal os (arrow) with the cervix (C) demonstrating uniform low signal intensity after radiotherapy.

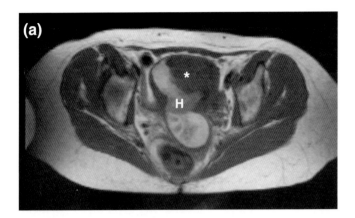

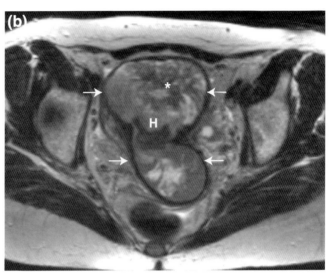

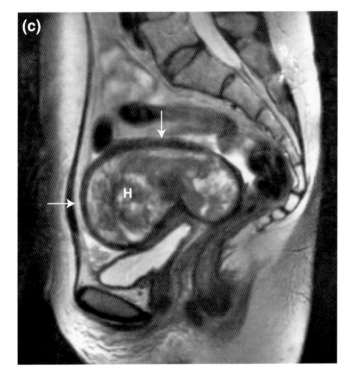

Figure 4.40. Post-radiotherapy haematometria.

Transaxial **(a)** T1WI, **(b)** T2WI and **(c)** sagittal T2WI. The uterus (arrows) is distended and contains altered blood (haematometria (H)) as shown by high signal intensity on T1WI and whorled intermediate and high signal intensity on T2WI. The apparent focal lesion (asterisk) in the left anterior uterine fundus represents haematoma of a different age to the rest of the uterine cavity. The patient went on to have a hysterectomy and altered blood filled the uterine cavity. There was no evidence of malignancy.

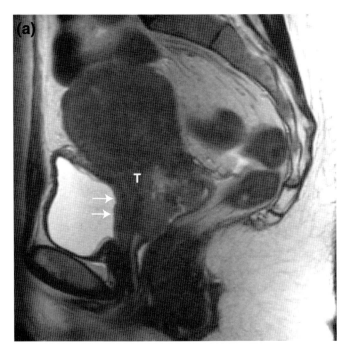
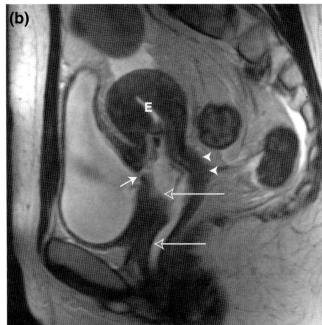

Figure 4.41. Radiotherapy induced vesico-uterine fistula.

(a) and **(b)** Sagittal T2WI. In (a) there is a large necrotic cervical tumour (T) involving the uterine body and extending through the bladder wall to involve the mucosa (arrows). In (b) 3 months post treatment a fistula (arrow) can be seen and the cervical cavity and vagina are fluid filled (open arrows). The uterus has decreased in size and the endometrial cavity (E) is visualised. The posterior cervix has reconstituted (arrowheads).

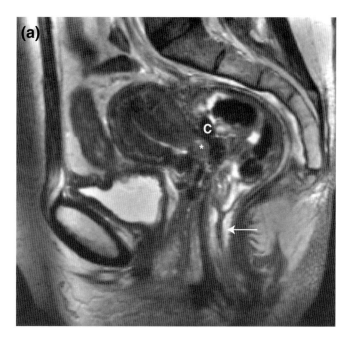

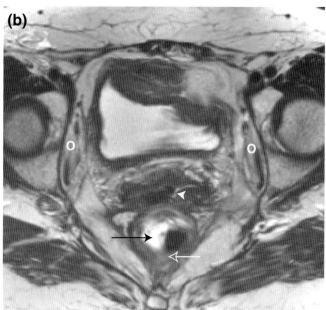

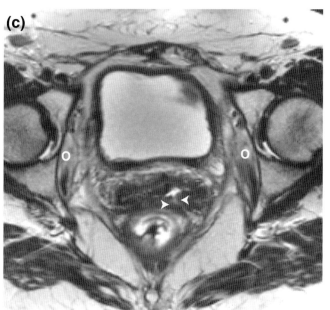

Figure 4.42. Evolution of complex post radiation fistula.

(i) 12 months after therapy. (a) Sagittal, **(b)** and **(c)** transaxial T2WI. There is high signal intensity within the cervix (asterisk) due to oedema and hypervascularity. The anorectum demonstrates treatment effect with high signal intensity of the mucosa (arrow) and a high signal intensity thickened lamina propria (open arrow in (b)). An extraluminal air-containing cavity (C) is present between the uterus and the proximal rectum in (a). A small tract (arrowhead) is seen extending through the posterior vaginal wall in (b) but no fistulous connection is identified with the rectum. In (c) there is a further tract (arrowheads) which extends through the posterior vaginal wall without involving the rectal wall.

(ii) 18 months after therapy. (d) Sagittal and **(e)** transaxial T2WI. There is complete necrosis of the cervix and a double fistula between the cervix / vagina and the proximal and mid rectum (arrows), whose anterior wall has largely necrosed with a small residual portion superiorly (asterisk). There is also a fistula between the vagina and the bladder (open arrow). The mucosa and muscle layers of the bladder wall are markedly thickened with increased signal intensity of portions of the muscle layer (arrowheads in (e)). Fluid is seen extending down the vagina and there is high signal intensity material (black arrows in (d)) on the patient's perineal skin because of the fistulous discharge per vaginum. On all transaxial images the obturator internus muscles (O) demonstrate high signal intensity due to radiation therapy.

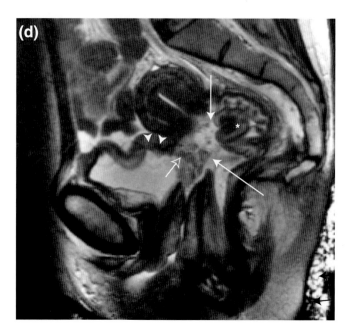

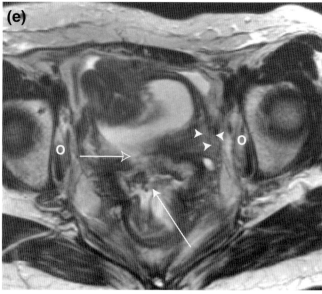

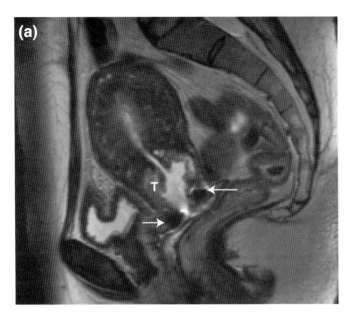

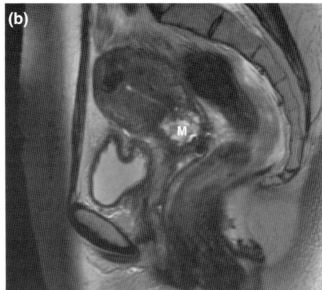

Figure 4.43. Residual cervical cancer.

Sagittal T2WI **(a)** pretreatment, **(b)** 6 months post-radiotherapy. A cavitating high signal intensity tumour (T) is present. Two metallic marker seeds (arrows) have been placed in the anterior and posterior lips of the cervix at examination under anaesthesia to guide the external beam radiotherapy. These clips demonstrate the bloom susceptibility artifact associated with metal. After treatment there remains a high signal intensity mass (M) in the cervix, which shows no evidence of reconstituting. The rest of the uterus has atrophied. One marker seed remains in the posterior lip. The patient underwent salvage hysterectomy with cystectomy (anterior pelvic clearance) and residual adenocarcinoma was confirmed. Residual high signal intensity within the cervix more than 6 months after radiotherapy warrants investigation. The abnormality may be due to tumour or occasionally radiation-induced oedema and telangiectasia. Dynamic contrast enhanced MR imaging may help differentiate between the two conditions.

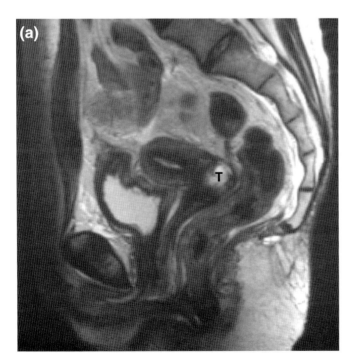

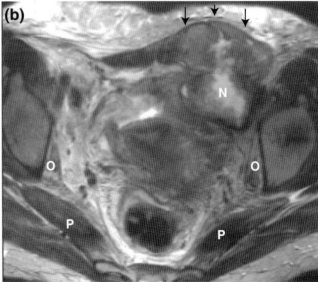

Figure 4.44. Recurrent cervical cancer.

(a) Sagittal and **(b)** transaxial T2WI demonstrating a central high signal intensity partially necrotic recurrent tumour (T) and necrotic left external iliac lymph node metastasis (N) invading the left anterior abdominal wall (arrows). There is abnormal high signal intensity of the obturator internus muscles (O) and portions of the piriformis muscles (P) which reflects oedema and hyperaemia, either due to local inflammation or the effect of radiation therapy.

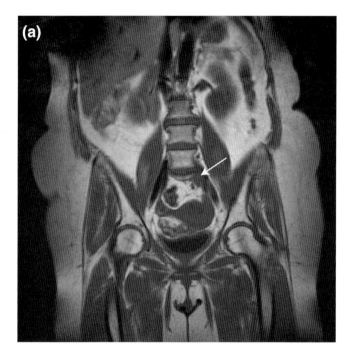

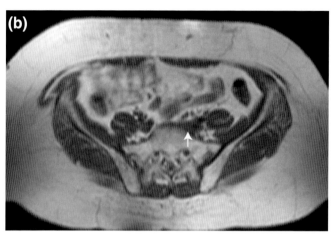

Figure 4.45. Recurrent common iliac lymph node metastasis.

(a) Coronal and **(b)** transaxial T1WI showing a small left common iliac nodal mass (arrows) which was producing back pain. The patient had undergone radiotherapy to the primary tumour and pelvic nodal stations two years before. In these circumstances, nodal recurrences are often at or above the margin of the field, here at L5/S1 level. The metastatic nodes may erode into adjacent bone, and produce severe pain. Note the high signal intensity of the pelvic marrow due to fat replacement, but preservation of haemopoietic marrow in L5 vertebral body.

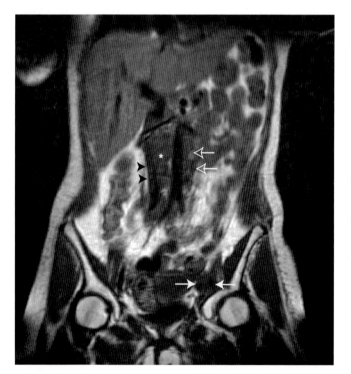

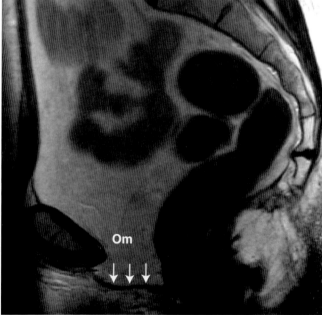

Figure 4.46. Recurrent pelvic sidewall and upper retroperitoneal lymph node metastases.

Coronal T1WI showing a small left external iliac nodal mass (arrows) and upper retroperitoneal lymph node metastases in a para-aortic (open arrows) and interaortocaval (asterisk) distribution. The IVC (arrowheads) is displaced laterally.

Figure 4.47. Anterior pelvic clearance.

Sagittal T2WI. The bladder, urethra, uterus and vagina have been removed and the levator ani muscles oversewn (arrows). The omentum (Om) has been placed in the surgical bed to prevent small bowel prolapsing inferiorly.

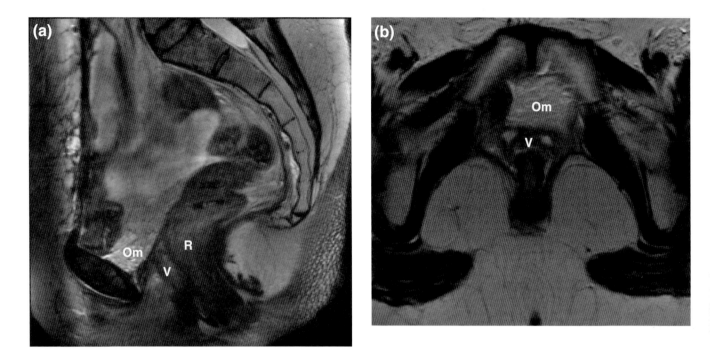

Figure 4.48. Anterior pelvic clearance with neovagina formation.

(a) Sagittal and **(b)** transaxial T2WI demonstrating absence of the anterior pelvic organs, retention of the rectum (R) and formation of a neovagina (V) from colon. Omentum (Om) has been placed in the surgical bed.

5 Endometrial Cancer

Jane M. Hawnaur

BACKGROUND INFORMATION

Epidemiology

In the United Kingdom, endometrial carcinoma has an incidence of 4850 new cases per year, compared to 6820 per annum for ovarian cancer and 3240 for cervical cancer. There are approximately 990 deaths per year from uterine cancer in the UK. Endometrial carcinoma is the commonest gynaecological malignancy in the USA, and the American Cancer Society estimates that 39 300 new cases and 6600 deaths will occur in 2002. The disease predominantly affects postmenopausal women, peaking in the decade 55–65 years. The most frequent presenting symptom is abnormal vaginal bleeding or discharge. Asymptomatic tumours may be detected by cervical smear or as an incidental finding during pelvic ultrasound. Women at high risk include those with the hereditary nonpolyposis colorectal cancer (HNPCC) gene who usually develop endometrial cancer before the age of 50 years. Women on long-term treatment with Tamoxifen for breast cancer also have an increased risk of developing endometrial malignancy. Other predisposing factors include chronic exposure to unopposed oestrogens, either extrinsic or as a result of obesity or ovarian malfunction, for example in polycystic ovarian disease. There is also an association between endometrial cancer and diabetes mellitus.

Histopathology

The majority of endometrial carcinomas arise within glandular epithelium and are adenocarcinomas of endometrioid type (75%). The less common papillary serous, adenosquamous and clear cell types are associated with a worse prognosis. Tumours are graded from Grade I (well differentiated) to Grade 3 (poorly differentiated). Rare tumours of stromal origin include endometrial sarcoma, mixed Müllerian tumour and leiomyosarcoma.

Patterns of tumour spread

Endometrial carcinoma arising in glandular epithelium commonly grows as a polypoidal mass, ulceration of which results in bleeding. Direct invasion into the myometrium may initially occur at the stalk of a polypoid tumour, eventually extending more widely and deeply into the myometrium. Tumour may eventually reach the serosa of the uterus and thence into the peritoneal cavity and adjacent organs. Tumour may spread down the cervical canal, with the potential for invasion of cervical glandular epithelium and stroma. Cervical stromal invasion may also occur directly from myometrial tumour invasion extending below the isthmus of the uterine corpus into the cervix. Extension of tumour at the uterine cornua into the Fallopian tubes provides another route of spread to the adnexal structures and peritoneal cavity. Peritoneal metastases can also occur as a result of lymphovascular or trans-myometrial spread from endometrial carcinoma. Lymphovascular space invasion is associated with lymph node metastasis. The endometrium and myometrium of the upper corpus and fundus of the uterus drain via lymphatics in the infundibulo-pelvic ligament to the common iliac and para-aortic lymph nodes. The mid and lower corpus and the uterine cervix drain to parametrial, para-cervical and obturator lymph nodes, and thence along the external iliac, internal iliac, common iliac and para-aortic/para-caval lymph node chains. Fallopian tube or ovarian tumour can also metastasise directly to para-aortic lymph nodes. Tumours extending via the cervix to the lower vagina can metastasise to the inguinal lymph nodes. Inguinal nodes may also be involved via spread along the round ligament from adnexal or pelvic sidewall tumour involvement. Distant haematogenous metastasis can occur to lungs, liver or bones, but is unusual at presentation.

Staging

The TNM staging classification and its equivalent FIGO staging is given in *Table 5.1*. Carcinoma of the endometrium is commonly staged in the UK using the International Federation of Obstetrics and Gynaecology (FIGO) staging classification (1994), which is surgico-pathological.

Prognostic indicators

The mortality rate in the UK for endometrial carcinoma is 3 per 100000 women per year. In the USA, the average mortality rate is slightly higher at approximately 4 per 100000 women. It is particularly high in American black women (7 per 100000). Although 5-year survival in endometrial carcinoma is better than that for other gynaecological cancers, this is because most (75%) present with FIGO Stage I disease. The patient's prognosis depends on the histological type and grade of tumour, and the patient's fitness for surgery, as well as tumour stage (see *Table 5.1*). The probability of lymph node metastases is closely related to histological grade and the depth of myometrial invasion. Survival rates at 5 years vary from 80% for Stage I to 5% for Stage IV, i.e. similar to that for cervical carcinoma. Poor prognostic indicators include papillary serous, clear cell or undifferentiated

Table 5.1. Clinical staging of carcinoma of the endometrium: correlation of TNM (2002) and FIGO classifications (FIGO 1994)

TNM Classification	FIGO Stage	Description of tumour extent
Tis	0	Carcinoma *in situ*, intraepithelial neoplasm
T1	I	Tumour confined to the uterine corpus.
T1a	IA	Tumour confined to the endometrium
T1b	IB	Invasion into the inner half of the myometrium
T1c	IC	Invasion into the outer half of the myometrium
T2	II	Invasion of the cervix. Does not extend beyond uterus
T2a	IIA	Endocervical glands only involved. No stromal invasion
T2b	IIB	Invasion of cervical stroma
T3	III	Extra-uterine spread $+/-$ positive peritoneal cytology
T3a	IIIA	Invasion of the uterine serosa, or adnexae
T3b	IIIB	Vaginal invasion or metastasis
T4	IVA	Invasion of bladder and/or bowel mucosa
N0		No regional lymph node metastasis
N1	IIIC	Regional lymph node metastasis to pelvic and/or para-aortic nodes
M0		No distant metastasis
M1	IVB	Distant metastases, including inguinal lymph node metastases

histological type, and high grade (poorly differentiated) tumours of any type. Tumour size, the depth of myometrial invasion, and the proximity of tumour to the serosal surface of the uterus are inter-related adverse factors. Invasion of the cervix, spread to the adnexae, and the presence of lymphovascular space invasion or lymph node metastases also correlate with reduced survival.

Treatment

The choice of treatment for endometrial carcinoma is guided by patient factors and the histological grade/FIGO stage of the tumour. For surgically fit patients with tumours at low risk of extrauterine spread (Grade I–II, FIGO stage IA–IB), total abdominal hysterectomy and bilateral salpingo-oophorectomy is performed. Pelvic and para-aortic lymph nodes are palpated and removed if enlarged, and peritoneal washings are obtained for cytology. For higher risk tumours (Grade 2 or higher, FIGO stage $>$1B) full pelvic lymph node resection should be considered. In patients with papillary serous type tumours,

the peritoneum should be thoroughly inspected and an omentectomy performed, since these tumours behave in a similar way to ovarian carcinoma. Simple hysterectomy may be performed in women with major surgical risk factors and an early stage tumour. Adjuvant radiotherapy is usually given to the vaginal vault if the tumour is any worse prognostically than a Grade 1 tumour with limited myometrial invasion. Metastatic tumour in pelvic or retroperitoneal lymph nodes is also an indication for adjuvant radiotherapy. Disseminated tumour can be treated by hormonal treatment with progestogens, but only about 25% of patients respond and only over the short term. Chemotherapeutic agents such as doxorubicin and cisplatin may also produce a significant tumour response in approximately 25% of patients with advanced disease.

MR IMAGING OF ENDOMETRIAL CANCER

Technique

A standard pelvic imaging protocol is used. One of the T2-weighted sequences should be angled parallel to the short axis of the uterine corpus, to assess depth of tumour invasion into the lateral myometrium. T2-weighted sections through the short axis of the cervix may also be helpful if cervical stromal invasion is suspected. If T2-weighted sequences are not diagnostic for tumour extent, useful tumour-myometrial contrast can be achieved using enhancement with a paramagnetic contrast agent. A dynamic acquisition T1-weighted Gradient Recalled Echo sequence is obtained during bolus intravenous injection of Gadolinium–chelate 0.1 mmolkg^{-1} body weight. The imaging plane should be the one best demonstrating the endometrial/myometrial interface of tumour.

Current indications

MRI is indicated in patients with endometrial cancer where pre-operative knowledge of the stage of tumour might affect the choice of treatment or the surgical approach used. Examples include patients with clinical or ultrasound evidence of a bulky or fixed uterus, cervical or adnexal abnormality, or peritoneal or extrapelvic disease. In such cases, there is a significant chance of tumour spread beyond the uterine corpus, for which adjuvant or alternative treatment to hysterectomy is indicated. Conversely, MRI may be used to replace full FIGO staging in unfit patients with early stage disease in whom a simple hysterectomy may be adequate for treatment. There is no evidence at present that the results of MRI have a significant impact on clinical outcome in endometrial cancer, but research is ongoing.

Staging accuracy

Published evidence to support the use of MR imaging for staging endometrial cancer has been recently reviewed. MRI is 80–90%

accurate for assessing depth of myometrial invasion and the presence of cervical involvement. Post-contrast T1-weighted sequences do not increase staging accuracy over T2-weighted sequences. Dynamic contrast-enhanced techniques may be useful in post-menopausal patients.

Imaging features

Primary tumour

Primary endometrial carcinoma appears on T2-weighted images as a mass or thickening of the endometrium, of intermediate signal compared to the high signal intensity of normal endometrium or intra-cavitary fluid, and the low signal of myometrium. Integrity of a smooth endometrial / myometrial interface in the presence of histologically proven endometrial carcinoma indicates a Stage Ia tumour. Myometrial invasion is indicated by replacement of the relatively hypointense myometrium by tumour contiguous with the primary tumour. The normal uterine low signal junctional zone increases the contrast between tumour and inner myometrium, but may not be present in post-menopausal women. The endometrial / myometrial interface should be assessed in at least two planes, with thin sections, and with contrast enhanced T1-weighted sequences if T2-weighted scans are inconclusive, to look for evidence of myometrial invasion. The relationship of the tumour to the cervix is important prognostically, and should be evaluated carefully on T2-weighted images in the sagittal and transverse oblique planes.

Lymph node metastases

Lymph nodes replaced by tumour metastasis often have a similar signal intensity to the primary tumour (on T2-weighted sequences) whereas reactive lymph node enlargement tends to be of lower signal intensity. The lower the value of short axis diameter used as a cut-off for normality, the higher the sensitivity and the lower the specificity of MRI. Lymph nodes exceeding 5 mm in short axis diameter should be examined carefully for other signs of metastasis (e.g. abnormal shape, margins and signal intensity), and the probability of involvement given the stage of the primary tumour (and grade if known) as well as knowledge of the patterns of lymph node spread.

Post treatment

Since hysterectomy is the usual treatment, imaging in the early post treatment period is rarely carried out. MRI can be used to assess tumour response to primary radiotherapy prior to surgery in advanced endometrial cancer. It may be difficult to evaluate changes in viable tumour volume due to associated radiotherapy-induced necrosis, inflammatory reaction and oedema, and MRI can only provide a very crude assessment under these circumstances.

Recurrent tumour

Recurrent endometrial cancer most frequently occurs at the vaginal vault, and is detected by clinical examination. The pelvic sidewall is also a common site for recurrence, and tumour here usually presents with symptoms such as pain or swelling of the ipsilateral leg. There is no evidence that routine surveillance by diagnostic imaging or clinical follow-up improves the outcome by detecting asymptomatic recurrence of endometrial cancer. However diagnostic imaging is indicated to assess salvageability of the patient with a known recurrence by evaluating the extent of local tissue invasion, lymph node metastases and extrapelvic spread.

Pitfalls of MRI

Identification of the primary tumour

- Thickening of the endometrium, without myometrial invasion, may be due to benign disease such as endometrial hyperplasia or polyps, causing false-positive MRI.

- Stage Ia carcinoma may be of too small a volume or too similar in signal intensity to normal endometrium to visualise on MRI, resulting in a false-negative examination.

Assessment of depth of myometrial invasion

- The integrity of the endometrial / myometrial interface may be difficult to assess in post-menopausal women where the low signal junctional zone is indistinct.

- Concentric stretching and thinning of myometrium by a large tumour makes it difficult to assess the proportion of myometrium infiltrated, i.e., whether less than or more than half of the normal thickness.

- Concomitant benign disease, such as fibroids or adenomyosis, can result in morphological and signal changes in the myometrium mimicking tumour infiltration.

- Distortion of the endometrial / myometrial interface at the base of the stalk of a polypoid tumour may be difficult to distinguish from infiltration.

Assessment of invasion of the cervix

- It can be difficult to distinguish between tumour prolapsing into the upper cervical canal and early glandular or stromal invasion.

- Glandular and early stromal invasion are difficult to differentiate.

- When there is invasive disease near the isthmus, it can be difficult to determine whether or not myometrial tumour infiltration extends into the cervical stroma.

- Benign disease, such as tunnel clusters of glands, or even normal mucosa, can be mistaken for tumour.

Assessment of lymph nodes

- Microscopic or very small macroscopic tumour deposits in lymph nodes may be occult on MRI.

- Reactive lymph node enlargement can cause false-positive calls on MRI.

- Metastatic lymph nodes may be indistinguishable from adnexal structures / bowel loops / peritoneal tumour.

- Cystic lymph nodes may be mistaken for fluid-filled bowel / ascites.

Other extra-uterine disease
- The sensitivity of MRI for small peritoneal deposits is low.

FURTHER READING

1. Endometrial Cancer. Diagnosis and pre-treatment staging and Endometrial Cancer. Treatment. (1999) In: *Guidance on Commissioning Cancer Services. Improving Outcomes in Gynaecological Cancers. The Research Evidence.* NHS Executive. Review of research evidence for current management of endometrial carcinoma.

2. Odieino F, Favalli G, Zigliani L, et al. (2001) Staging of gynecological malignancies. *Surgical Clinics of North America* 81(4): 753–770. *Describes the current staging system for endometrial carcinoma.*

3. *Making the best use of a Department of Clinical Radiology,* 5th Edn (2003). The Royal College of Radiologists. *Evidence-based recommendations for diagnostic imaging in uterine tumours- UK.*

4. Hricak H, Mendelson E, Bohm-Velez M et al. (2000) Endometrial cancer of the uterus. *ACR* Appropriateness Criteria. *Radiology* 215 Suppl: 947–953. *Evidence-based recommendations for diagnostic imaging in uterine tumours- USA.*

5. Kinkel K, Kaji Y, Yu KK, Segal MR, Lu Y, Powell CB and Hricak H. (1999) Radiologic staging in patients with endometrial cancer: a meta-analysis. *Radiology* 212(3): 711–718. *A comparison of imaging techniques for staging endometrial carcinoma.*

6. Frei KA and Kinkel K. (2001) Staging endometrial cancer: role of magnetic resonance imaging. *J. Magn. Reson. Imaging* 13(6): 850–855. *Up-to-date review of the topic.*

7. Ascher SM, Takahama J and Jha RC. (2001) Staging of gynecologic malignancies. *Top. Magn. Reson. Imaging.* 12(2): 105–129. *Another up-to-date review of the topic.*

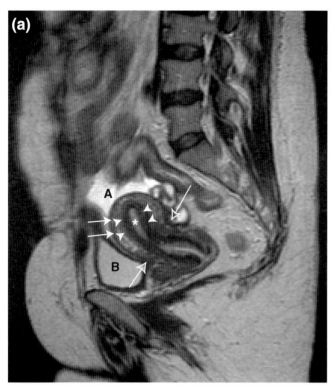

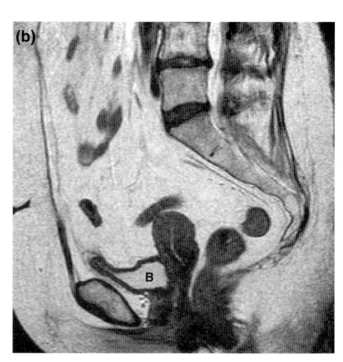

Figure 5.1. Normal uterine zonal anatomy.

Sagittal T2WI in **(a)** a pre-menopausal patient and **(b)** a post-menopausal patient. The zonal anatomy of the uterus is appreciated in the pre-menopausal patient. There is a central high signal intensity stripe (asterisk in (a)), which represents the endometrium and its secretions. The low signal intensity junctional zone (arrowheads) represents the inner portion of the myometrium and blends inferiorly with the fibromuscular stroma of the cervix. The outer myometrium (arrows) is heterogeneous intermediate and high signal intensity. The junction between the uterine corpus and the cervix is marked by waisting of the contour of the uterus (open arrows). Bladder (B). Ascites (A) from an incidental non gynaecological cause. In the post menopausal patient the endometrial stripe is thin and the entire uterus is of low signal intensity with loss of the junctional anatomy.

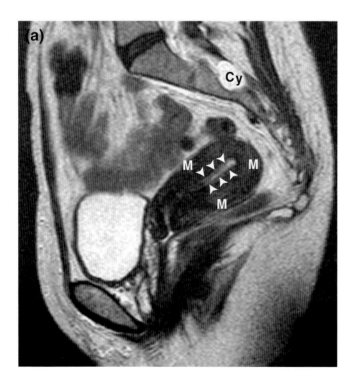

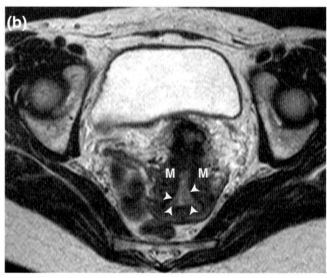

Figure 5.2. T1aN0/Stage IA endometrial cancer.

(a) Sagittal and **(b)** transaxial T2WI showing tumour (arrowheads) confined to the endometrium with minimal widening of the endometrial cavity, a smooth interface between the endometrium and the inner myometrium (M) and no sign of myometrial invasion. Incidental note is made of an arachnoid cyst (Cy) in the spinal canal.

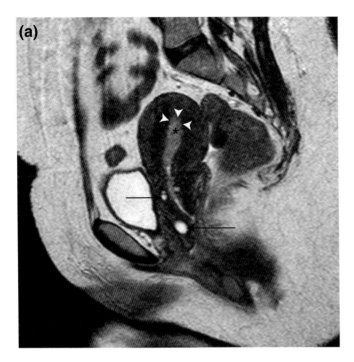

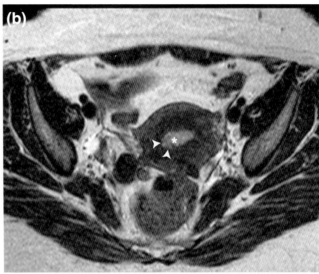

Figure 5.3. T1bN0/Early stage IB endometrial cancer.

(a) Sagittal and **(b)** transaxial T2WI of an endometrial tumour (asterisk) which demonstrates irregularity of the endometrial/myometrial interface (arrowheads) indicating myometrial invasion confined to the inner half of the myometrium. Incidental note is made of cervical Nabothian cysts (arrows in (a)).

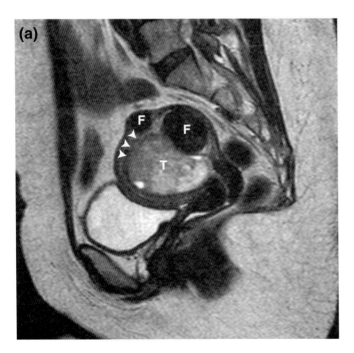

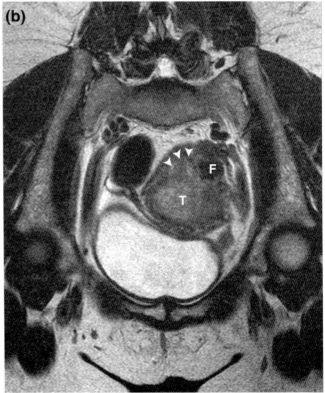

Figure 5.4. T1bN0/Late stage IB endometrial cancer.

(a) Sagittal and **(b)** oblique transaxial T2WI showing a large endometrial tumour (T) invading the inner half of the myometrium on its fundal aspect (arrowheads). Note hyperintense compressed myometrium surrounding the endometrial fibroids (F), which has a similar signal intensity to the tumour proper.

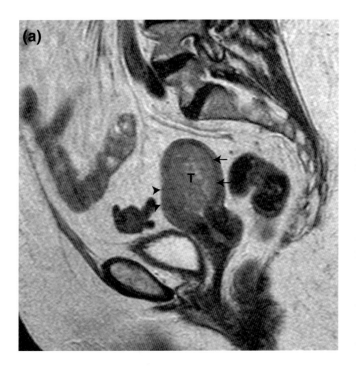

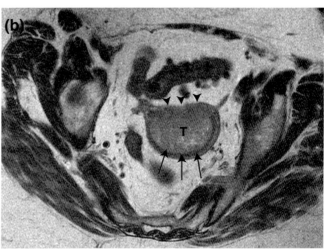

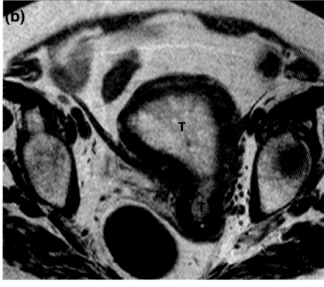

Figure 5.5. T1cN0/Stage IC endometrial cancer.

(a) Sagittal and (b) oblique transaxial T2WI showing a large endometrial tumour (T) invading the outer half of the myometrium on its anterior aspect (arrowheads). Note that the intact posterior myometrium is markedly stretched and thinned by the tumour but that the inner myometrial junctional zone retains its low signal intensity (arrows).

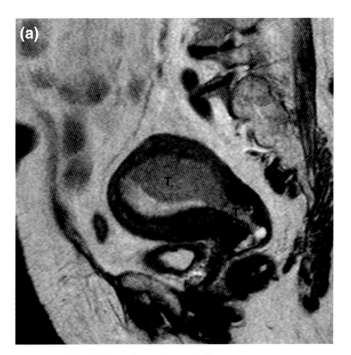

Figure 5.6. T2aN0/Stage IIA endocervical cancer.

(a) Sagittal and (b) transaxial T2WI showing myometrial invasion by an endometrial tumour (T), which is also extending into the cervix without stromal invasion.

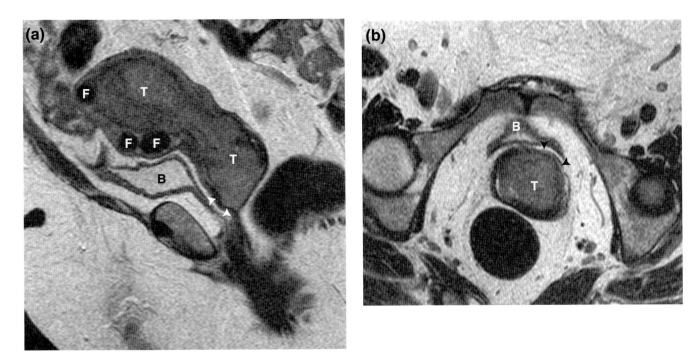

Figure 5.7. T2bN0/Stage IIB endometrial cancer.

(a) Sagittal and (b) oblique transaxial T2WI demonstrating a large endometrial tumour (T) extending down into and distending the endocervical canal. Tumour is invading the cervical stroma anteriorly (arrowheads). Note mural fibroids (F). Bladder (B).

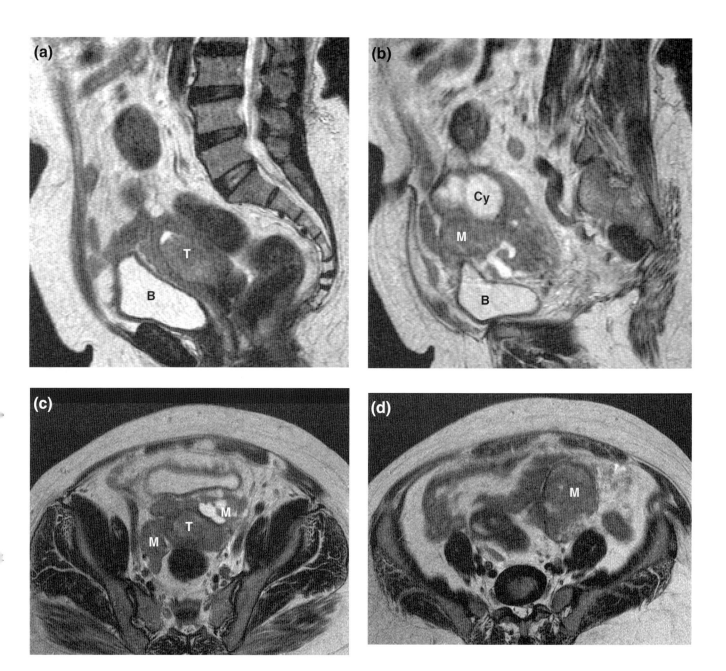

Figure 5.8. T3aN0/Stage IIIA endometrial cancer.

(a) and (b) Sagittal and (c) and (d) oblique transaxial T2WI demonstrating a large endometrial tumour (T) within the endometrial cavity but not involving the cervix. There are bilateral adnexal masses (M), larger on the left side, the solid portions of which have similar signal intensity to the endometrial tumour. There is a cystic component (Cy) on the left side. Bladder (B).

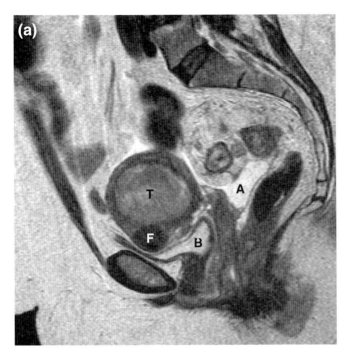

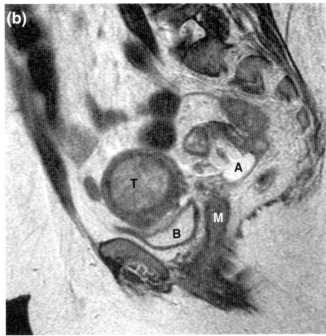

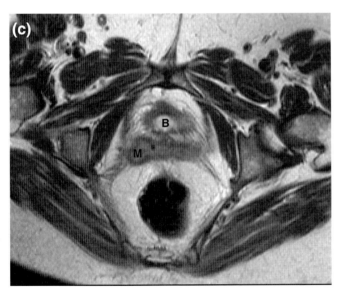

Figure 5.9. T3bN0/Stage IIIB endometrial cancer.

(a) and **(b)** Sagittal and **(c)** transaxial T2WI demonstrating a large endometrial tumour (T) distending the uterine cavity without evidence of myometrial or cervical invasion. There is a metastasis (M) in the right vagina which demonstrates similar signal intensity to the endometrial tumour proper.

Incidental note is made of an anterior wall uterine fibroid (F). There is small volume pelvic ascites (A). Bladder (B).

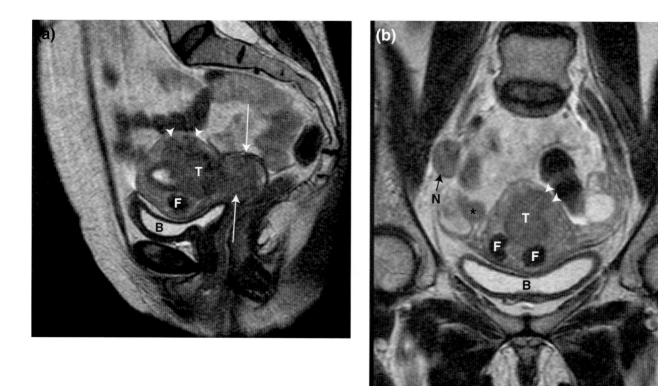

Figure 5.10. T3aN1/Stage IIIC endometrial cancer.

(a) Sagittal and **(b)** coronal T2WI showing an endometrial tumour (T) with myometrial invasion to the outer half (arrowheads) but also extension to the cervix with stromal invasion (arrows in (a)), and a tumour nodule on the right adnexa (asterisk in (b)). There is also a metastatic lymph node in the right external iliac chain (N in (b)). The MR stage is therefore T3aN1/IIIC. The patient also has intramural fibroids (F). Bladder (B).

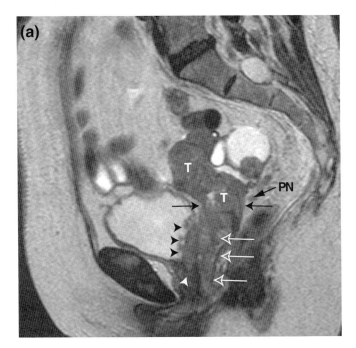

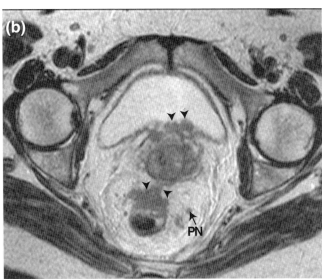

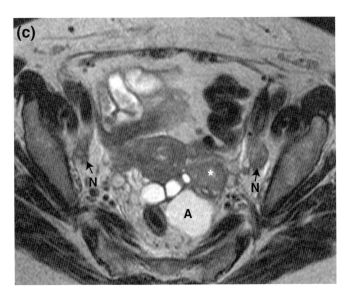

Figure 5.11. T4N1/Stage IVA endometrial cancer.

(a) Sagittal and (b) and (c) oblique transaxial T2WI showing an endometrial tumour (T) replacing the cervix (arrows) and extending into the left adenexal structures in (c) (asterisk), vagina in (a) (open arrows) and invading the posterior bladder wall in (a) and (b), the proximal urethra in (a) and the rectum in (b) (black and white arrowheads). The presence of bladder and rectal involvement makes the stage of this tumour T4N1/Stage IVA. There are bilateral metastatic surgical obturator nodes in (c) (N) and suspicious perirectal nodes (PN) in (a) and (b). A small volume of ascites (A) is present.

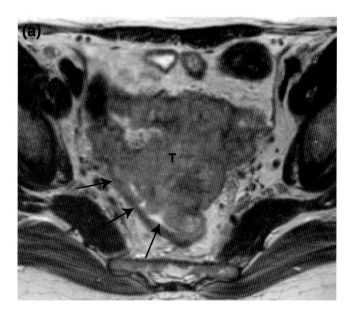
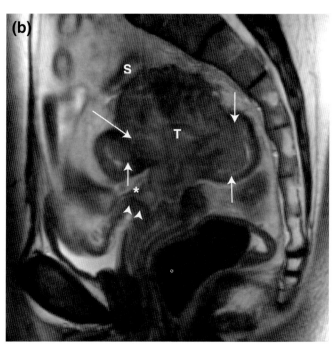

Figure 5.12. Central recurrence of endometrial cancer.

(a) Transaxial and **(b)** sagittal T2WI demonstrating a large central pelvic tumour recurrence (T). The mass, which is arising exophytically from the vaginal vault, extends to involve the recto-sigmoid colon (arrows) without extension to the pelvic sidewall. One small bowel loop (S) is seen to be adherent to the superior surface of the mass in (b). The postero-superior bladder wall is abnormal (arrowheads) due to small volume tumour infiltrating the remnant of the uterovesical ligament (asterisk). (Figure courtesy of Dr. Carrington, Christie Hospital).

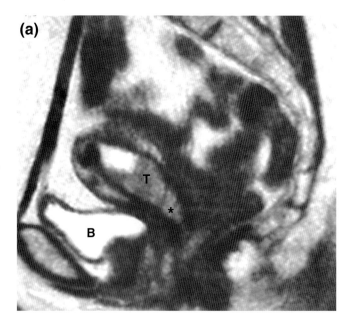
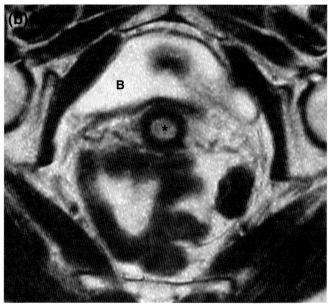

Figure 5.13. Pseudo invasion of cervix by endometrial cancer.

(a) Sagittal and **(b)** oblique transaxial T2WI demonstrating an endometrial tumour (T) extending into and distending the cervical canal (asterisk). The resected specimen demonstrated tumour prolapse into the cervix without invasion of the cervical mucosa or stroma. Tumour prolapse can result in overstaging. Bladder (B).

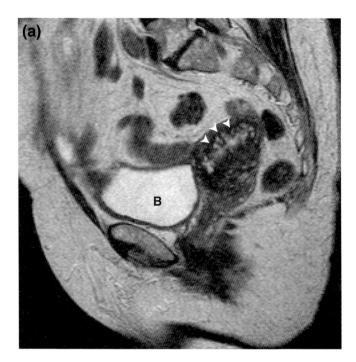

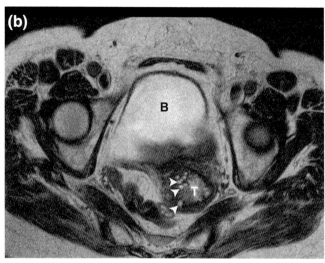

Figure 5.14. Adenomyosis and endometrial cancer.

(a) Sagittal and (b) transaxial T2WI demonstrating adenomyosis in a patient who also had a small T1a endometrial tumour (T). The adenomyosis mimics myometrial invasion (arrowheads). Bladder (B).

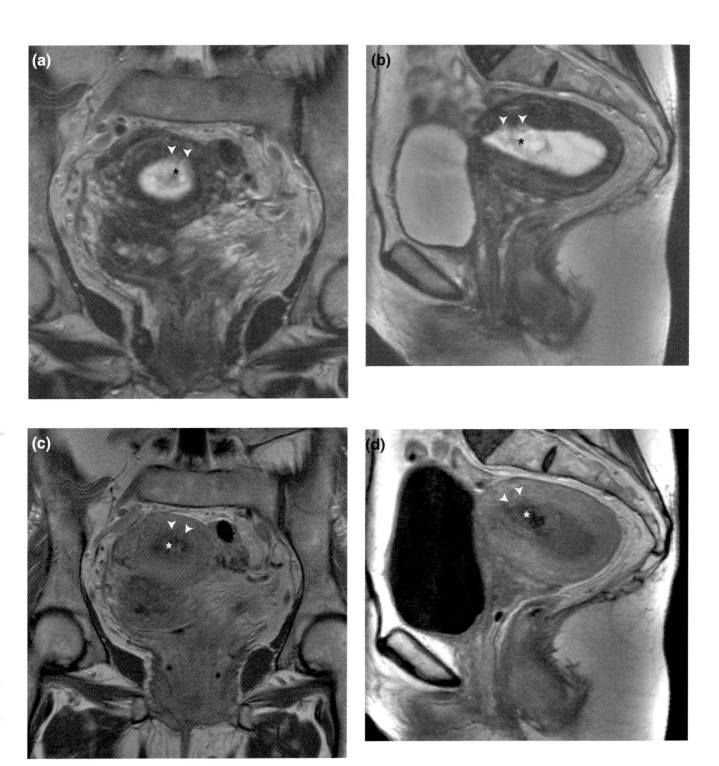

Figure 5.15. Endometrial polyp in a Tamoxifen uterus.

(a) Coronal and (b) sagittal T2WI, (c) contrast-enhanced coronal T1WI and (d) contrast-enhanced sagittal T1WI. The endometrial cavity is distended and there is high signal intensity material within it due to haemorrhage (also high signal on the T1WI). In the lower uterine cavity, a more ill defined abnormality (asterisk) is seen forming an irregular interface with the junctional zone (arrowheads). After intravenous Gd-DTPA, there was little enhancement of this region. At hysterectomy, the uterine cavity was distended with haemorrhage and a nonmalignant endometrial polyp was present at the site of the heterogeneous lesion. The junctional zone abnormalities correspond to the polyp's insertion. It is important to be aware that Tamoxifen treatment can predispose to an adenomyosis-like picture, endometrial polyps and endometrial carcinoma. (Figure courtesy of Dr. Carrington, Christie Hospital.)

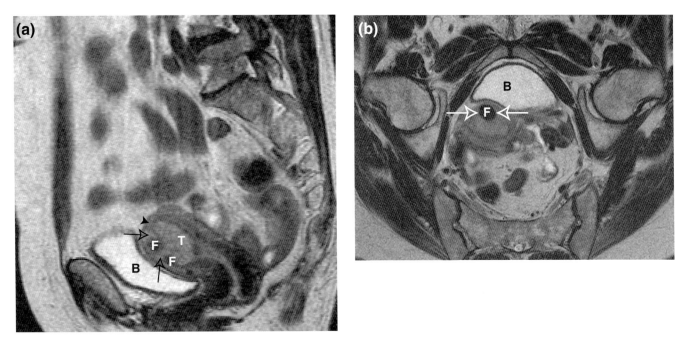

Figure 5.16. Pseudomyometrial invasion due to fibroids.

(a) Sagittal and **(b)** oblique transaxial T2WI demonstrating an endometrial tumour (T) infiltrating the anterior wall of the uterus (arrowhead). The intramural fibroids (F) incite high signal intensity within the adjacent myometrium (open arrows) which can result in difficulty in determining the true extent of tumour involvement of the myometrium. Intramural or submucosal fibroids can also distort the endometrial/myometrial interface adding to staging difficulty. Bladder (B).

6 Ovarian Cancer

Sue Roach and Paul A. Hulse

BACKGROUND INFORMATION

Epidemiology

Ovarian carcinoma makes up 4% of all female cancers. In the UK there are approximately 7000 new cases per year and there are 20 700 new cases in the USA where it is the commonest cause of death from gynaecological malignancy. Median age at diagnosis is 60 to 65 years and it is rare in women under 30 years old.

Aetiological factors include early menarche, nulliparity by 35 years and late menopause with the strongest risk factor being a family history of ovarian cancer. An individual with two or more first-degree relatives with ovarian cancer may have as much as a 50% chance of developing the disease. This risk is reduced in individuals who have had their first child by 25, are on the oral contraceptive pill and breast feed.

There are autosomal dominant forms of ovarian cancer inheritance. One example is the hereditary breast and ovarian cancer syndrome, which is linked to the BRCA 1 gene and another example is the Lynch 2 syndrome, which consists of colonic, endometrial, breast and ovarian cancer.

Histopathology

Ovarian tumours are categorised according to tissue of origin (*Figure 6.1*).

Epithelial tumours arise from the mesothelial layer covering the peritoneal surface of the ovary (*Table 6.1*) and can be benign, malignant or borderline malignant.

Borderline malignant tumours show some features associated with malignancy such as irregular architecture, nuclear stratification and polymorphism and mitotic activity but lack the most important feature of invasion. Their biological behaviour is intermediate between that of clearly benign and overtly malignant lesions. They occur in younger patients with a median age of 39 to 45 years.

Sex cord stromal tumours arise from those cells which are the adult derivatives of the primitive sex cords in the foetal ovary. They can differentiate in an ovarian, testicular or stromal direction (*Table 6.2*) and frequently secrete steroids. Unclassified tumours fail to differentiate in a clearly recognisable male or female direction and account for 10% of sex cord stromal tumours. Gynandroblastoma is a rare type of tumour that displays both male and female cell types.

Germ cell tumours arise from the primitive germ cells of the ovary (*Table 6.3*). They are most common in the first two decades of life, grow rapidly and often present with pain secondary to haemorrhage or torsion.

Ovarian neoplasms are also classified according to histological grade, from 1 to 4, according to degree of cellular differentiation, with grade 1 being well differentiated tumours and 4 being poorly differentiated tumours with the poorest outcome.

Patterns of tumour spread

Direct spread of ovarian cancer occurs along the Fallopian tubes to involve the broad ligaments and uterus. Direct invasion of the rectum, sigmoid colon, bladder and pelvic sidewalls also occurs in late disease.

Transcoelomic spread by tumour surface shedding and intraperitoneal dissemination is a characteristic feature of ovarian malignancy. Tumour cells are then carried up into the abdomen by the flow of peritoneal fluid. Common sites of seeding include the undersurface of the diaphragm (preferentially on the right due to flow), the omentum, the serosa of small and large bowel, the surface of liver and the pelvic *cul-de-sac*.

Lymphatic spread occurs to the para-aortic nodes from the primary lymphatic drainage of the ovaries, to the obturator, common and external iliac nodes due to secondary spread via the broad ligament and to the inguinal nodes by secondary involvement via the round ligament.

Haematogenous spread occurs as a late feature in advanced disease to the liver, lungs, pleura, kidneys and bone.

Prognostic indicators

An important prognostic feature is tumour stage at diagnosis (*Table 6.4*). For example, Stage 1 disease at presentation has an 85% and Stage 4 disease has a 4% 5-year survival.

Histological grade of tumour also affects prognosis with high-grade tumours having a poorer prognosis than Grade 1 disease.

The volume of residual tumour following initial staging laparotomy affects prognosis. It has been shown that initial optimal debulking, with residual disease measuring less than 1.5 to 2.0 cm in diameter, results in a better outcome by enhancing the effect of chemotherapy and prolonging survival.

Tumour markers

The tumour marker CA-125 is elevated in 80 to 85% of patients with ovarian cancer but only in 50% of patients with Stage 1 disease. In

Table 6.1. Epithelial tumours: make up 60–90% of all ovarian tumours; make up 90% of all malignant ovarian tumours

	Serous	Mucinous	Endometrioid	Clear cell	Brenner
Incidence	20–50% of malignant tumours	10% of malignant tumours	20% of malignant tumours	6% of malignant tumours	1–2% of malignant tumours
Aggression	Benign 60% Malignant 25%	Benign 80% Malignant 10%	Almost always malignant	Almost always malignant but 75% Stage 1	Rarely malignant
Bilateral	25% of benign 65% of malignant	5% of benign 20% of malignant	40%	40%	6%
Age	Post-menopausal	Post-menopausal	Post-menopausal	Post-menopausal	Any age, 50% over 50 yrs
Typical features	Predominantly cystic. Malignant lesions have more solid components. Psammoma bodies in 30%	Multilocular cysts containing haemorrhage or cellular debris	Variable cystic/solid components. Associated with endometrial hyperplasia and carcinoma	Usually unilocular cyst with few mural nodules protruding into the lumen	Solid and homogenous. Occasionally cystic. Usually small (1.0–2.0 cm). Extensive calcification common

Table 6.2. Sex cord stromal tumours: 5% of all ovarian malignancies; 85–90% synthesise steroid

	Fibroma	Thecoma	Granulosa cell	Sertoli-Leydig cell
Incidence	Rare	Commonest	5–10% of all ovarian malignancies	Less than 0.2% of all ovarian malignancies
Aggression	Benign	Benign	Malignant potential increases with size. 5yr survival is 90%	Aggressiveness depends on degree of differentiation. 5yr survival is 70%
Bilateral	Unilateral	Unilateral	Unilateral in >95%	Unilateral
Age	4th and 5th decades	Reproductive years	Any age but commonest in post-menopausal years	Reproductive years
Typical features	Solid. Associated with pleural effusion (Meigs syndrome)	Solid. Produces oestrogen and associated with abnormal vaginal bleeding, endometrial hyperplasia and carcinoma	Multi-cystic. May be haemorrhagic or necrotic. Can secrete oestrogen and is associated with abnormal vaginal bleeding, hyperplasia and carcinoma	Can be solid or cystic. Synthesise androgens resulting in masculinisation.

approximately 90% of patients doubling or halving of the CA-125 correlates with disease progression or regression respectively. In patients with treated early stage disease a rising CA-125 is predictive of recurrence regardless of imaging features. However, if the CA-125 falls to normal following treatment, this may not indicate complete response and up to 50% of patients will have residual disease discovered at laparotomy.

It is important to note that CA-125 is not exclusive to ovarian cancer and is also elevated in 40% of patients with advanced non-ovarian intra-abdominal malignancy, as well as other abdomino-pelvic conditions such as liver cirrhosis, pancreatitis, endometriosis, pelvic inflammatory disease, pregnancy and also in 1% of healthy individuals.

Treatment

Surgery

The initial treatment for all suitable patients is a staging laparotomy which includes total abdominal hysterectomy and bilateral salpingo-oophorectomy, infra-colic omentectomy, cytological analysis of ascites and peritoneal washings, biopsies of peritoneum and diaphragm and selective pelvic and para-aortic lymph node sampling. The aim is to remove all macroscopic tumour and is usually possible in Stage I and early Stage II disease. In more advanced disease the aim is for optimal cytoreduction, that is residual tumour deposits less than 1.5 to 2.0 cm in diameter. Patients with unresectable disease benefit from chemotherapy followed by surgical debulking. Some of the less aggressive germ cell tumours and sex cord stromal tumours, which occur in younger patients, can be treated with limited surgery to preserve fertility.

Table 6.3. Germ cell tumours: 15–20% of all ovarian malignancies; most common in the 1st and 2nd decades; 60–70% Stage I at diagnosis

| | Dysgerminoma | Teratoma | | | Yolk sac | Choriocarcinoma |
		Mature	Immature	Monodermal		
Incidence	Commonest malignant germ cell. 2–5% of primary ovarian malignancies	Commonest ovarian neoplasm	Less than 1% of ovarian malignancies	Rare	1% of ovarian tumours. 2nd commonest malignant germ cell tumour	Very rare
Aggression	Malignant. 90% 5yr survival	Benign	Malignant. 80–90% 5 yr survival	Variable	Malignant. 2 yr survival 60–70%	Malignant. Poor prognosis
Bilateral	10%	Usually unilateral	Usually unilateral	Usually unilateral	Unilateral	Unilateral
Age	2nd and 3rd decades	Any age	10–20 yrs	Any age	Under 30 yrs	Under 20 yrs
Typical features	Solid with cystic areas secondary to necrosis or haemorrhage	Fat/fluid or hair/fluid levels. Calcification, bone and teeth	Predominantly solid. Contain foetal / embryonal tissue	Solid. Thyroid tissue (Struma ovarii) or carcinoid tissue	Cystic or solid. Areas of haemorrhage	Usually solid. Often a component of other malignant germ cell tumour

Chemotherapy

Chemotherapy is routinely used in the adjuvant setting in patients with Stage IC and more advanced epithelial tumours. Recent trials have shown that adjuvant chemotherapy may also improve prognosis in patients with Stage IA and IB tumours. The agents used currently are carboplatin or a combination of carboplatin and paclitaxel and result in a complete or partial response in 70% of patients. The same agents are also used in patients with germ cell tumours that are greater than Stage I. Chemotherapy is rarely required for patients with sex cord stromal tumours but is used occasionally for poorly differentiated Sertoli-Leydig tumours.

Radiotherapy

Radiotherapy has only a very limited role in palliative care for symptom control and in patients with localised relapse that is unresectable.

MR IMAGING OF OVARIAN CANCER

Technique

A standard technique is employed for examination of the abdomen and pelvis (see Chapter 2). In addition, fat suppressed T1-weighted images post Gd-chelate aid in characterisation of the internal architecture of cystic ovarian lesions and improve detection of peritoneal and omental implants.

The use of a negative bowel contrast agent such as 2% barium allows distension of bowel and improves detection of enhancing serosal deposits. An anti-peristaltic agent such as glucagon or hyoscine butylbromide aids in detection of serosal and peritoneal deposits by reducing bowel movement artifact.

If available, breath-hold axial fast multiplanar Spoiled Gradient Recalled Echo images with fat suppression both before and after Gd-chelate should replace the T1 images and are superior due to reduced movement artifact and reduced scan times.

Current indications

Ovarian cancer staging is usually performed surgically and neither MR imaging nor CT have a role in most instances. CT is employed in the evaluation of post-operative tumour residuum prior to chemotherapy and in the assessment of tumour response to chemotherapy.

MRI may be useful in assessment and pre-operative planning in advanced ovarian cancer where pelvic spread is suspected or in cases of localised pelvic recurrence. It is the optimal method for evaluating spread to involve the uterus, bladder, rectum or pelvic sidewall and in determining if tumours can be optimally debulked.

MRI is indicated for treatment planning in patients who are allergic to iodinated contrast media, pregnant or have an inconclusive CT examination. It may also be indicated if the CT examination is negative but there has been a significant rise in the CA-125.

Other roles for MRI include the further characterisation of an ovarian mass where other imaging investigations have been nondiagnostic or equivocal.

Imaging features

Primary tumour

Certain features suggest malignancy in ovarian masses. Solid, non-fatty, non-fibrous tissue is the most powerful predictor of malignancy

Table 6.4. FIGO and TNM classification of ovarian carcinoma

TNM Stage	FIGO Stage	Extent of Disease
TI	I	Tumour limited to ovaries
TIa	IA	Tumour limited to one ovary; capsule intact, no tumour on ovarian surface; no malignant cells in ascites or peritoneal washings
TIb	IB	Tumour limited to both ovaries; capsule intake, no tumour on ovarian surface; no malignant cells in ascites or peritoneal washings
TIc	IC	Tumour limited to one or both ovaries with any of the following: capsule ruptured, tumour on ovarian surface; malignant cells in ascites or peritoneal washings
T2	II	Tumour involves one or both ovaries with pelvic extension
T2a	IIA	Extension and/or implants on the uterus and/or tubes; no malignant cells in ascites or peritoneal washings
T2b	IIB	Extension to other pelvic tissue; no malignant cells in ascites or peritoneal washings
T2c	IIC	Pelvic extension (2a or 2b); malignant cells in ascites or peritoneal washings
T3	III	Tumour limited to one or both ovaries with microscopically confirmed peritoneal metastasis outside the pelvis and/or regional lymph node metastasis
T3a ± NI	IIIA	Microscopic peritoneal metastasis beyond pelvis
T3b	IIIB	Macroscopic peritoneal metastasis beyond pelvis 2.0 cm or less in greatest dimension
T3c	IIIC	Peritoneal metastasis beyond pelvis more than 2.0 cm in greatest dimension and/or lymph node metastasis
N0		No regional lymph node metastases
NI	IIIC	Regional lymph node metastases
M0		No distant metastasis
MI	IV	Distant metastasis (excludes peritoneal metastasis)

Note: There is discontinuity in the TNM staging progression with respect to malignant ascites as Stage TIc indicates the presence of malignant ascites but it is absent in Stages T2a and T2b.

and other features include thick walls, septations and papillary projections. For example, papillary projections are seen in 92% of malignant ovarian tumours. Pelvic organ invasion, implants, ascites and enlarged lymph nodes increase the diagnostic confidence of malignancy.

The cystic components of malignant ovarian tumours have a variable signal intensity but are usually low to intermediate signal intensity on TI-weighted images and high signal intensity on T2-weighted images.

Local invasion
Uterine invasion is identified by localised distortion of the uterine contour, an irregular interface between the tumour and the myometrium and increased signal intensity of involved myometrium on T2-weighted images. In bladder or sigmoid colon invasion, there is loss of the normal intervening tissue plane between a solid component of the tumour and the wall of colon or bladder. Invasion can also be diagnosed if there is encasement of the sigmoid colon or direct tumour extension can be seen. Pelvic sidewall invasion can be diagnosed when tumour approaches the pelvic sidewall to within 3.0 mm or when the iliac vessels are surrounded or distorted.

Transcoelomic spread
Peritoneal deposits are seen as nodular or plaque-like lesions adjacent to or projecting from the peritoneal surfaces. They are high signal intensity on T2-weighted images and enhance on post Gd-chelate TI-weighted images. Omental involvement is identified as infiltrative, nodular or cake-like soft tissue within the usually fatty omentum which is of intermediate signal intensity on TI- and T2-weighted images and shows enhancement after administration of Gd.

Serosal bowel deposits are seen as plaques or nodules on the surface of bowel, which have the same signal characteristics as peritoneal deposits. There is usually also involvement of adjacent peritoneum and mesentery.

Nodal disease
As with other pelvic tumours lymph nodes with a short axis diameter of greater than 1.0 cm should be regarded as suspicious for metastatic involvement. Other features suggestive of nodal involvement are rounded shape and a signal intensity on T2-weighted images which is the same as the solid components of the primary tumour.

Haematogenous spread
Although haematogenous metastases are rare, the liver and bone marrow should be scrutinised. Bone metastases are so rare in ovarian cancer that if found, the possibility of a lobular breast cancer with peritoneal metastases or a second primary should be considered.

MRI staging accuracy

Overall accuracy of MR imaging for ovarian cancer staging is 75–78% with optimal technique and this is very similar to the results with CT. Studies comparing CT and MRI have had variable results. MRI is superior to CT for characterisation of the primary tumour and evaluating local spread to the colon, bladder and uterus. Accuracy of determining pelvic sidewall invasion is 67% for CT and 70% for MRI.

MRI has been shown to detect small (less than 1.0 cm) peritoneal deposits better than CT but there has been no statistical difference between the staging accuracy of CT and MRI demonstrated as a consequence. MRI has been shown to be superior to CT for peritoneal implants in the *cul-de-sac*, while CT is more accurate for the paracolic gutter and omentum. MRI and CT are similar in accuracy for detection of liver surface and diaphragmatic disease. The majority of mesenteric and small bowel implants are not detected with either modality.

Pitfalls of MRI

- Hydrosalpinx and peritoneal inclusion cysts can be mistaken for cystic ovarian masses. Hydrosalpinx has a characteristic thin-walled convoluted tubular structure most apparent on the T2W sagittal images. Peritoneal inclusion cysts typically have an extra-ovarian location remote from the peritoneal *cul-de-sac*, the expected location of ascites.

- No MR imaging characteristics are specific for malignant epithelial tumours. As described above certain features are suggestive of malignancy but thick walls and septations can also be seen in endometriosis, abscess, peritoneal cysts and benign neoplasms.

- Clot or debris in benign cystic masses such as haemorrhagic cysts can be mistaken for papillary projections but the use of Gd-chelate should eliminate this error, as genuine papillary projections will show enhancement.

- Metastases to the ovary result in a solid or partially cystic mass, which can be mistaken for a primary ovarian carcinoma. These typically arise from stomach or colon cancer when they are known as Krukenberg tumours.

- Peritoneal or bowel wall inflammation will enhance and appear identical to peritoneal or serosal tumour on Gd-enhanced images.

- In acute bowel obstruction, it is difficult to differentiate intestinal and mesenteric enhancement secondary to bowel obstruction from recurrent disease.

- Like all imaging techniques, MRI has a poor sensitivity for the detection of peritoneal deposits and the majority of deposits are not seen. Calcified deposits are particularly difficult to detect with MRI.

- Normal post-surgical appearances can be mistaken for disease. A haematoma within the medial end of the divided round ligament, or the normal post-operative vaginal vault can be confused with deposits of disease. Peritoneal thickening and enhancement at the site of the abdominal incision can also lead to confusion and be misinterpreted as peritoneal disease deposits.

FURTHER READING

1. Sohaib S, Reznek R and Husband JES. (1997) Ovarian cancer. In: *Imaging in Oncology* (eds Janet ES Husband and R Reznek). Isis Medical Media Ltd, Oxford, pp. 277–305. *A chapter summarising the imaging features of malignant ovarian diseases for all commonly utilised modalities. Also provides a summary of epidemiology and pathology.*

2. Forstner R, Hricak H, Occhipinti KA *et al.* (1995) Ovarian cancer: Staging with CT and MR Imaging. *Radiology;* 197:619–626. *Study to evaluate ovarian cancer staging and tumour resectability with CT and MR. Results showed that while the staging accuracy of both modalities is only moderate, the prediction of resectability is excellent.*

3. Ghossain MA, Buy JN, Ligneres C *et al.* (1991) Epithelial Tumours of the Ovary: Comparison of MR and CT Findings. *Radiology* 81: 863–870. *Retrospective study, looking at the characteristics of epithelial tumours on MR and CT. The accuracy for overall characterisation of benign as opposed to malignant tumours was better for MR than CT although no significant difference in sensitivity or specificity was identified.*

4. Semelka RC, Lawrence PH, Shoenut JP, *et al.* (1993) Primary Ovarian Cancer: Prospective Comparison of Contrast-enhanced CT and Pre- and Postcontrast, Fat-suppressed MR Imaging, with Histologic Correlation. *J. Magn. Reson. Imaging* 3: 99–106. *Prospective study comparing CT and MR staging of ovarian cancer. Results showed that MR is at least equivalent and may be superior to CT in the evaluation of ovarian cancer.*

5. Prayer L, Kainz C, Kramer J *et al.* (1993) CT and MR Accuracy in the Detection of Tumour Recurrence in Patients Treated for Ovarian Cancer. *J. Comput. Assist. Tomogr.* 17(4): 626–632. *Prospective study to evaluate the accuracy of clinical examination (including CA-125 level), CT and MR in the detection of tumour recurrence. Results showed that CA-125 is accurate in determining tumour recurrence and that CT is the primary imaging modality in the diagnosis of macroscopic disease. Neither CT nor MR can exclude microscopic disease.*

6. Jeong YY, Outwater EK and Keun Kang H. (2000) From the RSNA Refresher Courses. Imaging Evaluation of Ovarian Masses. *Radiographics* 20:1445–1470. *A review article summarising the features of both benign and malignant ovarian conditions on US, CT and MR.*

7. Kurtz AB, Tsimikas JV, Tempany CM *et al.* (1999) Diagnosis and Staging of Ovarian Cancer: Comparative Values of Doppler and Conventional US, CT, and MR Imaging Correlated with Surgery and Histopathological Analysis – Report of the Radiology Diagnostic Oncology Group. *Radiology* 212:19–27. *Large study aimed at determining the optimal imaging modality for diagnosis and staging of ovarian cancer. Conventional US, CT and MR were compared and results showed little variation between these modalities as regards staging of ovarian cancer but MR was shown to be superior for diagnosis.*

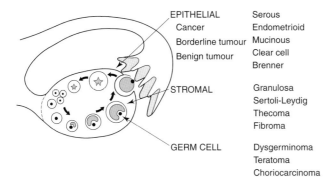

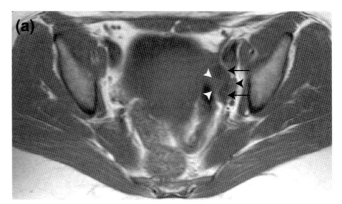

Figure 6.1. Schematic drawing showing sites of origin of ovarian cancer.

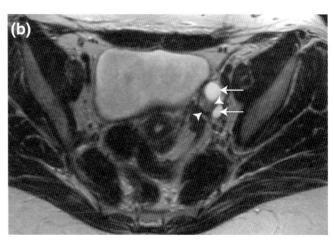

Figure 6.2. Normal ovarian anatomy in a woman of reproductive age.

(a) Transaxial T1WI and **(b)** transaxial T2WI showing normal follicular cysts in the left ovary. These appear thin-walled and of low signal intensity on T1WI and high signal intensity on T2WI (arrows). The ovarian stroma is low-intermediate signal intensity on T1WI and of higher signal intensity on T2WI (arrowheads).

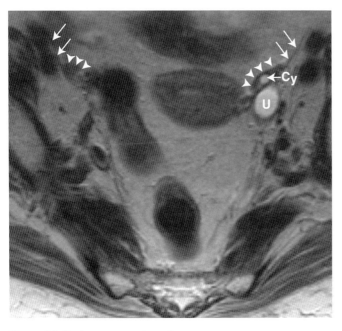

Figure 6.3. Post-menopausal ovaries.

Transaxial T2WI showing normal appearances of the ovaries in a post-menopausal woman. They are of small volume and reduced signal intensity (arrowheads), as the ovarian stroma is replaced by fibrous tissue. Note the round ligament lying in close proximity to the ovaries (arrows). The left ovary contains a persistent small follicular cyst (Cy). The left ureter (U) is dilated due to a distal obstructing mass.

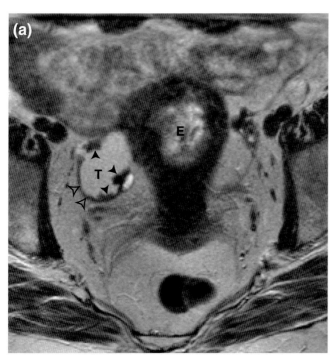

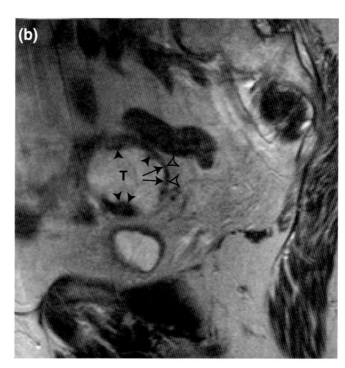

Figure 6.4. T1a Ovarian cancer.

(a) Transaxial T2WI and **(b)** sagittal T2WI showing right ovarian endometrioid carcinoma. There is a cystic mass (T) with an irregularly thickened wall (arrows) and vegetations (arrowheads). The outer surface of the mass is smooth (open arrowheads) indicating an intact ovarian capsule. Note the primary endometrial tumour (E). 15–20% of endometrioid ovarian carcinomas have a synchronous endometrial carcinoma.

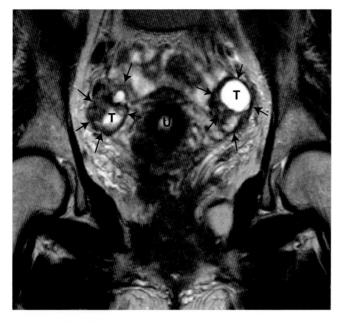

Figure 6.5. T1b Ovarian cancer.

Coronal T2WI showing bilateral ovarian cystic tumours (T). The capsules of the ovaries are intact (arrows). Note the absence of ascites. Uterus (U).

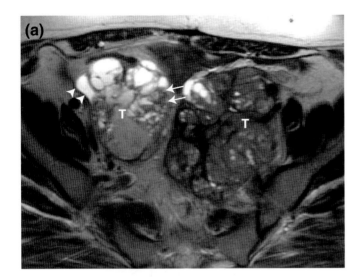

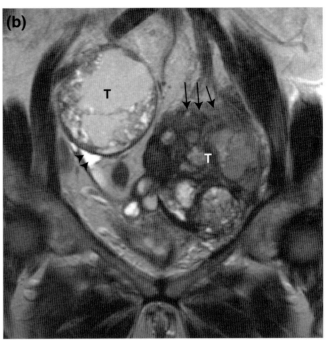

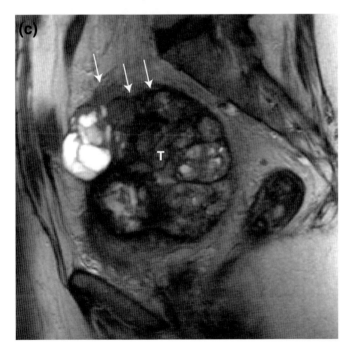

Figure 6.6. T1c Ovarian cancer.

(a) Transaxial T2WI (b) coronal T2WI and (c) sagittal T2WI showing bilateral mixed composition ovarian masses (T). The lesions are lobulated and incompletely encapsulated, with tumour on the medial ovarian surface of the right sided mass and the superior ovarian surface of the left sided mass (arrows). There is a small volume of malignant ascites (arrowheads).

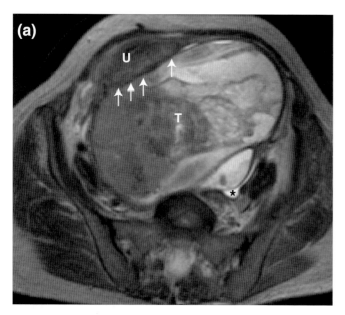

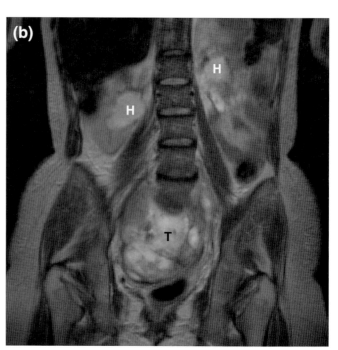

Figure 6.7.T2a Ovarian cancer.

(a) Transaxial T2WI and (b) coronal T2WI showing a large mixed composition tumour mass (T) filling the pelvis. The uterus (U) is displaced anteriorly and to the right and is inseparable from the tumour (arrows). The mass effect has resulted in bilateral hydronephrosis (H). Ureter (asterisk).

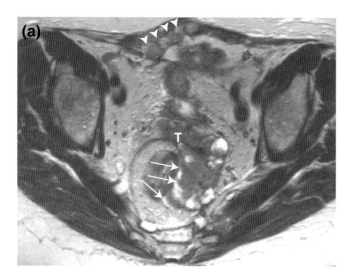

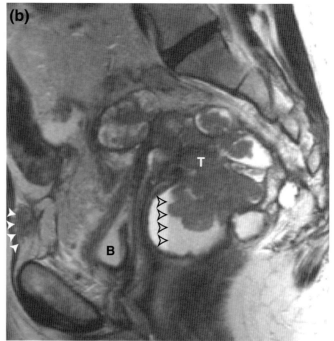

Figure 6.8.T2b Ovarian cancer.

(a) Transaxial T2WI and (b) sagittal T2WI showing a locally extensive ovarian tumour (T) which has spread posteriorly to penetrate the perirectal fascia and fat and adhere to the rectum (arrows). Anteriorly tumour extends to abut and infiltrate the posterior surface of the rectus sheath (arrowheads) and involve the bladder (B). Note the fluid/fluid level in part of the tumour mass representing layering of proteinaceous secretions and haemorrhage (open arrowheads) and the absence of ascites.

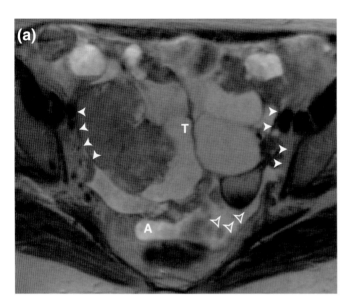

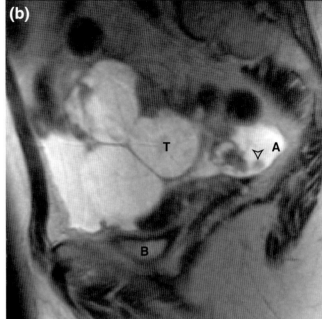

Figure 6.9. T2c Ovarian cancer.

(a) Transaxial T2WI and (b) sagittal T2WI showing mixed cystic and solid tumour mass (T) filling the central pelvis and extending to the pelvic sidewalls (arrowheads). The bladder (B) is displaced inferiorly by the mass. Malignant ascites (A) is present with a number of tumour nodules adherent to the peritoneum (open arrowheads).

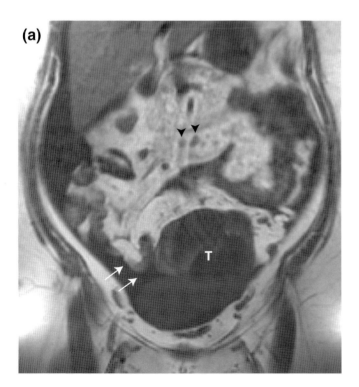

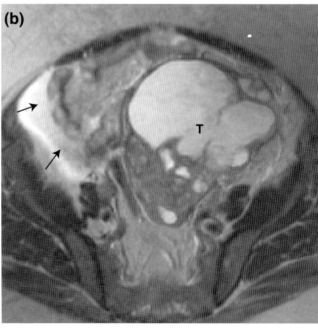

Figure 6.10. T3b Ovarian cancer.

(a) Coronal T1WI and (b) transaxial T2WI showing mixed solid and cystic central pelvic tumour mass (T). There are metastatic deposits (arrowheads) in the omentum. Note the presence of ascites (arrows).

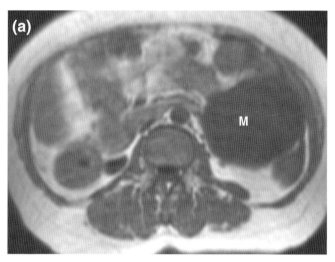

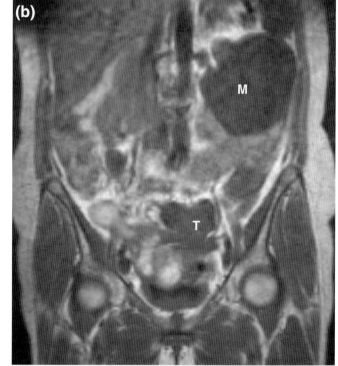

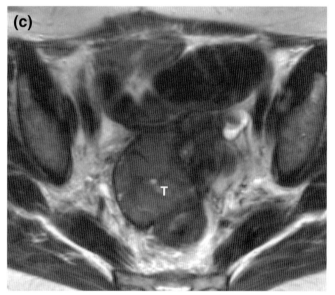

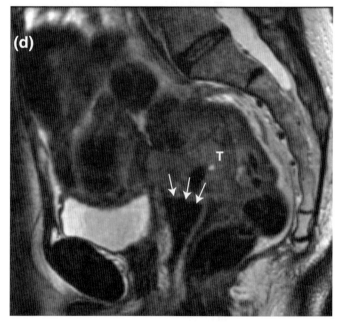

Figure 6.11. T3c Ovarian cancer.

(a) Transaxial T1WI, **(b)** coronal T1WI, **(c)** transaxial T2WI and **(d)** sagittal T2WI. There is a large mixed composition pelvic mass (T) involving the vaginal vault (arrows). A metastatic deposit (M) greater than 2.0 cm in diameter is present in the left mid abdomen.

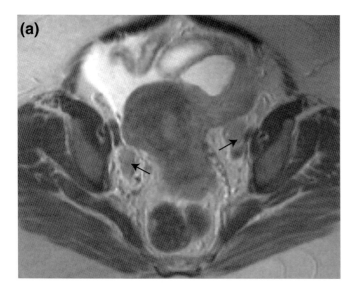

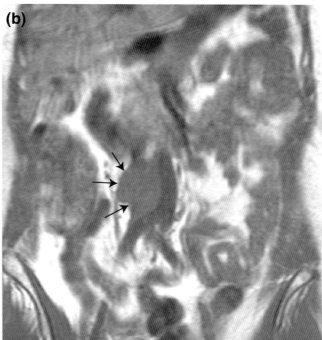

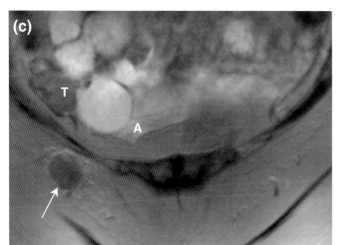

Figure 6.12. N1 Ovarian cancer.

(a) Transaxial T2WI (b) coronal T1WI (c) coronal T2WI showing lymph node metastases in various locations (arrows): (a) right obturator and left external iliac (b) interaortocaval and (c) right superficial inguinal sites. Tumour mass (T); ascites (A).

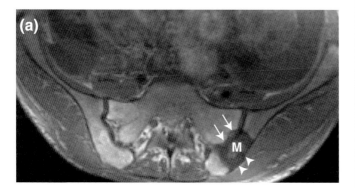

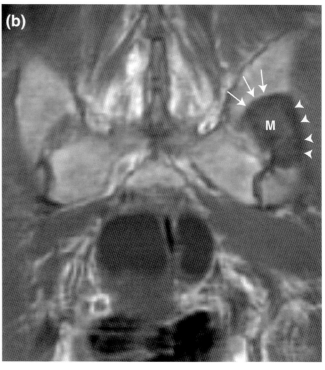

Figure 6.13. M1 Ovarian cancer.

(a) Transaxial T1WI and (b) coronal T1WI showing a metastatic deposit (M) centred on the left ilium. The tumour has crossed the sacro-iliac joint to invade the sacral ala (arrows) and extended into the soft tissues of the buttock breaching the low signal intensity line of the bone cortex (arrowheads). Bone metastases from epithelial ovarian cancer are rare; when they occur the diagnosis should be reconfirmed.

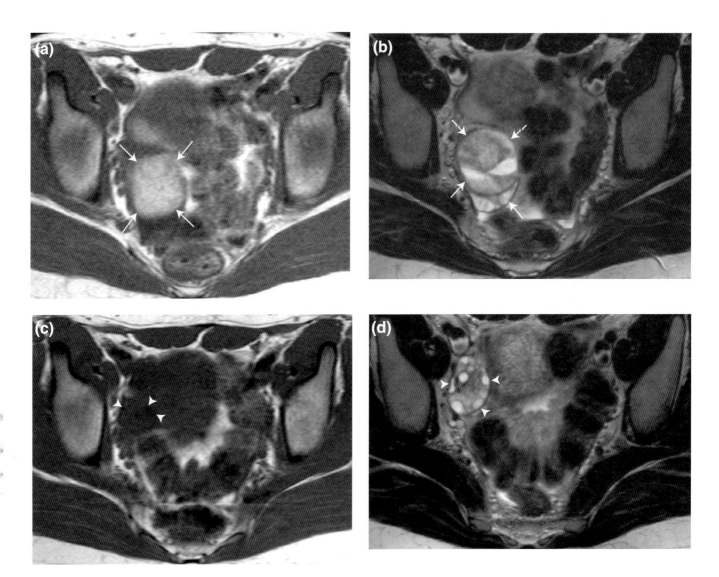

Figure 6.14. Haemorrhagic follicular cyst.

(a) Transaxial T1WI and (b) transaxial T2WI, (c) transaxial T1WI and (d) transaxial T2WI. (a) and (b) demonstrating the right ovary enlarged by a thin-walled follicular cyst containing subacute (greater than 1 week old) haematoma which appears high signal on T1WI and mixed high signal on T2WI (arrows). This signal pattern termed "shading" is due to the presence of intracellular methaemoglobin and is a finding more commonly seen in endometriomas (see *Figure 6.17*), (c) and (d) were obtained 3 months later and show resolution of the haematoma and a normal pattern of follicular cysts (arrowheads). Neoplasia cannot be excluded from an apparently haemorrhagic follicular cyst so that imaging after a 2–3 month interval using ultrasound or MRI is required.

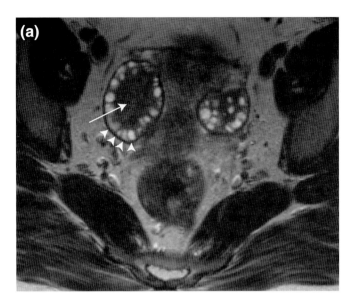 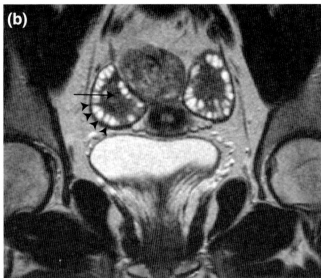

Figure 6.15. Polycystic ovary disease.

(a) Transaxial T2WI and (b) coronal T2WI showing enlarged ovaries with characteristically distributed multiple small peripheral cysts (arrowheads) with an hypertrophied low signal intensity central stroma (arrow). This condition should be recognised and distinguished from the normal appearance of follicular cysts seen in *Figures 6.2* and *6.14d* above.

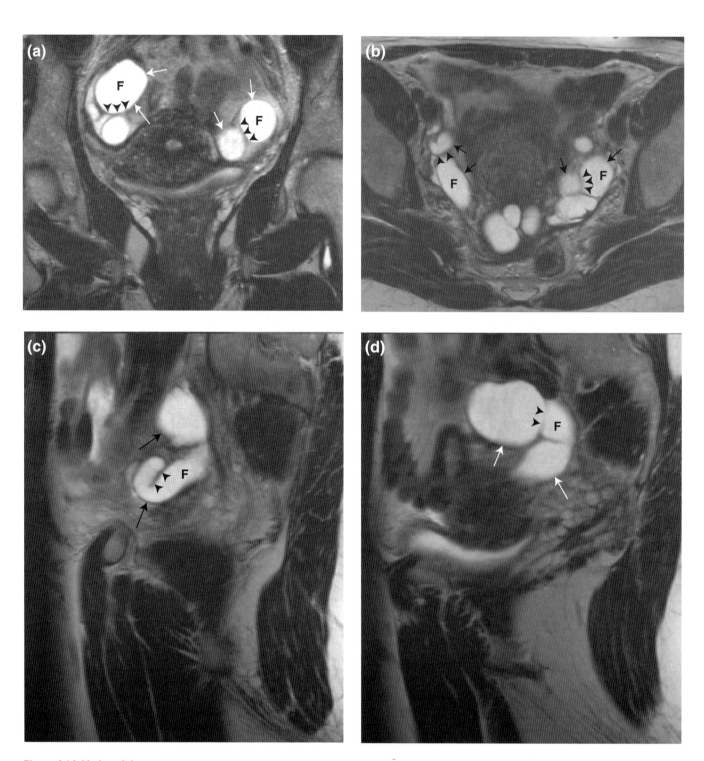

Figure 6.16. Hydrosalpinx.

(a) Coronal T2WI (b) transaxial T2WI (c) and (d) parasagittal T2W images showing bilateral hydrosalpinges. On initial inspection the coronal and transaxial images give the erroneous impression of bilateral adnexal cystic masses. Review of the parasagittal images confirms the presence of dilated Fallopian tubes (F) represented as thin-walled (arrows) convoluted tubular structures with mucosal folds (arrowheads).

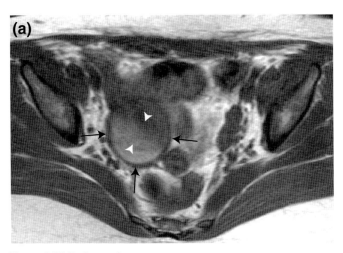

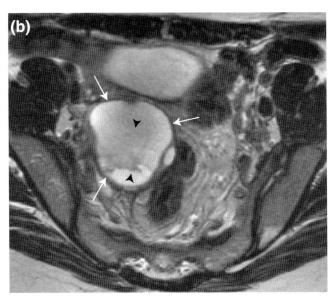

Figure 6.17. Endometrioma.

(a) Transaxial T1WI and (b) transaxial T2WI showing an endometrioma of the right ovary. Endometriomas typically have a uniformly thick low signal intensity rim (arrows) indicating a fibrous capsule and variable signal intensity contents on T1WI and T2WI due to haemoglobin breakdown products (arrowheads). A characteristic pattern is of high signal on T1WI and loss of signal on T2WI termed "shading" a finding indicating the presence of intracellular methaemoglobin.

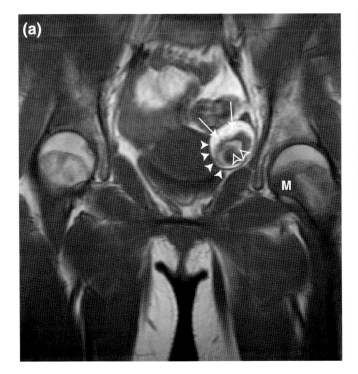

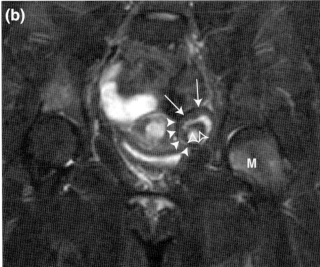

Figure 6.18. Benign cystic teratoma.

(a) Coronal T1WI and (b) coronal STIR image showing a left ovarian benign cystic teratoma (teratodermoid). The diagnostic feature of these tumours is fat (arrows) contained within a well-circumscribed wall (arrowheads) from which ectodermal elements (open arrowheads) with varying degrees of differentiation arise. Fat suppressed imaging usually differentiates between haemorrhagic cysts and benign cystic teratomas as the signal from fat in teratomas is suppressed as in (b). Note the metastasis (M) in the left femoral head from a facial rhabdomyosarcoma.

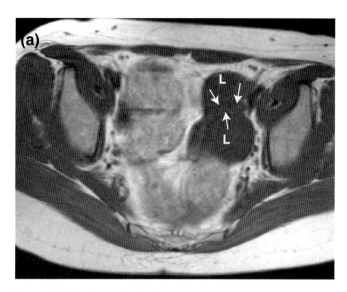

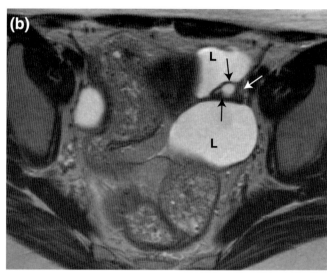

Figure 6.19. Peritoneal inclusion cysts.

(a) Transaxial T1WI and (b) transaxial T2WI in a 41-year-old woman with Crohn's disease. The left ovary (arrows) is partially surrounded by fluid-filled locules (L). These are derived from non-neoplastic mesothelial proliferation caused by retained ovarian fluid in patients with peritoneal adhesions. The extra-ovarian location of the cysts differentiates them from benign or malignant ovarian tumours. The shape and location remote from the peritoneal *cul-de-sac* differentiates the cysts from ascites.

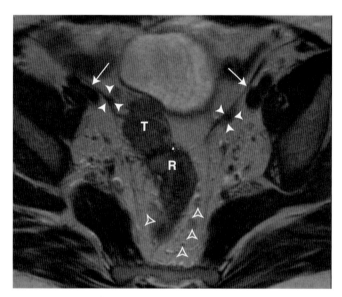

Figure 6.20. Post-operative swelling of round ligaments.

Transaxial T2WI demonstrating bilateral bulbous swelling (arrowheads) of the proximal ends of the transected round ligaments (arrows) 4 months following total abdominal hysterectomy and bilateral salpingo-oophorectomy for ovarian cancer. These changes usually resolve by 12 months after surgery. They should be recognised and differentiated from tumour masses. Note the residual tumour (T) arising from the vaginal vault and involving the rectum (R) with several perirectal tumour nodules (open arrowheads) likely in lymph nodes.

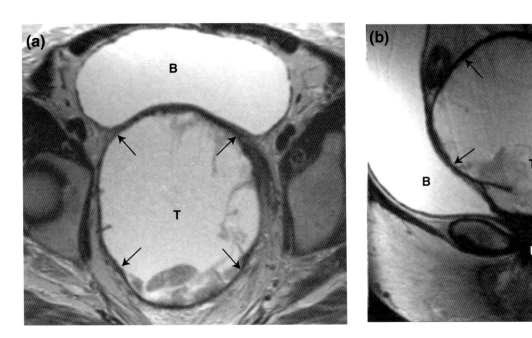

Figure 6.21. Recurrent ovarian cancer; suitable for surgical resection.

(a) Transaxial T2WI and (b) sagittal T2WI showing a large mixed composition pelvic tumour mass (T). The encapsulated nature of the mass (arrows) and the absence of metastases makes it suitable for surgical resection. Note the mass effect has caused descent of the pelvic floor and prolapse of the pelvic viscera with bladder (B) outlet obstruction due to compression of its neck. Anal canal (AC); vagina (V); urethra (U).

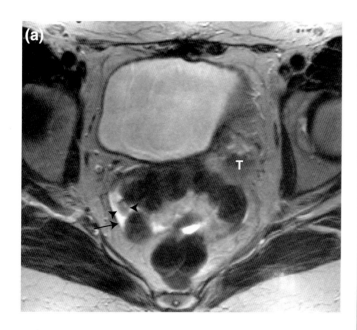

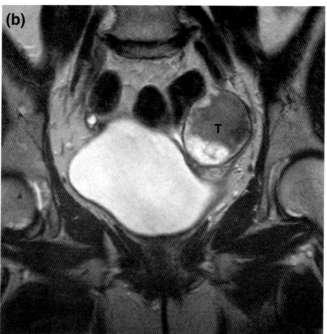

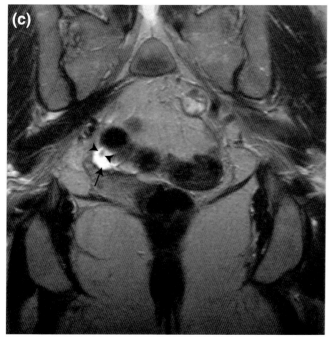

Figure 6.22. Recurrent ovarian cancer; unsuitable for surgical resection.

(a) Transaxial T2WI, **(b)** and **(c)** coronal T2WI following total abdominal hysterectomy and bilateral salpingo-oophorectomy for borderline ovarian tumour. There is a mixed composition pelvic tumour mass (T). In addition there is a small volume of ascites (arrows) outlining a serosal tumour nodule adherent to the sigmoid colon (arrowheads). The presence of serosal and peritoneal disease precludes curative surgery.

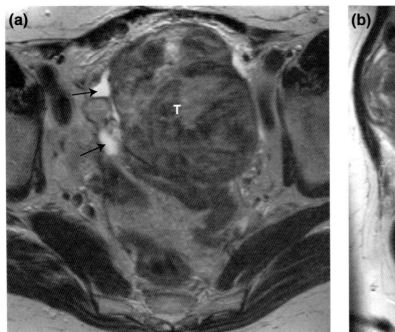
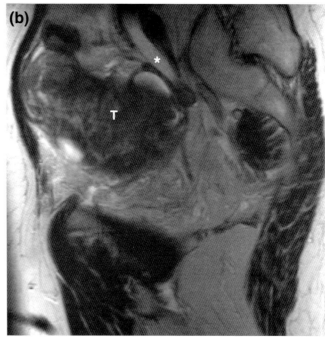

Figure 6.23. Krukenberg tumour.

(a) Transaxial T2WI and (b) sagittal T2WI in a patient with primary gastric adenocarcinoma. There is a large mixed composition tumour mass (T) arising from the left ovary and causing obstruction and dilatation of the left ureter (*). There is a small volume of ascites (arrows). The term Krukenberg tumour refers to ovarian metastases containing mucin filled signet ring cells usually from a primary gastric cancer. The only imaging feature described to help differentiate between Krukenberg tumours and primary ovarian cancer is that primary ovarian cancers are more frequently multilocular. Approximately 7% of ovarian cancers are metastatic from another primary site.

7 Vaginal Cancer

M. Ben Taylor and Neelam Dugar

BACKGROUND INFORMATION

Epidemiology

Vaginal carcinoma is a rare tumour, accounting for 2–3% of gynaecological malignancies. The incidence in the USA is around 0.6 per 100000. It is predominantly a disease of the elderly, with 70–80% of cases occurring in women over the age of 60.

In common with cervical carcinoma, invasive vaginal carcinoma is associated with vaginal intraepithelial neoplasia (VAIN), often induced by exposure to human papilloma virus. The rare clear cell carcinoma, which affects young women, is associated with maternal exposure to diethylstilboestrol.

Histopathology

Around 90% of tumours are squamous cell carcinomas and 5–10% are adenocarcinomas. Other tumour types are rare and include clear cell carcinoma, small cell carcinoma, melanoma and sarcomas.

Patterns of tumour spread

Most vaginal carcinomas arise in the upper vagina. Direct involvement of the cervix is common. This may lead to problems with classification as the FIGO classification system states that vaginal tumours that extend to the external cervical os should be considered cervical carcinomas.

Tumours breaching the vaginal wall commonly infiltrate around the urethra anteriorly and the rectovaginal fascia posteriorly. Larger tumours may directly involve the bladder or rectum. Laterally tumours extend into the paracolpol tissues and may extend to the pelvic side-wall. Lower vaginal tumours may extend onto the perineum and involve the vulva, urethra and anus.

The vagina has a rich lymphatic drainage. The lower vaginal lymphatics drain with those of the vulva to the inguinal nodes. Those of the mid and upper vagina drain predominantly to the obturator nodes, although the posterior wall may drain first to the perirectal nodes. Tumour spread is then usually contiguous, through the internal, external and common iliac chains and eventually to the upper retroperitoneum.

Haematogenous spread may occur and is most commonly to the lungs.

Prognostic indicators

The following factors affect prognosis:

- Tumour stage. Stage is the most important prognostic factor; in one large series, 10 year disease free survival was 80% for stage I, 38% for stage III and 0% for stage IV.

- Tumour size. Tumours > 4.0 cm in diameter have a worse prognosis, but this variable is not independent of tumour stage.

- Tumour position. In one series tumours of the lower $\frac{2}{3}$ of the vagina or involving the posterior wall had a worse prognosis.

- Tumour morphology. Stage I tumours with a superficially ulcerated exophytic morphology have a better prognosis than infiltrative or necrotic tumours of the same stage.

- Histological type. One series suggested that adenocarcinomas had a worse prognosis, but this has not been confirmed by other studies.

- Histological grade. Poorly differentiated tumours have a worse prognosis.

Table 7.1. Clinical staging of vaginal cancer: correlation of TNM (2002) and FIGO (1994) classifications

TNM	FIGO	
Tx		Primary tumour cannot be assessed
T0		No evidence of primary tumour
Tis	0	Carcinoma *in situ*
TI	I	Tumour limited to vagina
T2	II	Tumour involves the paravaginal tissues but does not extend to the pelvic wall
T3	III	Tumour extends to the pelvic wall
T4	IV	Tumour extends beyond the true pelvis or clinically involves the mucosa of the bladder or rectum
	IVA	Spread to adjacent organs, direct extension beyond the true pelvis, or both
Nx		Regional lymph nodes cannot be assessed
N0		No regional lymph node metastases
NI		Pelvic or inguinal lymph node metastases
Mx		Distant metastases cannot be assessed
M0		No distant metastases
MI	IVB	Distant metastases (includes lymph node metastases outside the pelvis or inguinal regions)

Treatment

Surgery

Surgical options include partial vaginectomy with radical hysterectomy for tumours of the upper vagina. Tumours of the mid or lower vagina may require total vaginectomy. Surgery will usually include bilateral pelvic lymph node resection. Pelvic exenteration is a valid option for selected patients, particularly when pelvic irradiation has been previously given or in patients with a rectovaginal or vesico-vaginal fistula. However, the role of surgery in vaginal carcinoma is not well defined and most patients are treated by radiotherapy.

Radiotherapy

External beam radiotherapy is used and must include the primary tumour and the local lymph nodes; in tumours of the lower vagina the inguinal nodes must be included. Brachytherapy, which is the local application of radiation sources, is particularly useful in earlier stage tumours.

Chemotherapy

There is no direct evidence of benefit from chemotherapy in vaginal carcinoma. However, chemoradiation (concurrent treatment with chemotherapy and radiation) is of value in squamous cell carcinoma of the cervix and may be justified in certain cases of primary vaginal carcinoma.

MR IMAGING OF VAGINAL CARCINOMA

Technique

As for other pelvic tumours, imaging is best performed with a phased array surface coil utilising turbo spin echo sequences. Thin section T2-weighted sequences in the transaxial and sagittal planes are most useful in the evaluation of local tumour extent. Transaxial images must include the entire vagina down to the vulva, this usually requires an additional image series. Off-axis imaging, perpendicular to the vagina, may be helpful to assess invasion of the bladder or rectum. Tampons may obscure detail of the vaginal mucosa and should not be used. T1-weighted images are acquired in the transaxial plane through the entire pelvis to include the upper pelvic lymph node groups. An additional coronal T1-weighted sequence to cover the entire abdomen is helpful in assessing for upper retroperitoneal lymph node metastases and hydronephrosis.

Intravenous contrast agents are not routinely used, but dynamic T1-weighted Gd-DTPA enhanced fat saturated sequences may be of value in delineating tumour extent, with tumour typically showing early enhancement. Delayed sequences, obtained after filling of the bladder with Gd-DTPA, can demonstrate small fistulae from the bladder.

Another interesting technique is MR vaginography, using saline or other positive contrast material, injected via a Foley catheter to distend the vagina. T2-weighted sequences are then performed in the standard planes. This technique has been used to determine vaginal extent of cervical carcinomas and could also be of use in primary vaginal carcinoma.

Imaging features

Vaginal carcinomas are typically of intermediate signal intensity on T1-weighted images and relatively high signal intensity on T2-weighted images. Small tumours may be difficult to distinguish from the high signal epithelial layer and central mucus on T2-weighted images. Larger tumours can be seen invading the low signal vaginal wall and extending into the paracolpol fat. Tumours typically show early phase enhancement following intravenous Gd-DTPA. Very large tumours will commonly show central necrosis.

Post treatment: radiotherapy

Following radiotherapy, the primary tumour will typically shrink and small tumours may no longer be visible. Larger tumours, if successfully treated, will show a low signal residuum representing fibrosis. In the acute stage there may be oedema of the mucosa and muscle layer, manifest as high signal on T2-weighted images, which usually develops 3 to 6 months following radiotherapy. This high signal typically subsides 12 to 24 months following radiotherapy, but may persist for many years. In the later stage the vaginal muscle wall is more typically of low signal on T1-weighted images and T2-weighted images due to fibrosis and the vagina may be shortened or stenosed. The vagina may also be distorted with tethering to structures previously involved with tumour.

Post treatment: surgery

For small tumours in the upper vagina, partial vaginectomy may be performed, with hysterectomy if the uterus has not previously been removed. The oversewn residual vagina has a linear or bow-tie shape and may have a nodular contour. The vaginal wall is normally of low signal on T2-weighted images due to fibrosis, this is a helpful feature in distinguishing post-surgical change from tumour, which is typically of intermediate to high signal.

MRI staging accuracy

Vaginal carcinoma is a rare tumour and there are no published series comparing MRI staging with either surgically resected specimens or clinical staging. MRI has better soft tissue discrimination than CT and is more sensitive in the detection of small tumours and in the identification of local invasion of the pelvic floor, perineum, urethra and anal canal. CT is a valid alternative to MRI in large tumours when assessment of bladder or rectal invasion is required.

Assessment of nodal status in pelvic malignancy is based on node size and shape, with nodes ≥ 10.0 mm in maximum short axis diameter or with a round shape being more likely to be involved by tumour. Accuracies are similar for CT and MRI. Nodes showing central necrosis, manifest as central high signal on T2-weighted images or lack of enhancement following Gd DTPA, are more likely to be metastatic.

Current indications

The role of MRI in the staging of vaginal carcinoma is not well defined. More studies are required, but are difficult due to the rarity of the tumour. In most cases initial management decisions are based upon clinical examination. However, clinical examination may be inaccurate and ideally MRI should also be performed as it may detect more advanced tumour than is suspected clinically and lead to alterations in management. MRI has an important role in selection of patients and surgical planning prior to pelvic exenteration.

The likelihood of pelvic lymph node metastases, determined by MRI or CT, will affect radiotherapy planning.

MRI is useful in detecting tumour recurrence, particularly in patients with vaginal stenosis secondary to radiotherapy who cannot be adequately examined clinically. In addition, in patients with symptoms suggestive of colovaginal or vesicovaginal fistula, MRI is the imaging investigation of choice for delineation of the extent of the fistula and for surgical planning.

Pitfalls of MRI

- **Following biopsy** differentiation of tumour from inflammation and haemorrhage is often difficult, particularly if the primary tumour is small.

- **The introitus** is difficult to assess on MRI, as it is often asymmetrical and the superficial perineal structures are of similar signal to tumour on T2-weighted images. Fortunately, superficial tumour extent is usually apparent clinically. Dynamic T1-weighted Gd-DTPA enhanced fat saturated sequences may be of value in the perineum and vulva, with enhancing tumour seen well against the saturated vulval fat.

- **Following radiotherapy** it is often difficult to discriminate between a sterile tumour residuum and recurrent tumour. Inert post treatment residuum is fibrotic and typically of low signal, whereas tumour is more commonly of intermediate to high signal on T2WI. However, there is overlap in the appearances and both may show Gd-DTPA enhancement. Consequently, biopsy is often required to diagnose recurrence. Alternatively, enlargement of a mass on serial examinations is almost invariably due to recurrence.

FURTHER READING

1. Hricak H, Chang YCF and Thurnher S. (1998) Vagina: Evaluation with MR imaging. Part 1. Normal anatomy and congenital anomalies. *Radiology* 169: 169–174.

2. Chang YCF, Hricak H, Thurnher S and Lacey CG. (1988) Vagina: Evaluation with MR imaging. Part 2. Neoplasms. *Radiology* 169: 175–179.

3. Siegelman ES, Outwater EK, Banner MP, Ramchandani P, Anderson TL and Schnall MD. (1997) High-resolution MR imaging of the vagina. *Radiographics* 17: 1183–1203. *Beautifully illustrated article including normal anatomy, congenital anomalies and neoplasms.*

4. Chang SD. (2002) Imaging of the vagina and vulva. *Radiol. Clin. North Am.* 40: 637–658. *Includes discussion of imaging in vaginal and vulval carcinoma.*

5. Chyle V, Zagars GK, Wheeler JA, Wharton JT and Delclos L. (1996) Definitive radiotherapy for carcinoma of the vagina: outcome and prognostic features. *Int. J. Radiat. Oncol. Biol. Phys.* 35: 891–905. *A clinical review of 301 patients treated with radiotherapy.*

6. Brown JJ, Guitierrez ED and Lee JK. (1992) MR appearance of the normal and abnormal vagina after hysterectomy. *Am. J. Roentgenol.* 158: 95–99. *A description of post-surgical appearances.*

7. Van Hoe L, Vanbeckevoort D, Oyen R, Itzlinger U and Vergote I. (1999) Cervical Carcinoma: Optimized Local Staging with Intravaginal Contrast-enhanced MR Imaging – Preliminary Results. *Radiology* 213: 608–611. *A description of MR vaginography in cervical carcinoma.*

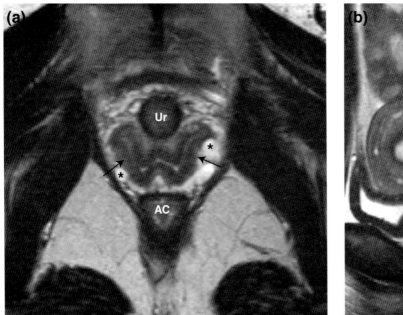

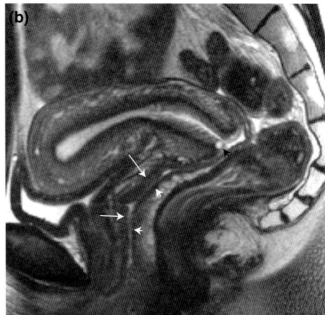

Figure 7.1. Normal appearance of the vagina.

(a) Transaxial T2WI through the lower vagina showing normal anatomy. The collapsed vagina is seen as a 'W-shaped' structure with a low signal fibromuscular wall (black arrows). A thin layer of high signal within the vagina represents the vaginal mucosa and intraluminal mucus. The high signal of the paracolpol adventitia surrounding the vagina (asterisk) is due to slow flowing blood within the vaginal venous plexus. Urethra (Ur), Anal canal (AC).

(b) Sagittal T2WI through the pelvis showing normal anatomy. The anterior (long arrows) and posterior (short arrows) fibromuscular walls of the vagina are of low signal. The vaginal mucosa and intraluminal mucus are visible as a thin layer of high signal. A small Nabothian cyst is seen in the anterior cervix as a well defined rounded area of high signal (*Short black arrow*).

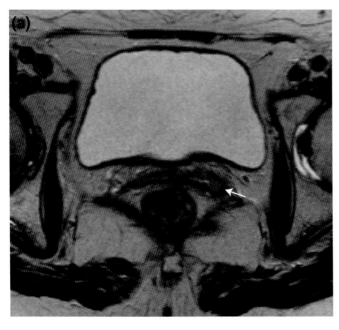

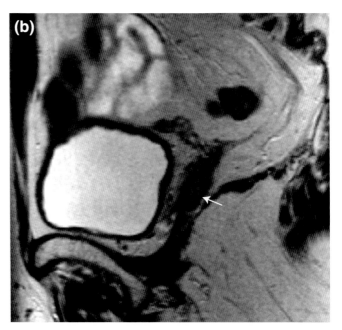

Figure 7.2. T1 N0 Vaginal carcinoma.

(a) Transaxial T2WI and (b) sagittal T2WI showing a small tumour (arrow) in the left mid vagina. The tumour is constrained by the low signal vaginal wall.

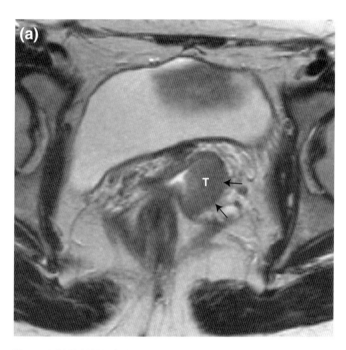

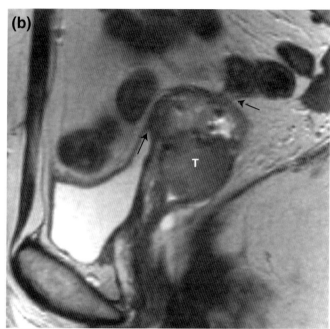

Figure 7.3. T2 N0 Vaginal carcinoma (clear cell tumour).

(a) Transaxial T2WI and **(b)** sagittal T2WI showing a heterogenous soft tissue tumour (T) in the upper and mid vagina in a patient with previous hysterectomy. Tumour expands the vaginal lumen and breaches the low signal vaginal wall laterally to involve the paracolpol fat (small arrows). The sigmoid colon is tethered to the vaginal vault (black arrow in (b)), but this may be a normal post-operative finding. Anteriorly the tumour is fixed to the bladder muscle wall (white arrow in (b)).

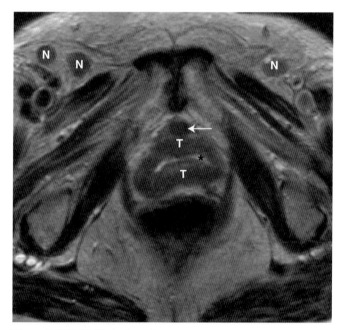

Figure 7.4. T2 N1 Vaginal carcinoma.

Transaxial T2WI of tumour (T) circumferentially thickening the lower vagina, but not extending to the pelvic floor nor involving the urethra (arrow). There is a small amount of fluid in the vaginal lumen (asterisk). There are bilateral inguinal lymph node metastases (N) of similar signal intensity to the primary tumour.

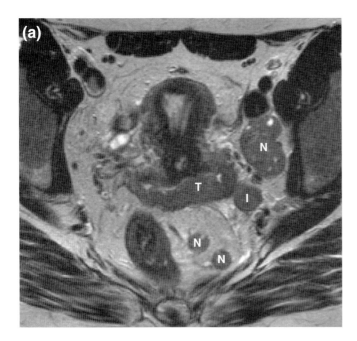

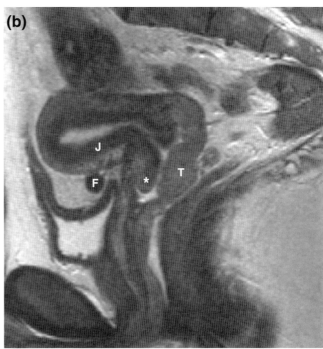

Figure 7.5. T2 N1 Vaginal carcinoma with posterior pelvic lymph node metastases.

(a) Transaxial T2WI and (b) sagittal T2WI showing tumour (T) predominantly involving the posterior wall of the upper vagina but also within the anterior fornix (*). There are enlarged internal iliac (I), perirectal and obturator nodes (N) which show signal intensity similar to the primary tumour. The uterus is anteverted with a prominent junctional zone (J) and a small subserosal fibroid (F).

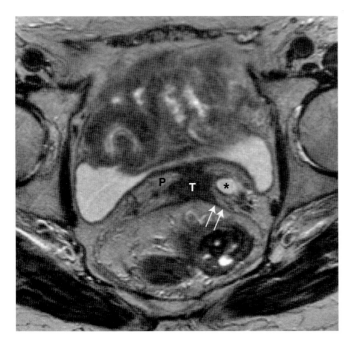

Figure 7.6. T2 N0 Vaginal carcinoma with ureteric obstruction and adherence to the posterior bladder wall.

Transaxial T2WI showing spiculated tumour (T) at the vaginal vault with low signal tumour extending into the parametrium (P), onto the posterior bladder wall (arrowheads) and onto the perirectal fascia (arrows). The left ureter (*) is obstructed by tumour but this, unlike the staging system for cervical carcinoma, does not increase the tumour stage to T3. Involvement of the bladder muscle wall is not sufficient to classify the tumour as T4, for this stage to apply tumour must extend to the bladder mucosa.

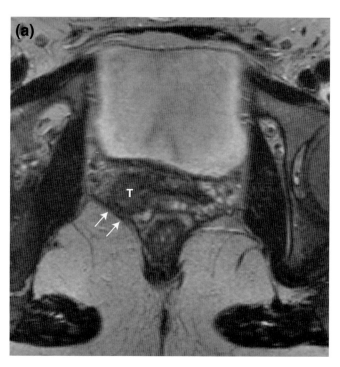

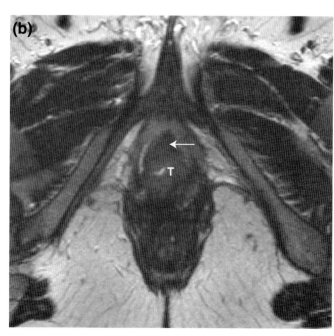

Figure 7.7. T3 N0 Vaginal carcinoma involving the pelvic floor.

(a) Transaxial T2WI showing tumour (T) extending through the right lateral vaginal wall to involve the levator ani muscle (arrows). (b) Transaxial T2WI at the level of the vaginal introitus showing tumour (T) around the introitus and involving the urethral meatus (white arrow).

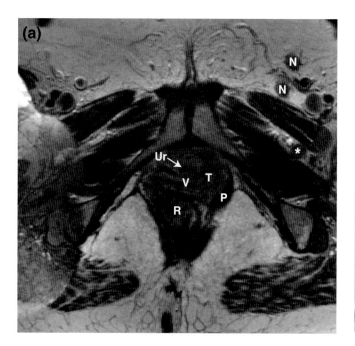

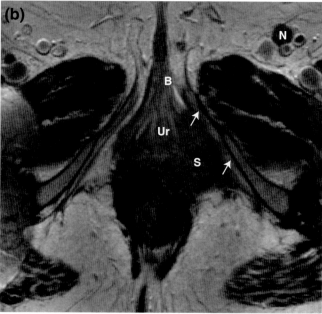

Figure 7.8. T3 N1 Vaginal carcinoma invading the perineal structures.

(a) Transaxial T2WI at the level of the lower vagina (V) showing tumour (T) on the left side invading the left anterior pubo-rectalis muscle (P). There is circumferential involvement of the urethra (Ur) with loss of its normal zonal anatomy. There are left inguinal lymph node metastases (N) and a metastatic left anatomical obturator node (asterisk), these lymph nodes lie between the obturator externus and pectineus muscles and are not normally visible. Lower rectum (R).
(b) Transaxial T2WI at a slightly lower level than (a) showing tumour extending through the left superficial perineal space (S) to involve the left ischiocavernosus muscle and crus of clitoris (arrows). The urethral meatus (Ur) and left bulbospongiosus muscle (B) are also invaded. There are left inguinal lymph node metastases (N).

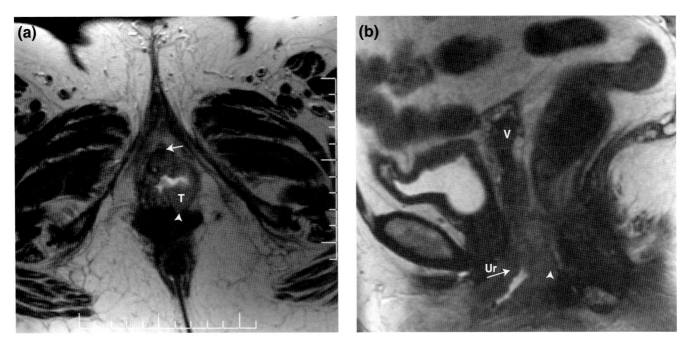

Figure 7.9. T3 N0 Vaginal carcinoma involving the urethra and perineal body.

(a) Transaxial T2WI showing circumferential tumour (T) involving the lower vagina with direct invasion of the urethra (arrow). Posteriorly, tumour involves the perineal body on the left (arrowhead). **(b)** Sagittal T2WI showing tumour involving the anterior (arrow) and posterior (arrowhead) walls of the lower vagina. Anteriorly, tumour involves the urethral meatus (Ur). Note previous hysterectomy with fibrosis at the vaginal vault (V).

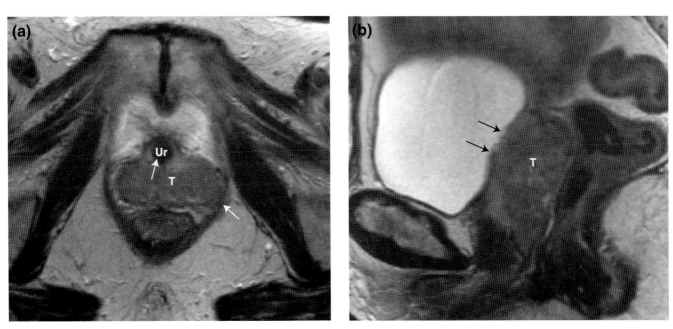

Figure 7.10. T4 N0 Vaginal carcinoma involving the posterior bladder wall.

(a) Transaxial T2WI showing a large tumour (T) filling the lower vagina and breaching the left vaginal wall with involvement of the left levator ani muscle (white arrow). There is circumferential involvement of the urethra (Ur) (black arrow). **(b)** Sagittal T2WI showing tumour (T) involving the entire length of the anterior vaginal wall. The low signal bladder muscle wall is destroyed and tumour involves the bladder mucosa (arrows).

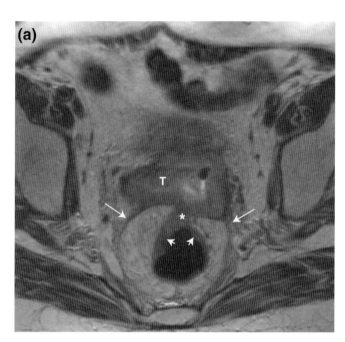
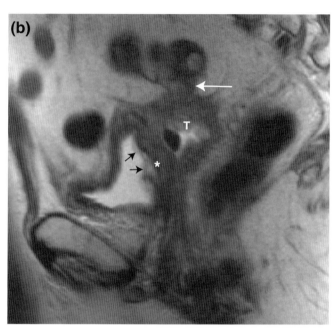

Figure 7.11.T4 N0 Vaginal carcinoma involving the bladder muscle layer, rectum and sigmoid colon.

(a) Transaxial T2WI showing an upper vaginal tumour (T) which infiltrates the paracolpol tissues and extends along the perirectal fascia bilaterally (arrows). In the midline there is breach of the perirectal fascia with tumour extension to the rectum (asterisk), including the rectal mucosa (short white arrows). **(b)** Sagittal T2WI showing upper vaginal tumour (T) with invasion of the posterior bladder wall, the low signal bladder muscle wall is interrupted (asterisk) and there is bladder mucosal oedema (small black arrows). Superiorly, the tumour is invading loops of sigmoid colon (large white arrow).

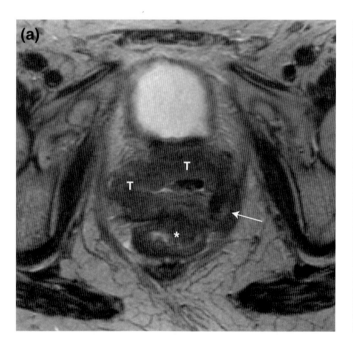
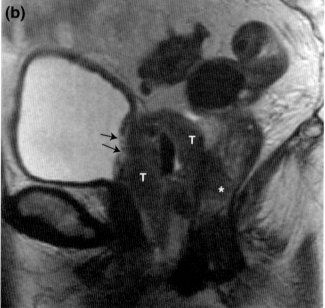

Figure 7.12.T4 N0 Vaginal carcinoma involving the bladder, rectum and pelvic floor.

(a) Transaxial T2WI and **(b)** sagittal T2WI showing a large tumour (T) with circumferential involvement of the entire length of the vagina. Tumour extends posteriorly to invade the rectum (asterisk) and laterally to invade the left levator ani muscle (large white arrow). Anteriorly, there is tumour invasion of the posterior bladder wall with tumour extension to the bladder mucosa (small black arrows).

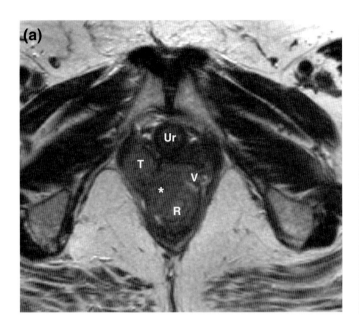
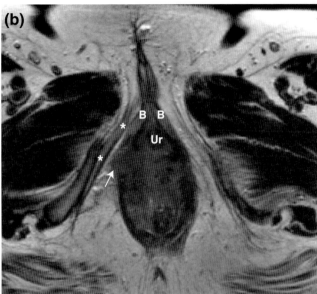

Figure 7.13. T4 N0 Vaginal carcinoma invading the ischioanal fossa.

(a) Transaxial T2WI showing lower right vaginal tumour (T) which extends into the paracolpol space and invades (asterisk) the lower rectum (R). Urethra (Ur), low signal vaginal muscular wall (V). **(b)** Transaxial T2WI showing extensive tumour infiltration of the perineum with involvement of the right puborectalis muscle (arrow) and circumferential involvement of the lower urethra (Ur). The bulbospongiosus muscles (B) and right ischiocavernosus muscle (asterisk) are well seen.

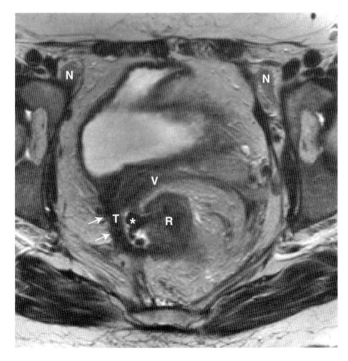
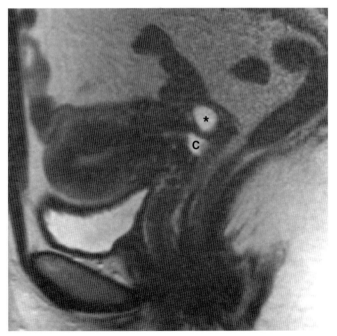

Figure 7.15. T1 N0 Vaginal carcinoma, post-biopsy change.

Sagittal T2WI showing high signal in the cervix (C) and posterior vaginal fornix (*) following biopsy of a small vaginal primary. The abnormalities are well defined and of high signal intensity suggestive of locules of fluid, rather than tumour which is typically less well defined and of intermediate to high signal intensity. In this patient there was residual tumour, which was not visible on MRI.

Figure 7.14. T4 N1 Vaginal carcinoma with rectovaginal fistula.

Transaxial T2WI showing upper vaginal tumour which presented with rectovaginal fistula. Low signal tumour (T) extends from the right lateral vagina (V) along the right utero-sacral ligament (short arrows) and is tethered to the sacrum posteriorly (arrow). Tumour extends through the right perirectal space to invade the rectum (R). Fluid and locules of gas are seen within the fistula tract (asterisk). There are bilateral enlarged external iliac lymph nodes (N).

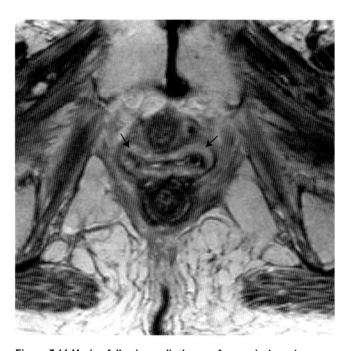

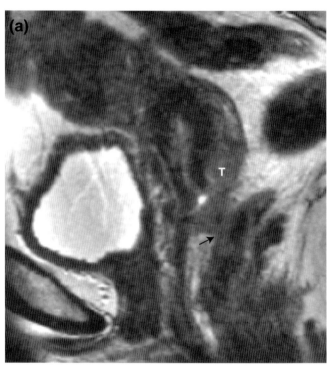

Figure 7.16. Vagina following radiotherapy for cervical carcinoma.

Transaxial T2WI showing high signal thickening (arrows) of the lower vagina, principally involving the muscular component, in a patient treated with radiotherapy for cervical carcinoma 20 years previously. High signal in the vaginal wall typically resolves within 12 to 18 months after radiotherapy, but may persist long term.

Figure 7.17. T4 N0 Vaginal carcinoma showing response to radiotherapy.

(a) Sagittal T2WI before and **(b)** 3 years following radiotherapy. Before radiotherapy, tumour (T) is seen involving the posterior vaginal fornix and extending through the posterior vaginal wall to involve the rectal wall (arrow). Following radiotherapy, the tumour is no longer visible. The vaginal wall shows very low signal, the posterior vaginal wall appears adherent to the posterior lip of the cervix with obliteration of the posterior vaginal fornix (arrows).
(c) Transaxial T2WI at the level of the mid vagina 3 years following radiotherapy. The vaginal wall is thickened, irregular and of low signal following radiotherapy (arrows). There is a small low signal nodule (arrowhead) between the posterior vaginal wall and the rectum representing fibrosis at the site of previous tumour invasion.

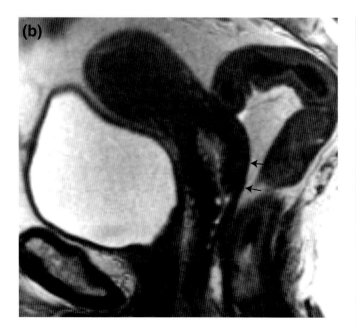

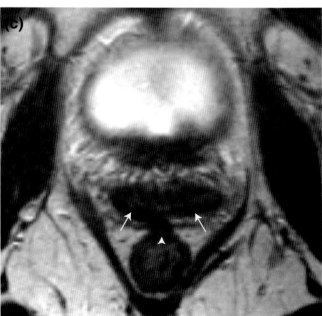

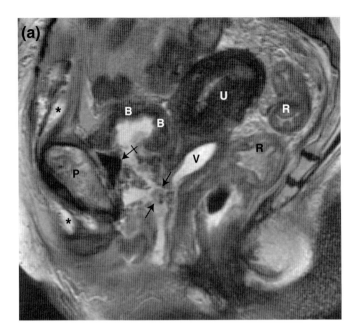

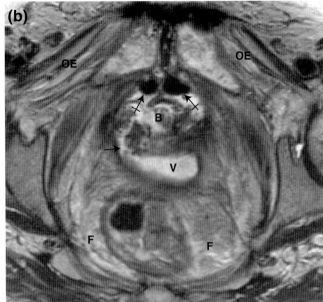

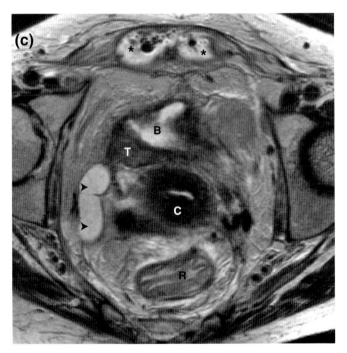

Figure 7.18. Vesico-vaginal fistula and recurrent tumour following radiotherapy for T4 vaginal carcinoma.

(a) Sagittal T2WI showing vesico-vaginal fistula (black arrows). The bladder wall (B) is thickened and irregular. There is air (crossed arrows) in the anterior bladder and urine in the upper vagina (V). There is also a defect in the anterior bladder wall and urine (asterisks) tracks around the pubis (P) into the anterior abdominal wall. High signal is seen in the rectal submucosa (R) due to radiotherapy. Uterus (U). **(b)** Transaxial T2WI showing vesico-vaginal fistula on the right (arrow) with urine in the upper vagina (V). There is air (crossed arrows) and debris in the bladder lumen (B). There is high signal in the pelvic fat (F) due to previous radiotherapy. High signal in the obturator externus muscles (OE) may either be radiotherapy related or due to inflammation induced by the anterior urine leak. **(c)** Transaxial T2WI in the same patient showing recurrent tumour (T) at the right vesico-ureteric junction obstructing the right ureter (arrowheads). A collection containing urine and air due to bladder rupture is seen anteriorly within the rectus abdominis muscle (asterisk). The rectum (R) shows high signal in the submucosa and perirectal fat due to previous radiotherapy. Cervix (C); bladder (B). Differentiation of recurrent tumour from post treatment fibrosis or inflammatory tissue may be difficult. Tumour is typically of intermediate to high signal and has a solid appearance with mass effect. Fibrosis is typically of low signal with tethering and retraction of adjacent structures. Inflammatory masses are less common but may be indistinguishable from recurrent tumour.

8 Vulval Cancer

Jane M. Hawnaur

BACKGROUND INFORMATION

Epidemiology

Vulval carcinoma occurs most frequently in elderly women, peaking in incidence in the sixth and seventh decades, but with 30% of cases arising in premenopausal women. There are approximately 900 new cases per year in the UK. The American Cancer Society estimates the incidence of vulval cancer in the USA will be 3800 new cases in 2002, with 800 deaths expected. Symptoms of vulval malignancy include a mass, pruritus, pain and discharge. Human papilloma virus (HPV) infection is believed to predispose to malignant transformation in the vulval epithelium. Women presenting with invasive squamous carcinoma often have a history of vulval intraepithelial neoplasia (VIN) with histological evidence of viral infection in the vulval epithelial cells. As with the relationship between cervical intraepithelial neoplasia and invasive cervical carcinoma, there is postulated to be a progression from low grade VIN (dysplasia) to high grade VIN (carcinoma *in situ*) with eventual development of invasive carcinoma. Chronic vulvitis from any cause may also predispose to VIN and invasive squamous carcinoma.

Histopathology

Clinical examination and colposcopically directed biopsy are used to diagnose the cause of diffuse vulval abnormality. Excision biopsy is carried out for well-circumscribed masses or naevi. Vulval tumours are usually squamous cell carcinomas (80% of total) but malignant melanoma, basal cell carcinoma and Paget's disease also occur on the vulval skin. Bartholin's glands or glands in the urethra may give rise to adenocarcinoma, and there are other rare forms of cancer arising within intraepithelial structures.

Patterns of tumour spread

Invasive lesions extend in breadth and depth within the vulval skin, and may eventually invade the urethra, vagina or anus. Multifocal disease is not unusual. Lymphovascular space invasion is associated with metastases to the regional lymph nodes, the superficial and deep inguinal nodes. Tumours on the labia majora, labia minora, fourchette and clitoris drain to the superficial and deep inguinal nodes and thence to the pelvic lymph nodes. Although lateral tumours usually involve the ipsilateral groin nodes initially, contralateral or bilateral nodal metastases can occur because of communication in the lymphatic network across the vulva. Central tumours, and those invading the urethra, vagina or anus may metastasise directly to pelvic lymph nodes. The obturator nodes are most frequently involved, followed by the external iliac, internal iliac and common iliac lymph nodes. Distant metastases, for example to liver, lung or bone, are uncommon.

Staging

Carcinoma of the vulva is commonly staged in the UK using the International Federation of Obstetrics and Gynaecology (FIGO) staging classification, which is based on surgico-pathological findings. The FIGO staging classification (1994) and its equivalent TNM staging is given in *Table 8.1*.

Prognostic indicators

The patient's prognosis is most dependent on the tumour size, depth of invasion and the number of metastatic inguinal lymph nodes. The tumour stage (see *Table 8.1*) and the site of the tumour on the vulva are other prognostic factors. Central tumours (involving the clitoris) have a worse prognosis than lateral (labial) tumours, and are more difficult to treat. The probability of lymph node metastases is closely related to the depth of invasion into the vulval skin, and bilateral metastases are more likely to occur from a central tumour than a lateral one. Patients with Stage I or II disease and negative lymph nodes have a five-year survival of 80–90%. Five-year survival in node-positive tumours is 30–55%, depending on the number of nodes involved.

Treatment

Treatment of invasive vulval carcinoma is by radical local excision or vulvectomy, and inguinal lymph node resection. The surgeon attempts to resect the tumour completely while leaving sufficient vulval skin to allow reconstruction. Skin flaps may have to be created if conservation of sufficient vulva is not feasible. T1a tumours do not require inguinal node dissection and unilateral lymph node dissection is adequate for lateral T1 tumours if the ipsilateral lymph nodes are negative. Adjuvant radiotherapy is usually given if the inguinal lymph nodes contain metastatic tumour. Inguinal lymph node dissection inevitably causes some degree of lymphatic stasis, and in some women postoperative lymphoedema in the legs and lower pelvis may be chronic and disabling.

Table 8.1. Clinical staging of vulval cancer: correlation of TNM (2002) and FIGO (1994) classifications

TNM Classification	FIGO stage	Clinical description of tumour extent
Tis	0	Carcinoma *in situ*, intraepithelial neoplasm
T1	I	Tumour confined to the vulva and/or perineum ≤ 2.0 cm diameter
T1a	IA	Depth of stromal invasion not exceeding 1.0 mm
T1b	IB	Depth of stromal invasion exceeds 1.0 mm
T2	II	Tumour confined to the vulva and/or perineum >2.0 cm diameter
T3	III	Tumour of any size, contiguous spread to lower urethra and/or vagina and/or anus
T4	IVA	Tumour invades upper urethra and/or bladder and/or rectal mucosa and/or fixed to pubic bone
N0		No regional lymph node metastasis
N1	III	Unilateral regional lymph node metastasis
N2	IVA	Bilateral inguinal lymph node metastases
M0		No distant metastasis
M1	IVB	Distant metastasis (including pelvic lymph node metastasis

MR IMAGING OF VULVAL CANCER

Technique

Vulval carcinoma can be imaged using a standard MRI pelvic tumour protocol to show the extent of primary tumour and assess the lymph nodes. High spatial resolution scans of the inguinal regions may be helpful to increase the sensitivity for lymph node metastases. A 20.0 cm diameter surface coil is positioned over the groins, centred over the symphysis pubis. Alternatively, a phased array body coil can be used, using all elements for the pelvic images and the anterior elements alone for the inguinal regions. Coronal T1-weighted and fat-suppressed T2-weighted fast spin echo sequences are obtained through the inguinal regions using a 20.0 cm field of view, 256×256 imaging matrix, and 3.0 mm slice thickness.

Current indications

There is little published evidence to support the use of MR imaging for staging vulval cancer, and limited data regarding its accuracy. From personal experience, MR imaging may be useful to assess the depth of invasion of the primary tumour, particularly to identify deep invasion of the urethra, vagina or anus. The extent of involvement of these structures may be difficult to determine on clinical examination; such knowledge is helpful to optimise treatment. MRI can also identify clinically occult metastatic lymph nodes in the inguinal regions and in the pelvis, the presence of which upstages the disease, irrespective of the size of the primary tumour (see *Table 8.1*).

Staging accuracy

There are limited prospective data published on the accuracy of MR staging in carcinoma of the vulva. A small retrospective series suggests a staging accuracy of 70% for the T stage of the primary tumour. Sensitivity for detection of superficial inguinal lymph node metastases ranges from 40% to 90% depending on the techniques used.

Imaging features

Primary tumour

This is best seen on T2-weighted scans as an intermediate signal intensity mass or thickening of the vulval skin. The relationship of the tumour to the clitoris, urethra, vagina and anus are important prognostically, and if deep invasion is suspected, T2-weighted images in the sagittal or coronal planes can be helpful to assess the cranial extent of tumour. Invasion is indicated by replacement of the relatively hypointense muscular coats of the urethra, vagina or anorectum by intermediate signal intensity tumour, contiguous with the vulval primary tumour. The axial T2-weighted sequence is also helpful to assess the other genital tract organs, since occasionally, a vulvo-vaginal tumour is metastatic from endometrial or ovarian carcinoma.

Lymph node

Lymph nodes can be assessed on all sequences, the T1-weighted sequences providing morphological information (size, shape, margin, presence of a fatty hilum) and the T2-weighted sequences a degree of tissue characterisation (nodal signal intensity, presence of cystic areas) which together can improve the discrimination between reactive and metastatic nodes over that achieved using lymph node diameters alone. Inguinal lymph nodes having a long axis diameter > 21 mm, short axis diameter >10 mm, long : short axis ratio <1.3, irregularity of contour (including clumping of nodes), or cystic changes are abnormal. Contour irregularity and cystic change are the most reliable predictive signs of metastasis, indicating respectively extranodal spread and squamous cell carcinoma deposits.

Post-operative/recurrent tumour

Assessment of the vulva for residual tumour is difficult in the early post-operative period due to inflammatory changes and anatomical distortion. Reactive changes may cause false-positive assessment of inguinal lymph nodes if imaging is carried out soon after significant vulval resection. Recurrent tumour usually arises in the residual vulval tissue, or in the inguinofemoral lymph nodes because deep inguinal and femoral nodes frequently remain after inguinal lymph node resection.

Pitfalls of MRI

Staging the primary vulval tumour

The superficial extent of vulval tumour is assessed clinically; MRI has advantages in identifying deep tumour extension.

- Stage I carcinoma may be too small to visualise on MRI.

- Larger stage I or II tumours that are *en plaque* may be difficult to identify, or distinguish from chronic inflammatory changes on the vulva.

- Superficial invasion can be difficult to exclude in tumours confined to the labia, but lying adjacent to the urethral orifice, introitus or anal margin.

Staging the inguinal lymph nodes

- In obese patients, with a large fatty apron, surface coils may be a significant distance from the inguinal lymph node chains, reducing signal : noise ratio.

- In obese patients, it may be difficult to judge the depth of lymph nodes from the surface, requiring careful positioning of the FOV to ensure complete coverage of superficial and deep inguinal lymph nodes.

- Hip replacements or other orthopaedic hardware in the pelvic region, may interfere with signal : noise in the inguinal regions, reducing image quality.

- The field of view should be centred over the symphysis pubis and should extend to the lateral end of the inguinal ligament, to cover the lateral group of superficial inguinal nodes.

- Lymph node enlargement can be secondary to inflammatory changes in the perineum or lower limb.

- Microscopic metastases are not visible by MRI.

FURTHER READING

1. Marsden DE and Hacker NH. (2001) Contemporary management of Primary carcinoma of the Vulva. *Gynecologic Oncology.* 81: 799–813. *Review of the clinical management of vulval carcinoma.*

2. Vulval Cancer (1999). In: *Guidance on Commissioning Cancer Services. Improving Outcomes in Gynaecological Cancers. The Research Evidence.* NHS Executive, pp.131–133. *Summary of the research evidence for current management of vulval carcinoma.*

3. Odicino F, Favalli G, Zigliani L and Pecorelli S. (2001) Staging of Gynecologic malignancies. *Gynecologic Oncology.* 81 (4): 753–770. *Describes the current staging system for vulval carcinoma.*

4. Sohaib SA, Richards PS, Ind T, Jeyarajah AR, Shepherd JH, Jacobs IJ and Reznek RH. (2002) MR imaging of carcinoma of the vulva. *Am. J. Roentgenol.* 178(2): 373–377. *Retrospective review of MRI findings in 22 patients with vulval carcinoma.*

5. Hawnaur JM, Reynolds K, Wilson G, Hillier V, Kitchener HC. (2002) Identification of inguinal lymph node metastases from vulval carcinoma by magnetic resonance imaging: an initial report. *Clin. Radiol.* 57: 995–1000. *Describes the technique and results of high resolution MRI for staging the inguinal lymph nodes in vulval cancer.*

6. Grey AC, Carrington BM, Hulse PA, Swindell R and Yates W. (2000) Magnetic resonance appearance of normal inguinal nodes. *Clin. Radiol.* 55: 124–130. *Defines normal values for inguinal lymph node measurements on pelvic MRI.*

7. Moskovic EC, Shepherd JH, Barton DP, Trott PA, Nasiri N and Thomas JM. (1999) The role of high resolution ultrasound with guided cytology of groin lymph nodes in the management of squamous cell carcinoma of the vulva: a pilot study. *Br. J. Obstet. Gynaecol.* 106(8): 863–867. *Study using ultrasound to stage the inguinal lymph nodes in vulval cancer.*

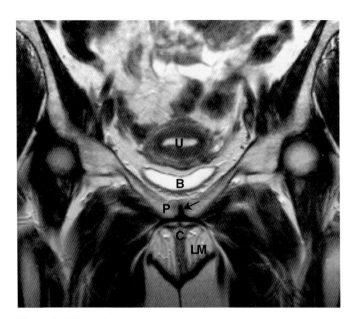

Figure 8.1. Normal vulval anatomy.

Coronal T2WI showing normal vulval anatomy. Clitoris (C); labium majora (LM); body of pubis (P); bladder (B); uterus (U); symphysis pubis (arrow).

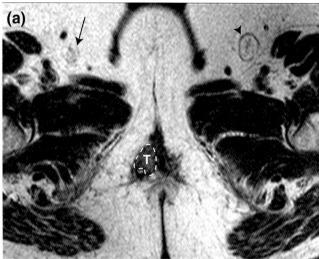

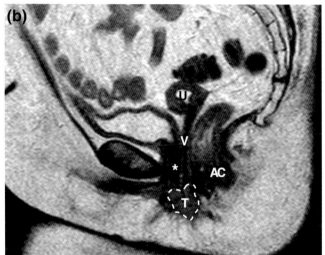

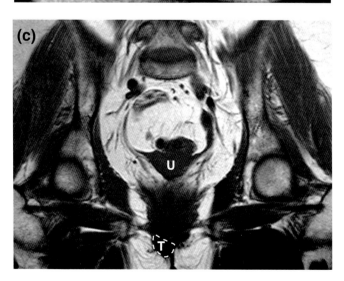

Figure 8.2. T1 Vulval carcinoma.

(a) Transaxial T2W (b) sagittal T2W and (c) coronal T1W images showing a small (<2.0 cm) tumour (T) (enclosed by hatched line) confined to the right side of the vulva, adjacent to but not invading the perineal structures. Normal lymph node (arrow), normal lymph node with fatty replacement (arrowhead), uterus (U), vagina (V), anal canal (AC), urethra (asterisk).

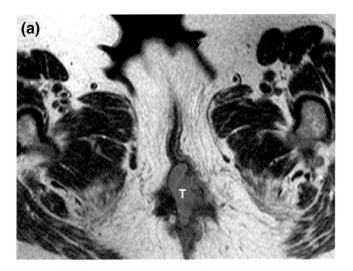

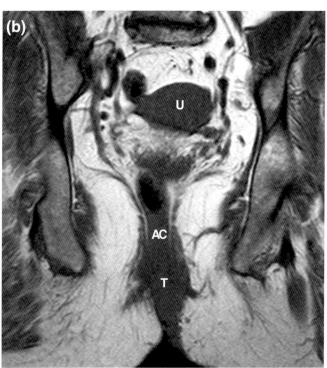

Figure 8.3. T2 Vulval carcinoma – posterior tumour.

(a) Transaxial T2WI and (b) coronal T1WI showing tumour (T) exceeding 2.0 cm in diameter centred on the posterior aspect of the left side of the vulva. Uterus (U); anal canal (AC).

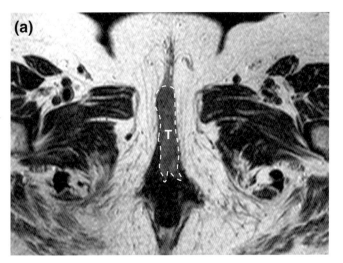

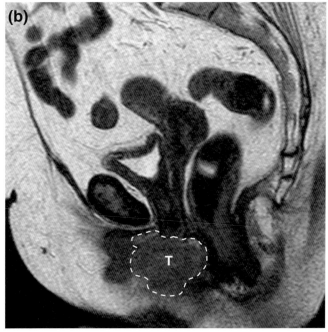

Figure 8.4. T2 Vulval carcinoma – anterior tumour.

(a) Transaxial T2WI and (b) sagittal T2WI showing tumour (T) (enclosed by hatched line) exceeding 2.0 cm in diameter centred on the anterior aspect of the left side of the vulva. There is possible vaginal and urethral involvement suggested on the sagittal image but this was excluded by interrogation of more cranially located transaxial images.

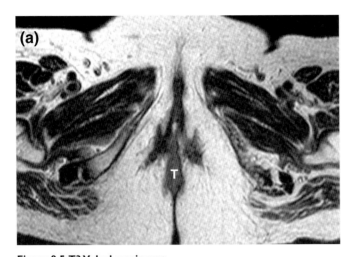

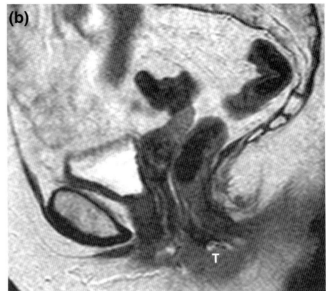

Figure 8.5.T3 Vulval carcinoma.

(a) Transaxial T2WI and (b) sagittal T2WI showing posteriorly located vulval tumour (T), which has spread to anal margin.

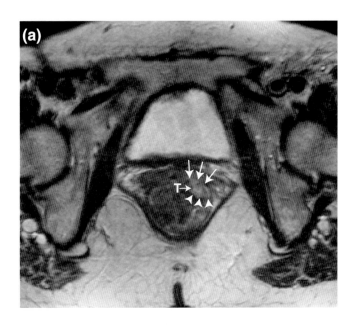

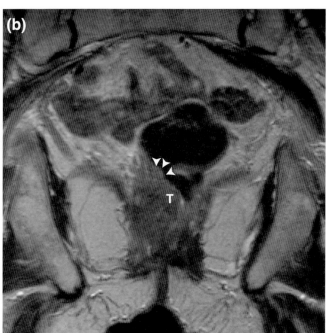

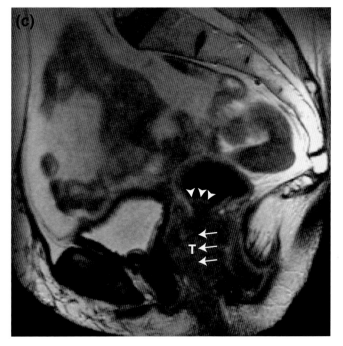

Figure 8.6. T4 Vulval carcinoma.

(a) Transaxial T2WI (b) coronal T2WI and (c) sagittal T2WI showing extensive vulval carcinoma. The tumour (T) has extended through the vagina (arrows) to infiltrate the anal canal and rectum at the ano-rectal junction (arrowheads), staging this as T4 disease. With such large tumours differentiation between those of vulval and vaginal origin can be difficult. Locating the epicentre of the lesion and review of the clinical history and examination findings are useful indicators.

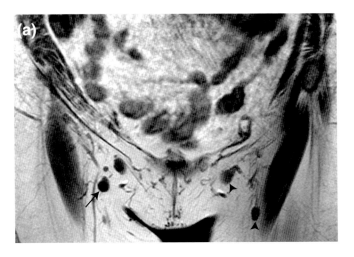
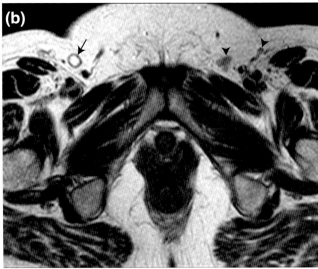

Figure 8.7. N1 Vulval carcinoma.

(a) Coronal T1WI and (b) transaxial T2WI showing a cystic metastasis in a right superficial inguinal lymph node (arrows). There are normal left inguinal nodes (arrowheads). The T1WI demonstrates that the metastatic node is not composed of fat.

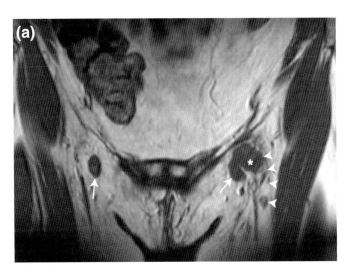
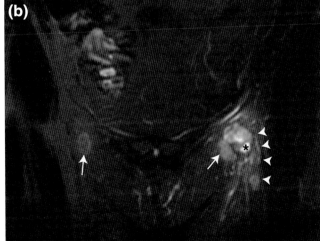

Figure 8.8. N2 Vulval carcinoma.

(a) Coronal T1WI and (b) coronal T2W fat-suppressed image showing bilateral enlarged metastatic superficial inguinal lymph nodes (arrows). On the left side there is extranodal spread (arrowheads) shown to advantage in (b) and a cystic area (asterisk) due to nodal necrosis.

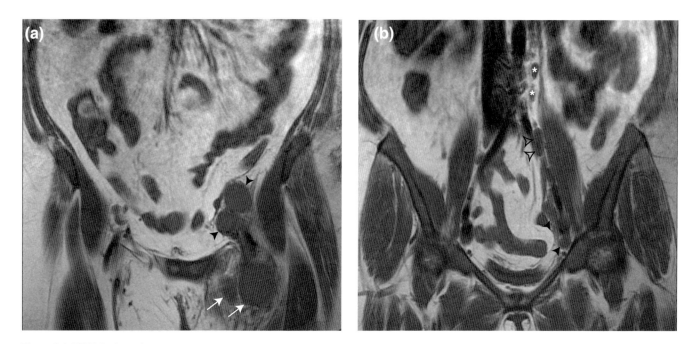

Figure 8.9. N2 Vulval carcinoma

(a) and (b) Coronal T1W images showing left inguinal (arrows), left external iliac (arrowheads), left common iliac (open arrowheads) and left para-aortic lymph node (asterisk) metastases.

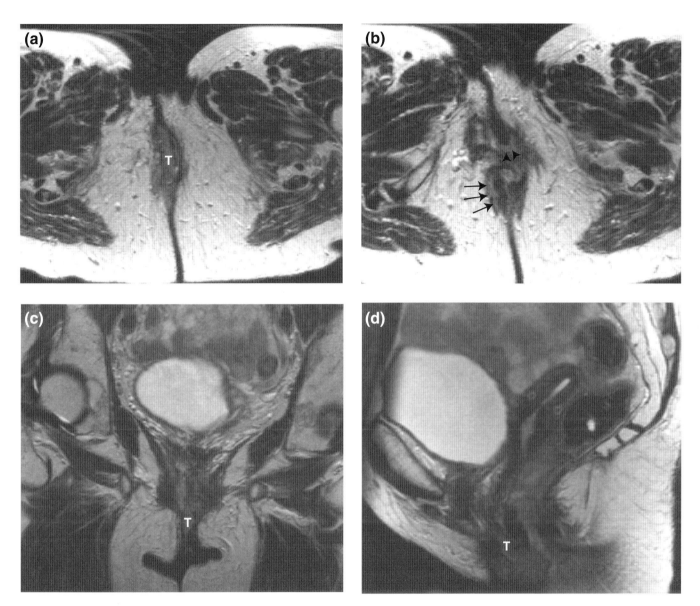

Figure 8.10. Recurrent vulval carcinoma.

(a) and (b) Transaxial T2WI (c) coronal T2WI and (d) sagittal T2WI showing recurrent vulval cancer following radiotherapy. The tumour (T) is centred on the right side of the natal cleft. It infiltrates the external anal sphincter (arrows) and vagina at the introitus (arrowheads). Surgical treatment of this lesion would involve an extended radical vulvectomy and colonic stoma formation. (Figure courtesy of Dr. Hulse, Christie Hospital.)

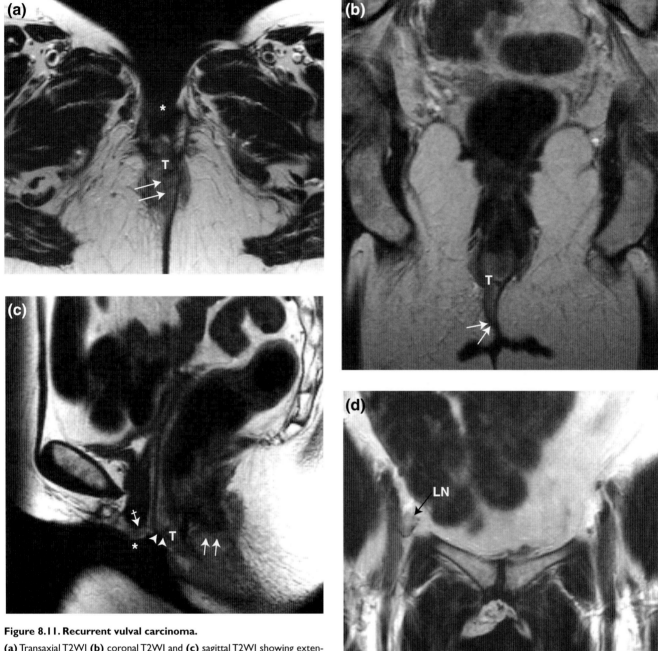

Figure 8.11. Recurrent vulval carcinoma.

(a) Transaxial T2WI (b) coronal T2WI and (c) sagittal T2WI showing extensive recurrent vulval carcinoma, following radical vulvectomy. The vulvectomy void (asterisk) is evident in (a) and (c). The tumour (T) has infiltrated the anus (arrows), posterior margin of the vagina (arrowheads) and the perineal aspect of the distal urethra (crossed arrow). (d) Coronal T2WI in the same patient showing a right inguinal lymph node metastasis (LN) which has an irregular margin indicating extranodal extension of tumour. (Figure courtesy of Dr. Carrington, Christie Hospital.)

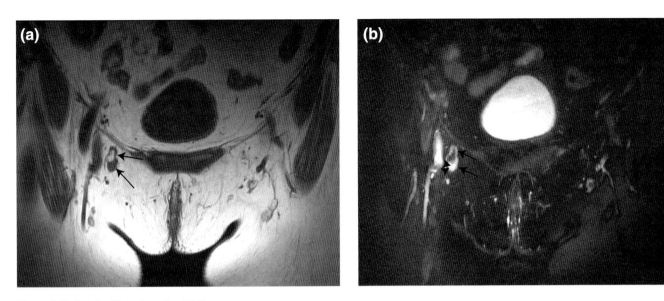

Figure 8.12. Inguinal lymph node pitfall

(a) Coronal T1WI and (b) coronal fat-suppressed T2WI in a patient who had a vulvectomy for vulval carcinoma a few weeks previously. There is an enlarged right inguinal lymph node (arrows) which has a hyperintense focus in its lower pole (arrowheads) in (b). This is an equivocal finding for a metastatic or hyperplastic node, although the high signal focus favours metastatic disease. On histology it was benign.

9 Rectal Cancer

Michael Dobson

BACKGROUND INFORMATION

Epidemiology

Colorectal cancer is the fourth most common cancer worldwide. There are approximately 130000 cases per year in the USA, causing 56000 deaths. More than 35000 new cases are diagnosed each year in the UK, making colorectal cancer the second commonest malignancy in women and the third commonest in men. Over thirty percent of colorectal cancer arises in the rectum.

Aetiological factors include:

- Diet: genetically mediated susceptibility to dietary mutagens (e.g. heterocyclic amines in cooked red meats); bile acids; low dietary folate in combination with high alcohol intake.

- Pre-existing polyps: these may be sporadic (especially villous adenomas) or relate to hereditary polyposis syndromes. The familial polyposis gene on chromosome 21 and the p53 gene on chromosome 17 have also been implicated in a substantial number of sporadic carcinomas.

- Prolonged ulcerative colitis.

- Smoking tobacco.

Protective factors against colorectal cancer include: increased dietary fibre, reduced animal fat, supplements of vitamin D, folate, and anti-oxidants such as vitamin E.

There is increasing evidence in favour of screening for colorectal cancer using combinations of faecal occult blood testing, sigmoidoscopy, colonoscopy, and double contrast barium enema. Research is ongoing into the role of CT colonography as a diagnostic and screening tool.

Histopathology

Most colorectal cancers are moderately well differentiated gland-forming adenocarcinomas. Less common cell types include signet ring adenocarcinoma (see *Linitis Plastica* in Pitfalls section), adenosquamous carcinoma, squamous cell carcinoma, small cell carcinoma, choriocarcinoma and medullary cell carcinoma. Colorectal carcinoid tumours occasionally occur (more commonly in the rectum) and arise in the submucosa. Sarcomas (usually leiomyosarcoma) are more rare, comprising up to 0.3% of colorectal tumours.

Patterns of tumour spread

Rectal cancers arise in the mucosa, usually in a pre-existing adenomatous polyp. Tumours advance radially through the layers of the bowel wall, longitudinal spread is uncommon. Following breach of the bowel wall, spread occurs directly into the meso-rectum (see below) and then progressively into adjacent pelvic structures.

Lymphatic spread occurs initially to the meso-rectal and pre-sacral nodes adjacent to the tumour, and thence along the course of the superior rectal vessels. More advanced lymph node spread involves the internal and external iliac chains, and the para-aortic nodes. The current staging system (*Tables 9.1* and *9.2*) only accounts for loco-regional nodal disease.

Haematogenous spread is apparent in up to 15% of patients at presentation and occurs most commonly to the liver by the portal venous route and lungs via the systemic circulation. Spread to the lungs is more common for tumours of the lower rectum because of systemic (middle and inferior rectal veins) drainage compared with

---

Table 9.1. TNM (2002) System for staging rectal cancer

Primary tumour (T)
TX:	Primary tumour cannot be assessed
T0:	No evidence of primary tumour
Tis:	Carcinoma *in situ*
T1:	Tumour invades submucosa
T2:	Tumour invades muscularis propria
T3:	Tumour invades through the muscularis propria into the subserosa, or into the nonperitonealised peri-rectal tissues
T4:	Tumour directly invades other organs or structures and/or perforates visceral peritoneum

Regional lymph nodes (N)
NX:	Regional lymph nodes cannot be assessed
N0:	No regional lymph node metastasis
N1:	Metastasis in 1 to 3 regional lymph nodes
N2:	Metastasis in 4 or more regional lymph nodes

Distant metastasis (M)
MX:	Distant metastasis cannot be assessed
M0:	No distant metastasis
M1:	Distant metastasis

Note: Even in the absence of identifiable lymph node tissue, a tumour nodule larger than 3.0 mm diameter in the peri-rectal fat is classified as a peri-rectal lymph node metastasis. A nodule ≤ 3.0 mm is classified as noncontiguous tumour extension (i.e. T3 disease).

the upper rectum, which drains into the portal system, by the superior rectal vein. Metastases to the brain and skeleton occur less commonly.

Table 9.2. Combined modified Dukes' and TNM systems for staging rectal cancer

	TNM		Modified Dukes'
Tis	N0	M0	
T1,T2	N0	M0	A
T3,T4	N0	M0	B
Any T	N1, N2	M0	C*
Any T	Any N	M1	D

Note: * Dukes' C stage is divided into C1 and C2. C1 indicates peritumoural lymph node infiltration, but not up to the point of surgical ligation. C2 indicates nodal involvement at the highest point of ligation and has a significantly worse prognosis.

Prognostic indicators

- Advancing tumour stage. Tumour confined to the bowel wall has an average 80% 5-year survival, falling to 50% if there is transmural disease without lymph node involvement. This figure falls as low as 12% where there is lymph node involvement up to the point of surgical ligation (Dukes' C2).
- Tumour involving the circumferential resection margin is associated with increased risk of local recurrence and a 5-year survival of 15%.
- High tumour grade.
- Perineural, vascular or lymphatic invasion.
- Mucinous histology.
- Infiltrative (as opposed to well defined) margin of extra-mural spread.
- *Linitis Plastica*.
- Age below forty years at presentation.

Treatment

Surgery
Best surgical practice for rectal cancer is total meso-rectal excision (TME), that is, removal of the tumour *en bloc* with the surrounding meso-rectum invested in the visceral meso-rectal fascia. The meso-rectum comprises the peri-rectal fat, containing the rectal vessels and perirectal lymph nodes, extending from the region of the aortic bifurcation to the inter-sphincteric groove. The plane of resection lies between the inner (visceral) and outer (parietal) layers of the meso-rectal fascia. Radial growth of tumour (primary or nodal) close to or into this plane greatly increases the risk of a positive circumferential resection margin at histology with associated increased risk of local

recurrence, and a reduced 5-year survival. A positive circumferential tumour margin is defined as tumour involving or lying within 1.0 mm of the resected visceral meso-rectal fascia.

Radiotherapy
Short course (5 days) neo-adjuvant (pre-operative) radiotherapy has been shown to reduce the rate of local recurrence for rectal cancer even if the patient has an expert TME. There is concern, however, that treating patients with early T3 or lesser stage disease would lead to unnecessary irradiation for a large number of patients. Research is ongoing into the development of evidence based, stage-related therapeutic protocols. Patients with a clinically fixed tumour or with evidence of meso-rectal fascial infiltration on MR imaging are generally referred for a long course (typically 5 weeks) of neo-adjuvant radiotherapy.

Chemotherapy
There is clear evidence of survival benefit for post-operative chemotherapy in patients with N1 or N2 (Dukes' C) tumours. Research is ongoing into the role of chemotherapy for patients with N0 (Dukes' B) lesions.

MR IMAGING OF RECTAL CANCER

Technique

The tumour is localised using a T2-weighted turbo (or fast) spin echo (TSE or FSE) sequence in the sagittal plane. High resolution (3.0 mm) T2-weighted images are then acquired *perpendicular to the tumour* to allow assessment of the circumferential extent of the lesion. A pelvic phased array coil is required for images of suitable quality. Endo-rectal coils are not required and may have inherent problems (see below). Smooth muscle relaxants improve image quality, though not necessarily staging accuracy. Similarly, intravenous contrast enhancement and endo-rectal contrast agents may increase the conspicuity of the tumour though not influence tumour staging.

Current indications

There is no routine indication for MR imaging in the staging of colon cancer. However, pre-operative staging of rectal cancer with pelvic phased array coil MR imaging is rapidly evolving as a routine procedure. MR accurately determines the proximity of tumours to the meso-rectal fascia, allowing identification of patients who may benefit from neo-adjuvant radiotherapy. Conversely, MR accurately defines earlier stages of disease, preventing unnecessary use of neo-adjuvant radiotherapy in these patients.

Staging accuracy

Staging accuracy of up to 82% for local tumour staging has been reported. This, however, takes into account studies that used inherently low-resolution body coil techniques. More recently, 100% correlation with histological staging was demonstrated using a pelvic phased array coil and high-resolution technique. Local staging accuracy of 84% has been quoted for endo-rectal coil techniques. However, acquisition of an image plane perpendicular to the tumour may not always be possible using endo-anal MRI and technical difficulties may also arise with high rectal tumours or a tightly stenotic lesion. Near-field flaring may also occur with endo-rectal techniques, although most manufacturers have developed software to overcome this problem.

Sensitivity for nodal infiltration has been reported as 65%, though this may improve with higher resolution techniques and detailed assessment of nodal morphology. Research is ongoing into the efficacy of super-paramagnetic iron oxide contrast agents in identifying malignant nodes in a variety of pelvic tumours including rectal cancer.

MRI has been shown to be superior to CT for the identification and characterisation of malignant liver lesions, when current techniques have been compared in most reports since 1990. A recent study comparing super-paramagnetic iron oxide MRI and dual-phase CT demonstrated a better sensitivity for MR (80.6%) than CT (73.5%) in the demonstration of colorectal liver metastases. In addition, MRI has been shown to be more sensitive than CT in the identification of extra-hepatic disease.

Imaging features

Primary tumour

There are five layers of the normal rectal wall, namely: mucosa, muscularis mucosa, submucosa, circular and longitudinal muscle (muscularis propria). Although all five layers may be seen on high resolution T2WI, this is rarely the case. In most cases, the mucosa and submucosa are seen as a single high signal layer deep to the low signal muscularis propria. The normal rectal wall should be no more than 6 mm thick in the distended state. Rectal tumours are usually of intermediate intensity compared with the muscularis propria of the bowel wall on T2WI. Mucinous tumours return a high signal due to high fluid content. Important features to be assessed are:

- T stage;
- proximity of tumour to the meso-rectal fascia;
- proximity of tumour to the anal sphincter;
- presence of meso-rectal nodes and peri-rectal tumour deposits and their proximity to the meso-rectal fascia;
- peri-vascular infiltration.

Lymph node disease

In common with various other tumour types, enlarged nodes in the presence of rectal cancer may be simply inflammatory and non-enlarged nodes may contain tumour. Pointers towards malignancy include an overtly infiltrative gland margin, nodal necrosis and signal intensity similar to the primary tumour (such as high signal nodes infiltrated by mucinous tumour). Proximity of suspicious nodes to the meso-rectal fascia should be noted as this may compromise the surgical plane and the patient may benefit from neo-adjuvant radiotherapy.

Post treatment appearances

Radiotherapy. The effects of rectal irradiation depend upon the total radiation dose, and will be more pronounced following a long (five weeks) course of treatment compared with the shorter five day regime. In the acute and sub-acute post treatment phases (up to twelve months post therapy) changes on MRI reflect cell death and inflammation. Hence, there may be visceral mural thickening (e.g. bowel, bladder, vagina, urethra), increased mucosal and submucosal signal on T2WI, and mucosal enhancement with intravenous contrast agents. The chronic effects of radiotherapy reflect fibrosis. Therefore, there may still be visceral mural thickening, though this will usually return low signal on T1 and T2WI and show little or no intravenous contrast enhancement. Other changes include peri-rectal fascial and peritoneal thickening, inflammation and atrophy of adjacent pelvic muscles and fatty marrow change (high signal on T1WI) in involved bone. More severe changes may include strictures of bowel and fistulation (e.g. recto-vaginal or recto-vesical).

Surgery. Both anterior resection and abdomino-perineal (APR) total meso-rectal excision may produce pre-sacral and peri-rectal fibrotic change. This is usually more pronounced following an APR. Also, post APR, there may be a pre-sacral 'pseudo-mass' on CT and T1WI due to the uterus, prostate or seminal vesicles occupying the void in the rectal bed. This should be readily discernible on T2WI.

Recurrent disease

Pelvic recurrence has been reported in up to 50% of patients with rectal cancer, though following TME with negative circumferential resection margins, this figure falls to less than 10%. Recurrent tumour usually manifests as a mass returning intermediate signal intensity on T2WI compared with muscle. However, radiation fibrosis may also return intermediate signal especially within the first two years following irradiation. Also, although fibrotic tissue returns low signal on T1 and T2WI, the same may apply to desmoplastic foci of tumour. Dynamic intravenous contrast-enhanced MR imaging may add to the specificity of diagnosing recurrent disease. MR imaging is accurate in assessing the extent of proven recurrent tumour and can significantly aid the planning of further 'salvage' surgery (see chapter 14).

Pitfalls of MRI

- **Tumour identification on the planning T2-weighted sagittal view:** This may be difficult, though it is crucial to further imaging. Knowledge of the tumour site at sigmoidoscopy is very important and should be included in the clinical information. Tumour is usually of intermediate signal intensity relative to the muscularis propria and flatus. At the site of tumour, there is often loss of detail of the different layers of the rectal wall, which is thickened, except in the case of T1 lesions. Other useful pointers may be the presence of blood vessels entering the tumour, or occasionally, bowel wall retraction at the tumour site. Smooth muscle relaxants and intravenous contrast enhancement may increase tumour conspicuity, but, with experience, are seldom required. There may be synchronous tumours in the rectum or colon. Careful review of the sagittal MR image should exclude the former, though the patient will also require formal colonic evaluation by colonoscopy ('virtual' or fibre-optic) or barium enema.

- **Over-staging due to peri-tumoural fibrosis:** This appears as linear, low signal stranding into the meso-rectal fat, as opposed to tumour, which has a nodular interface with the meso-rectum, and usually returns intermediate signal.

- **Over-staging due to partial volume artifact:** This should be minimised by meticulous attention to detail when planning the high-resolution sequence perpendicular to the tumour.

- **Intra-vascular tumour infiltration:** This is defined as tumour tissue extending to infiltrate a vessel or as satellite deposits in the meso-rectal fat.

- **Adjacent visceral infiltration:** This is clear evidence of the primary tumour extending *into* the adjacent viscera. Contiguity of the tumour with an adjacent organ does not necessarily indicate invasion and peri-tumoural fibrosis or inflammation may cause over-staging in these cases.

- **Nodal disease:** MR imaging remains inaccurate in the assessment of meso-rectal lymph node metastasis, though there are some useful discriminating features such as round shape, irregular margin or increased signal intensity on T2WI indicating central nodal necrosis or a mucinous tumour deposit.

- **Recurrent disease:** Radiation effect and/or surgical changes may give rise to an intermediate signal pre-sacral mass, mimicking tumour recurrence. Recurrent disease may return low signal due to desmoplasia, mimicking simple fibrosis. Biopsy may be required to clarify this although sampling errors can be problematical. Alternatively, repeat interval imaging and observation for recurrent disease outside of the pre-sacral area is valuable.

- **Intussuscepted tumour** makes it difficult to precisely T stage the tumour as the interface with adjacent fat is not evident. However, an intussuscepted tumour cannot be fixed and should be evident on the sagittal view. The key feature on the perpendicular image is the presence of several layers of muscularis propria.

- *Linitis Plastica.* This is a rare form of rectal cancer where malignant 'signet ring' cells or undifferentiated carcinoma diffusely infiltrate the submucosa and muscularis propria, with relative sparing of the mucosa. On T1WI there is marked thickening of the rectal wall and meso-rectal fascia. On T2WI there may be a ring pattern in the rectal wall due to a combination of tumour infiltration and fibrosis around intact layers of the muscularis propria. Early

recognition is important as it may guide the physician to perform deep biopsies (if the mucosa is spared). Also, because the prognosis is very poor, the patient may be spared unnecessary major surgery.

FURTHER READING

1. Skibber JM, Minsky BD and Hoff PM. (2001) Cancer of the colon. In: *Cancer. Principles and Practice of Oncology*, 6th Edn (eds DeVita VT Jr., Hellman S, Rosenberg SA). Lippincott, Williams and Wilkins, Philadelphia, Pensylvania, USA, pp. 1216–1271. *This is a definitive, comprehensive and up to date text on all aspects of rectal cancer and its management.*

2. Souhami R and Tobias J. (1995) Tumours of the small and large bowel. In: *Cancer and its management*, 2nd Edn. Blackwell Science, Oxford, UK, pp. 305–316. *A more concise though equally authoritative chapter on all aspects of rectal cancer.*

3. Heald RJ. (1995) Total mesorectal excision is optimal surgery for rectal cancer: a Scandinavian Consensus. *Br. J. Surg.* 82: 1297–1299. *This paper defines the best surgical practice for patients with operable rectal cancer.*

4. Adam IJ, Mohamdee MO, Martin IG, Scott N, Finan PJ, Johnston D, Dixon MF, Quirke P. (1994) Role of circumferential margin involvement in the local recurrence of rectal cancer. *Lancet* 344: 707–711. *This paper highlights the increased risk of local tumour recurrence in patients with positive circumferential resection margins following rectal cancer surgery.*

5. Bissett IP, Fernando CC, Hough DM et al. (2001) Identification of the fascia propria by magnetic resonance imaging and its relevance to pre-operative assessment of rectal cancer. *Dis. Colon Rectum* 44(2): 259–265. *Elegant confirmation of the MR appearances of the meso-rectal fascia by cadaveric imaging.*

6. Kapiteijn E, Marijnen CAM, Nagstegaal ID et al. (2001) Preoperative radiotherapy combined with total mesorectal excision for resectable rectal cancer. *N. Engl. J. Med.* 345(9): 638–646. *Large controlled trial proving that short-course pre-operative radiotherapy reduces the risk of local recurrence in patients with rectal cancer who have had a standardised TME.*

7. Beets-Tan RG, Beets GL, Vliegen RF et al. (2001) Accuracy of MR imaging in the prediction of tumour–free resection margins in rectal cancer surgery. *Lancet* 357: 497–504. *This paper demonstrates that the distance of tumour from the meso-rectal fascia can be accurately predicted on pre-operative MR imaging, allowing identification of patients at risk for positive resection margins.*

8. Brown G, Richardson CJ, Newcombe RG et al. (1999) Rectal carcinoma: thin-section MR imaging for staging in 28 patients. *Radiology* 211(1): 215–222. *Seminal paper on the method and accuracy of high resolution MR imaging in defining the stage and depth of extra-mural invasion of rectal cancer extent using surface phased array coils.*

9. Kwok H, Bissett IP and Hill GL. (2000) Pre-operative staging of rectal cancer. *Int. J. Colorectal Dis.* 15: 9–20. *A large meta-analysis of almost 5000 patients in 83 studies comparing CT, MRI and endoanal ultrasound for staging rectal cancer.*

10. Okizuka H, Sugimura K, Yoshizako et al. (1996) Rectal Carcinoma: Prospective comparison of conventional and gadopentate dimeglumine enhanced fat-suppressed MR imaging. *J. Magn. Reson. Imaging* 6: 465–471. *A study of thirty two patients showing that fat-suppressed, Gd-enhanced T1-weighted images give excellent rectal cancer detection though do not improve staging accuracy compared with non-enhanced images.*

11. Dicle O, Obuz F and Cacmakci H. (1999) Differentiation of recurrent rectal cancer and scarring with dynamic MR imaging. *Br. J. Radiol.* 72: 1155–1159. *This small study (n=19) supports the use of quantitative dynamic contrast enhanced MR imaging in distinguishing locally recurrent rectal cancer from benign tissue.*

12. Hawnaur JM, Zhu XP and Hutchinson CE. (1998) Quantitative dynamic contrast-enhanced MRI of recurrent pelvic masses in patients treated for cancer. *Br. J. Radiol.* 71(851): 1136–1142. *This study (n=32) showed that the combination of quantitative dynamic MR imaging, signal intensity and tissue morphology on conventional MR Images may be helpful in distinguishing recurrent pelvic tumour from benign disease.*

13. Robinson P, Carrington BM, Swindell R et al. (2002) Recurrent or residual bowel cancer: Accuracy of MRI Local Extent Before Salvage Surgery. *Clin. Radiol.* 57: 514–522. *The most thorough assessment to date of the ability of MRI to detail the extent of recurrent tumour, and its usefulness in pre-operative surgical planning.*

14. Semelka RC and Helmberger TK. (2001). Contrast agents for MR Imaging of the liver. *Radiology* 218: 27–38. *Excellent review of state-of-the-art MRI contrast liver imaging.*

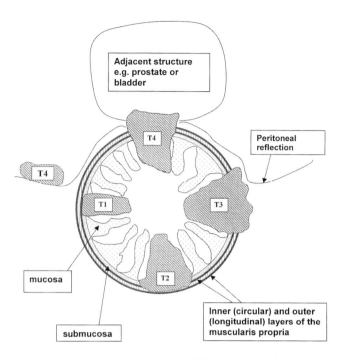

Figure 9.1. Schematic diagram of the T-Staging of rectal cancer.

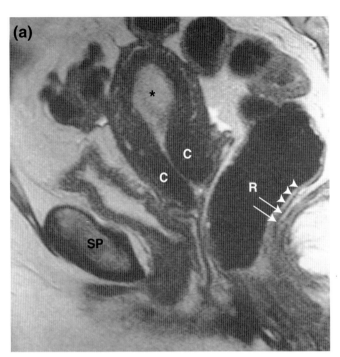

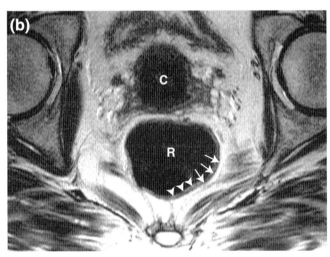

Figure 9.2. Normal rectum.

(a) Sagittal T2WI and **(b)** Transaxial T2WI of normal rectum. Note signal void due to gas in the rectal lumen (R), high signal combination of mucosa and submucosa (arrowheads) and the low signal muscularis propria (arrows). Symphysis pubis (SP). Intermediate signal endometrial tumour (asterisk), cervix (C).

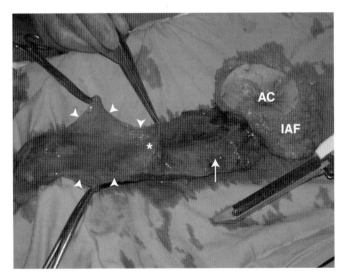

Figure 9.3. Lateral view of a surgical specimen from an abdomino-perineal TME.

Note the peritoneal reflection (arrowheads) and the Pouch of Douglas (asterisk), the uterus having been removed. Peritoneum covers the anterior and lateral aspects of the upper two thirds of the rectum. The lower third of rectum is circumferentially invested by meso-rectal fascia the visceral surface of which (arrow) invests the surgical specimen. Note the anus (AC) and the ischio-anal fossa fat (IAF).

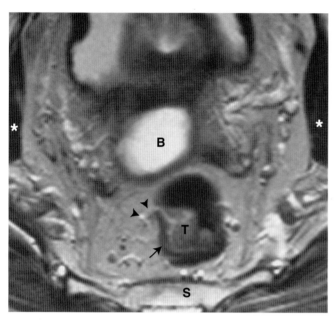

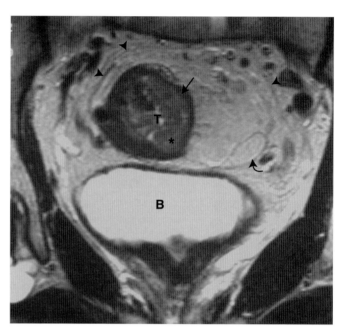

Figure 9.4. T1 Rectal cancer.

Transaxial T2WI of the lower third of rectum. Note the intact muscularis propria (arrow). The tumour (T) can be distinguished from faecal residue by the fact that there is a vessel entering the mass (arrowheads). Bladder (B), obturator internus muscles (asterisk) and sacrum (S).

Figure 9.5. T2 Rectal cancer.

T2WI perpendicular to an upper rectal tumour (T). Note the muscularis propria (arrow), which is focally infiltrated (asterisk) by the tumour. Note the peritoneal reflection (curved arrow) and piecemeal depiction of the meso-rectal fascia (arrowheads). Bladder (B)

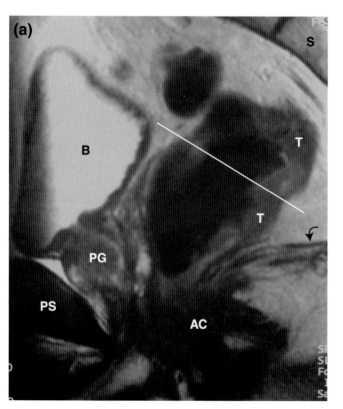

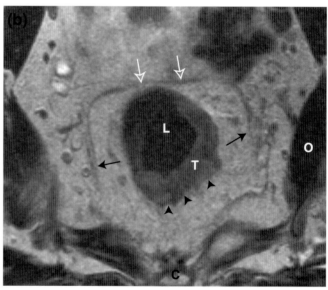

Figure 9.6. T3 Lower third rectal cancer.

(a) Sagittal T2WI demonstrating a posterior wall lower third rectal tumour (T) and (b) high resolution T2WI perpendicular to the tumour. Note the axis planned for the subsequent high-resolution off axis sequence (line). There is a broad front of infiltration into the meso-rectal fat (arrowheads) making this a T3 lesion, though the meso-rectal fascia (circumferential resection margin) is well clear (arrows). Note the peritoneal reflection anteriorly (open arrows), rectal lumen (L), obturator internus muscle (O), coccyx (C) anal canal (AC), levator ani (curved arrow), prostate gland (PG), bladder (B), sacrum (S), pubic symphysis (PS).

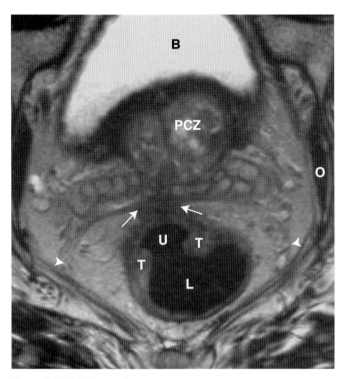

Figure 9.7. T3 Mid-rectal cancer.

High resolution T2WI perpendicular to a tumour (T) of the anterior and right mid-rectal walls. The tumour demonstrates central ulceration (U) and is contiguous anteriorly with the retro-prostatic or Denonvilliers' fascia (arrows) making this T-stage 3 with an involved anterior margin. This patient would benefit from a long course of pre-operative radiotherapy to reduce the risk of a positive anterior resection margin. Note how little space there is between the rectal wall and the meso-rectal fascia anteriorly compared with laterally, making anterior tumours at particular risk for resection margin involvement. Meso-rectal fascia (arrowheads), rectal lumen (L), bladder (B), prostate central zone (PCZ), obturator internus muscle (O).

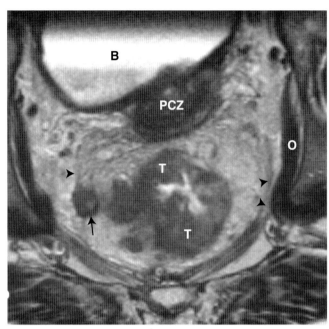

Figure 9.8. T3 Rectal cancer with lateral meso-rectal fascia infiltration.

T2WI perpendicular to an extensive T3 stage mid-rectal tumour (T). There is a broad front of nodular tumour extending into the right side of the meso-rectum with a tumour nodule (arrow) infiltrating the right meso-rectal fascia. This nodule may in fact reflect an infiltrated lymph node. This patient would require a long course of neo-adjuvant radiotherapy to reduce the risk of a positive lateral resection margin. Note the normal meso-rectal fascia elsewhere (arrowheads). Bladder (B), prostate central zone (PCZ), obturator internus muscle (O). An infiltrative tumour edge such as this carries a poorer prognosis than tumours with a better-defined margin such as in *Figure 9.7*.

Figure 9.9. (right) T3 Rectal cancer with intra-vascular infiltration.

T2WI perpendicular to a mid-third rectal tumour (T). Intact muscle is shown around the tumour (closed arrowheads), though there is histologically proven intra-vascular infiltration on the left side (open arrowheads) making this a T3 stage tumour. The intra-vascular infiltration describes a cigar shape extending around the blood vessel. This is in contrast to the more usual broad front of tumour infiltration seen in *Figure 9.8* and the nodular tumour infiltration and fine stranding of peri-tumoural fibrosis seen in *Figure 9.10*. Seminal vesicle (SV), bladder (B), piriformis muscle (P), coccyx (C), obturator internus muscle (O).

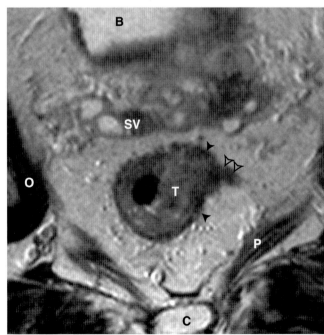

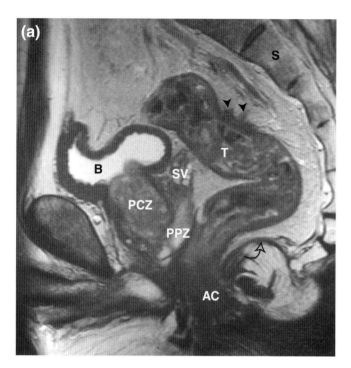

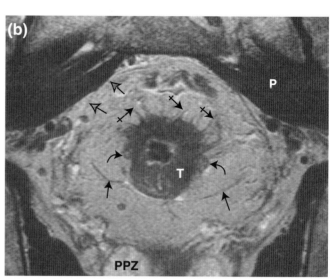

Figure 9.10. T3 Rectal cancer contrasted against peri-tumoural fibrosis.

(a) Sagittal T2W planning image through a bulky upper and mid- third rectal tumour (T) and **(b)** high resolution T2WI perpendicular to the tumour. Note focal infiltration dorsally into the meso-rectum (arrowheads). There is quite extensive fine stranding (crosssed arrows) extending into the dorsal meso-rectal fat. This has been shown to represent peri-tumoural fibrotic change. Additionally however there is a nodular front of infiltrative tumour from the right and left walls (curved arrows) making this a stage T3 lesion. Note the anterior peritoneal reflection (straight arrows), and the meso-rectal fascia (open arrows), which are not infiltrated. Seminal vesicle (SV), prostate central zone (PCZ), prostate peripheral zone (PPZ), bladder (B), levator ani muscle (curved open arrow), anal canal (AC), sacrum (S), piriformis muscle (P).

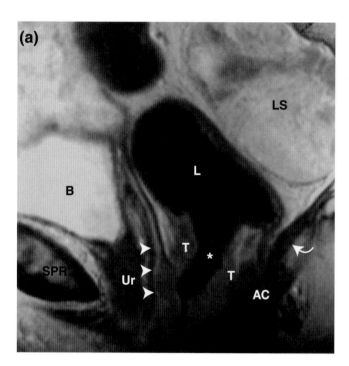

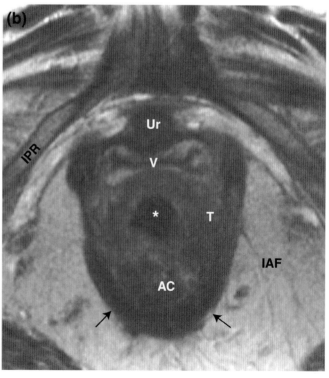

Figure 9.11. T3 Ano-rectal junction cancer.

(a) Sagittal T2WI showing an unusual tumour (T) anteriorly at the ano-rectal junction and **(b)** high resolution T2WI perpendicular to the tumour. The tumour has infiltrated anteriorly into the plane between the vagina (arrowheads) and the anal canal (AC). The vagina (V) is not overtly infiltrated so this is an advanced T3 stage lesion. Urethra (Ur), bladder (B), levator ani (curved arrow), superior pubic ramus (SPR), lower rectal lumen (L), ischio-anal fossa (IAF), inferior pubic ramus (IPR), anal canal (AC). Note the incidental pre-sacral liposarcoma (LS).

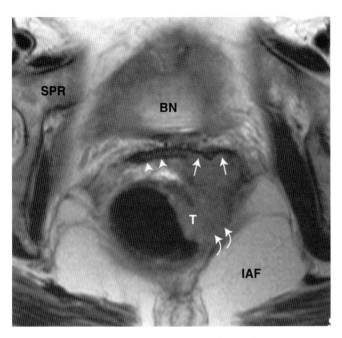

Figure 9.12. T4 Lower rectal cancer infiltrating vagina.

T2WI perpendicular to a tumour of the left side of lower rectum (T) just above the ano-rectal junction. Tumour extends anteriorly to infiltrate the left posterior vaginal wall where the muscle layer is destroyed (arrows). Note the intact posterior vaginal muscle on the right (arrowheads). This is therefore a T4 lesion. There is a broad base of contiguity with the left levator ani muscle (curved arrows), which was also infiltrated. Ischio-anal fossa (IAF), right superior pubic ramus (SPR), bladder neck (BN).

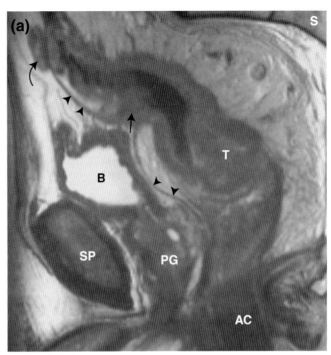

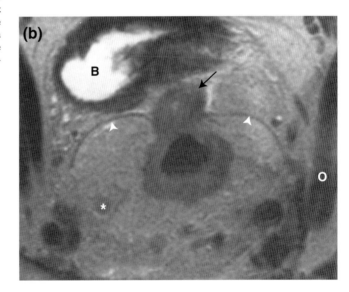

Figure 9.13. T4 mid- and upper rectal cancer with peritoneal infiltration.

(a) Sagittal T2WI through an extensive mid- and upper third rectal tumour (T) and (b) T2WI perpendicular to the more caudal part of the tumour. The peritoneal reflection (arrowheads) is thickened with focal nodular peritoneal deposits (arrows) making this a T stage 4 lesion. Note the enlarged mesorectal node (asterisk), Prostate gland (PG), anal canal (AC), symphysis pubis (SP), bladder (B), sacrum (S). left obturator internus muscle (O).

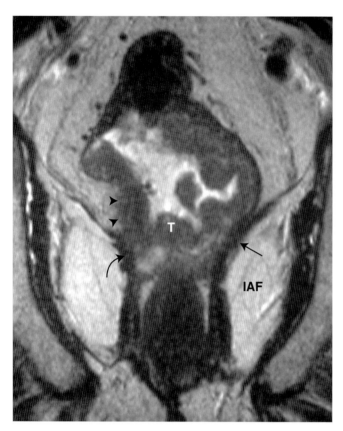

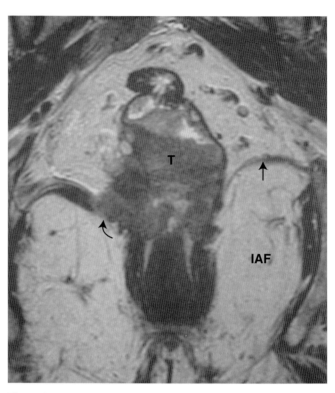

Figure 9.15. T4 Lower rectal cancer infiltrating levator ani muscle.

Coronal T2WI showing a large lower rectal tumour (T) which clearly infiltrates the right levator ani muscle (curved arrow). Left ischio-anal fossa (IAF) and left levator ani muscle (straight arrow).

Figure 9.14. T3 lower rectal cancer abutting right levator ani muscle.

Coronal T2WI of a large lower rectal tumour (T) that infiltrates through the right rectal wall (arrowheads) and is contiguous with the right levator ani muscle (curved arrow). However, it retains its normal morphology and is not infiltrated. Left ischio-anal fossa (IAF) and left levator ani muscle (arrow).

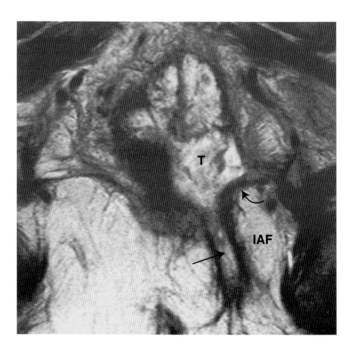

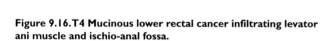

Figure 9.16. T4 Mucinous lower rectal cancer infiltrating levator ani muscle and ischio-anal fossa.

Off-axis T2WI of a large, high signal mucinous tumour (T) which has formed a sinus track (straight arrow) through the left levator ani muscle. Left ischio-anal fossa (IAF), left levator ani muscle (curved arrow).

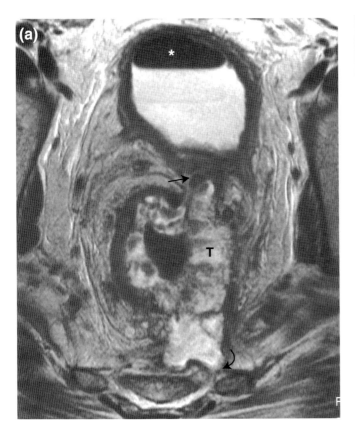

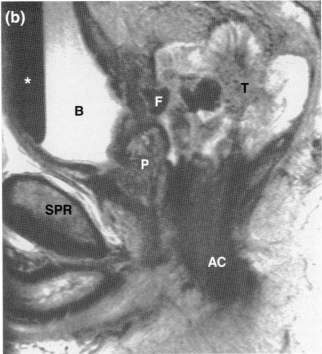

Figure 9.17. T4 Mid-rectal cancer infiltrating a left sacral foramen and the posterior bladder wall.

(a) T2WI perpendicular to a mucinous mid-rectal tumour (T) and (b) sagittal T2WI of the tumour. Note posterior extension into a lower left sacral foramen (curved arrow). Anteriorly, the tumour is contiguous with the posterior bladder wall (straight arrow) and there is gas in the bladder (asterisk) indicating recto-vesical fistulation (F). The tumour is contiguous over a wide area with the prostate (P) and bladder (B). Anal canal (AC), right superior pubic ramus (SPR).

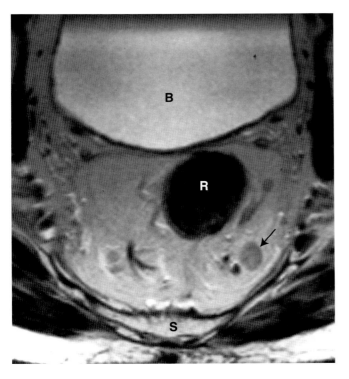

Figure 9.18. Enlarged benign meso-rectal lymph node.

Transaxial T2WI through the mid rectum (R) showing a clearly enlarged left meso-rectal lymph node (arrow). This was benign on histology. Bladder (B) and sacrum (S).

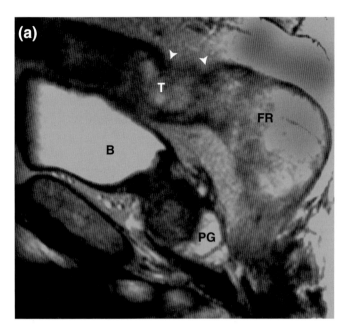
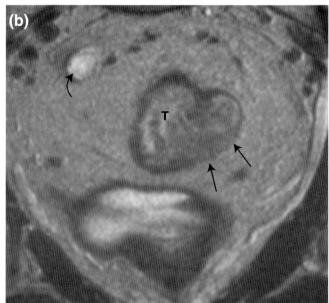

Figure 9.19. N1 Rectal cancer.

(a) Sagittal T2WI showing a high signal mucinous tumour (T) on the posterior upper rectal wall and **(b)** T2WI perpendicular to the tumour. The signal intensity of the tumour is similar to that of adjacent faecal residue (FR), though the tumour is defined by adjacent mural retraction (arrowheads). There is focal infiltration of the muscularis propria (arrows) making this a T2 lesion. In addition, there is a large right-sided meso-rectal lymph node (curved arrow). This returns high signal, which is abnormal, and is consistent with mucinous tumour infiltration. Bladder (B), prostate gland (PG).

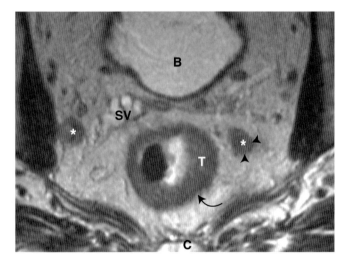

Figure 9.20. N2 Rectal cancer.

Transaxial T2WI showing a left sided mid-rectal tumour (T). The muscularis propria (curved arrow) is poorly defined though there is no overt meso-rectal infiltration. There are enlarged nodes in the left side of the meso-rectum and right internal iliac territory (asterisks). The right internal iliac node demonstrates inhomogeneous signal intensity and the meso-rectal node on the left demonstrates an irregular margin (arrowheads) both highly suggestive of lymph node tumour infiltration, which was subsequently proven. Bladder (B), right seminal vesicle (SV), coccyx (C).

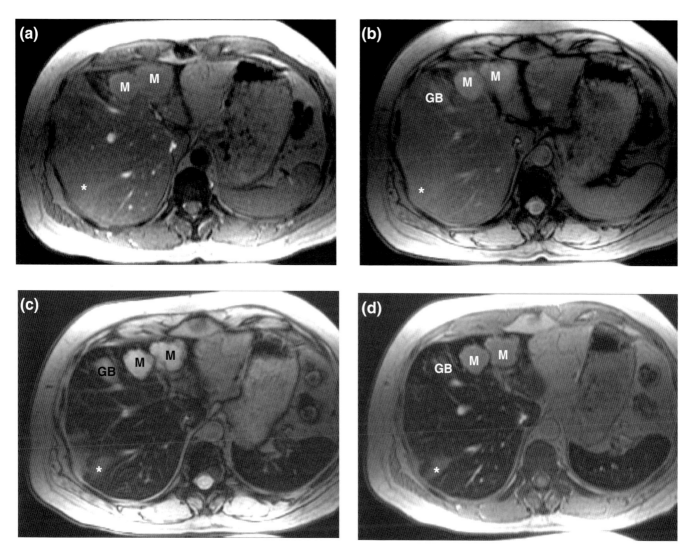

Figure 9.21. M1 Rectal cancer.

(a) Transaxial gradient echo proton density image (GEPDI) of liver and (b) transaxial gradient echo (GE) T2WI of liver showing two separate metastatic deposits (M) in segment 4A. Also note amorphous increased signal in segment 8 (asterisk). (c) Transaxial GEPDI and (d) transaxial GET2WI of liver obtained 60 minutes following infusion of super-paramagnetic iron oxide particles (SPIO) (Endorem 15 mmol kg^{-1}). There is marked increase in contrast between the metastases (M) and background liver. The lesion in segment 8 (asterisk) is now seen to represent further metastatic disease.

SPIOs are taken up by Kupffer cells, which are present in normal liver but absent from metastatic deposits. Therefore SPIOs cause signal drop out in normal liver but not in metastases. The lesion / background contrast is greatest using moderately T2W / proton density images at high field strengths of 1–1.5 T. Gallbladder (GB).

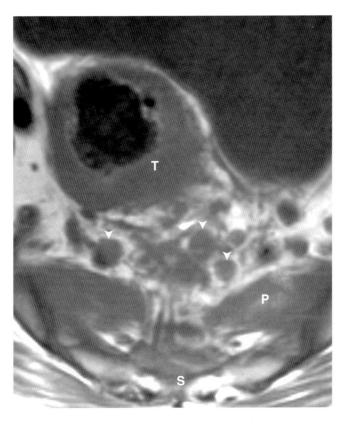

Figure 9.22. Advanced local lymph node metastasis.

Transaxial T1WI showing multiple enlarged lymph nodes (arrowheads) in the upper meso-rectum in the distribution of the superior rectal vessels. Note the T3 rectal tumour (T), sacrum (S) and piriformis muscle (P).

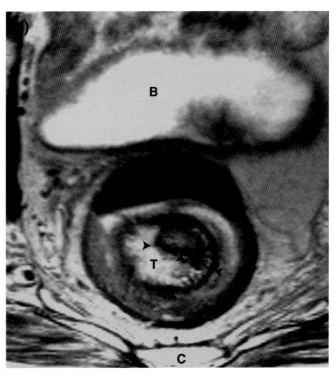

Figure 9.23. Intussuscepted tumour.

(a) Sagittal T2WI through an intussuscepted mid-rectal tumour (T) and **(b)** T2WI perpendicular to the lesion. This was pathological Stage T2 disease though the intussusception makes it very difficult to accurately define the stage on MR imaging. Note the multiple layers of muscularis propria (arrowheads) and intussuscepted meso-rectal fat (asterisk). Anal canal (AC), urethra (Ur), bladder (B), superior pubic ramus (SPR), sacrum (S), coccyx (C).

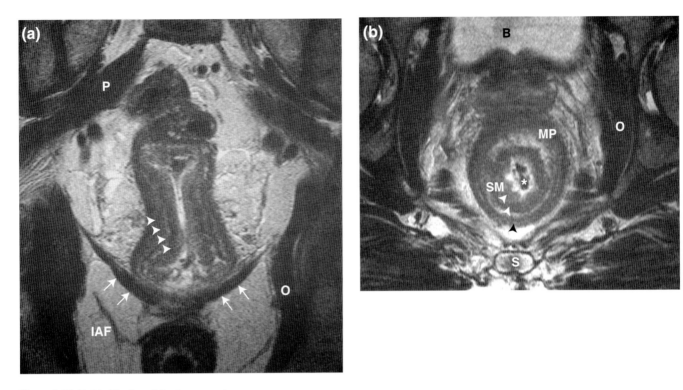

Figure 9.24. *Linitis Plastica* of the lower rectum.

(a) T2WI parallel to and (b) T2WI perpendicular to the lower rectum. In (a) there is mural thickening with a stratified appearance and in (b) a concentric mural ring pattern (arrowheads). There is a superficial resemblance to the intussusception shown in *Figure 9.23*. However, in this case, the ring pattern is due to undifferentiated tumour infiltrating between the different layers of the rectal wall, with the muscularis propria (MP) remaining essentially intact. Also, a florid desmoplastic response causes low signal in the submucosa (SM). Piriformis muscle (P), ischio-anal fossa (IAF), obturator internus muscle (O), levator ani muscle (arrows). Bladder (B), rectal lumen (asterisk), sacrum (S). (Reproduced with permission of American Journal of Roentgenology.)

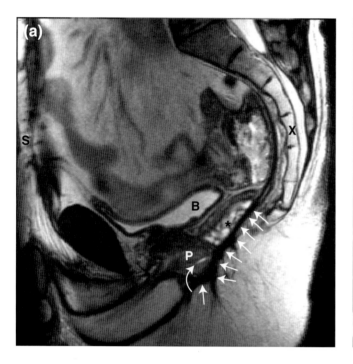

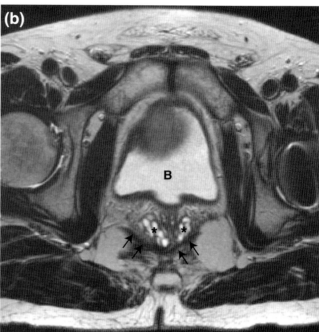

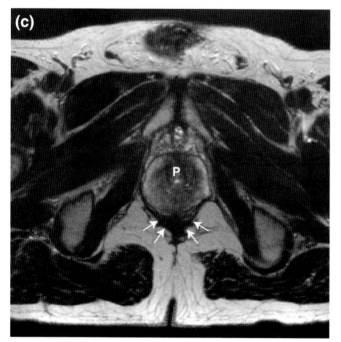

Figure 9.25. Appearances following APR in males.

(a) Sagittal T2WI, **(b)** and **(c)** transaxial T2WIs in a male following APR. The bladder (B), prostate (P) and seminal vesicles (asterisk) prolapse into the pelvic void left by the excised rectum. A fibrotic band (arrows) binds the prostate and seminal vesicles to the pelvic floor. In (a) note the high signal of the fatty marrow of the lower sacro-coccygeal segments following radiotherapy (X) and the post-surgical changes in the anterior abdominal wall (S). The small area of high signal in the prostate (curved arrow) is secondary to needle biopsy. (Images courtesy of Dr. Carrington, Christie Hospital.)

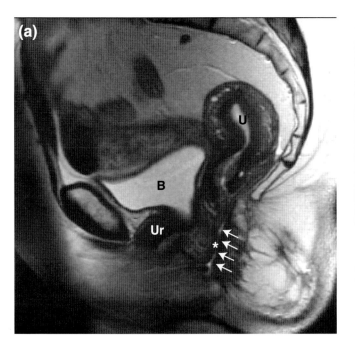

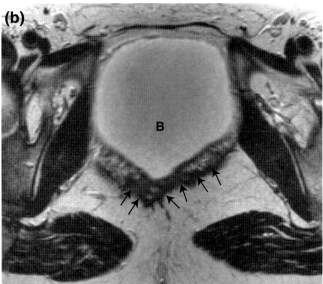

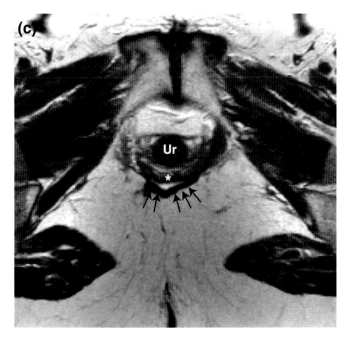

Figure 9.26. Appearances following APR in females.

(a) Sagittal T2WI in a female following APR and **(b)** and **(c)** transaxial T2WIs in a different female following hysterectomy and APR. The bladder (B), uterus (U) and vagina (asterisk) prolapse into the pelvic void left by the excised rectum. A fibrotic band (arrows) binds the vagina and cervix in (a) and the vagina and bladder in (b) and (c) to the pelvic floor. Note the posterior angulation of the urethra (Ur) in (a). (Images courtesy of Dr. Carrington, Christie Hospital.)

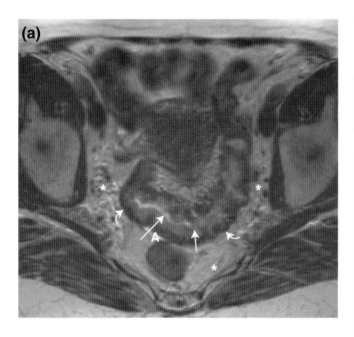

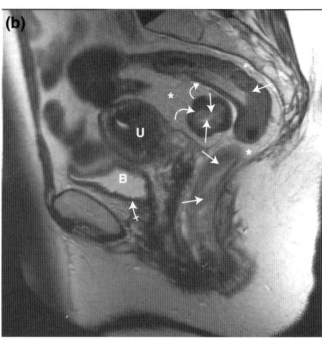

Figure 9.27. Appearances following radiotherapy.

(a) Transaxial T2WI and **(b)** sagittal T2WI in a female 8 months following intra-cavitary treatment for endometrial cancer. There is thickening and increased signal in the mucosa and submucosa of the rectum and sigmoid colon (arrows). The outer muscularis propria (curved arrows) is also thickened. There is abnormal stranding, nodularity and oedema in the pelvic fat (asterisks) and a trace of ascites (A). Radiation change is also present in the cervix and body of the uterus (U), which is of reduced size and almost uniform low signal intensity, and in the bladder (B) which has a thickened wall and mucosal oedema (crossed arrow). (Images courtesy of Dr. Hulse, Christie Hospital.)

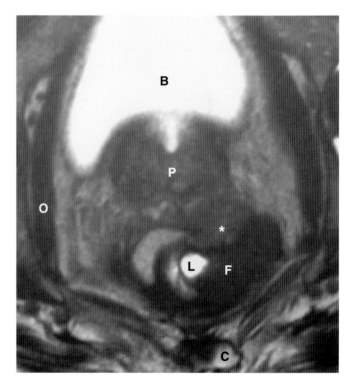

Figure 9.28. Recurrent rectal tumour.

T2WI perpendicular to the lower rectum. This patient had previously had an anterior lower third rectal tumour resected and there was clinical evidence of recurrent disease at the anastomotic site. Repeated biopsies through the left wall of the rectum revealed fibrotic tissue (F) only, which characteristically returns low signal on T2-weighted imaging as shown here. This image however, also shows an intermediate signal mass more anteriorly (asterisk) extending into the prostate gland (PG) which is much more suggestive of recurrent tumour. This allowed a guided biopsy, which confirmed the diagnosis of recurrent disease. Rectal lumen (L), bladder (B), coccyx (C) and right obturator internus muscle (O).

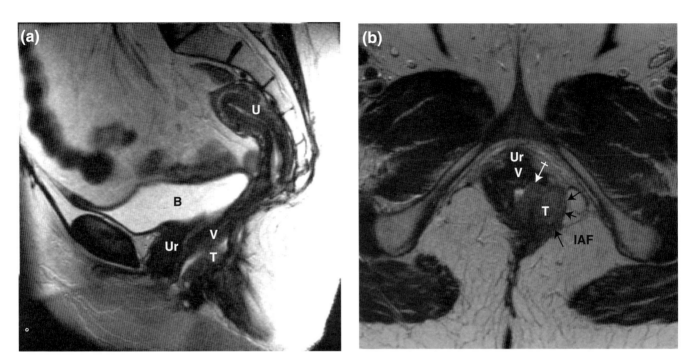

Figure 9.29. Recurrent rectal cancer following APR.

(a) Sagittal T2WI and (b) transaxial T2WI showing recurrent rectal tumour (T) following APR. The tumour has traversed the pelvic floor (arrows) and extends into the ischio-anal fossa (IAF), laterally, and the posterior wall of the vagina and vaginal lumen anteriorly (crossed arrow). Note the posterior prolapse of the uterus (U), vagina (V), bladder (B), and urethra (Ur) due to the previous APR (see *Figure 9.26*). (Images courtesy of Dr. Carrington, Christie Hospital.)

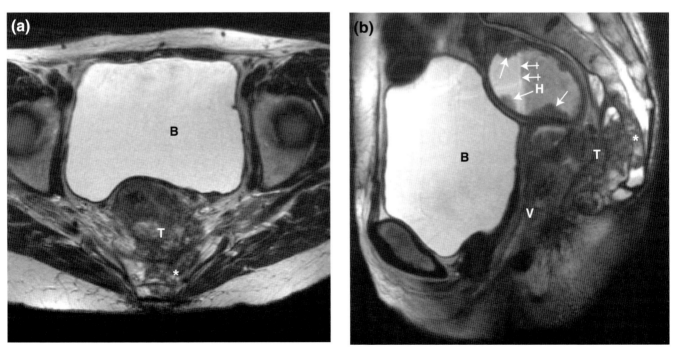

Figure 9.30. Recurrent rectal cancer following APR with haematometria.

(a) Sagittal T2WI and (b) transaxial T2WI showing a mixed composition recurrent tumour (T) in the pre-sacral space following APR. Tumour has invaded the vagina (V) and cervix of the uterus with consequent haematometria (H). Note the fluid/fluid level in the endometrial cavity (crossed arrow). There are tumour nodules adherent to the endometrium (arrows). Tumour has also invaded the sacrum (asterisk), Bladder (B). (Images courtesy of Dr. Hulse, Christie Hospital.)

10 Anal Cancer

Paul A. Hulse and Bernadette M. Carrington

BACKGROUND INFORMATION

Epidemiology

Cancers of the anal canal are rare, accounting for approximately 1.5% of gastrointestinal tract malignancies. In the United States, there were an estimated 3400 new cases in 2000. In England, there were 245 new cases in men (1.0/100000) and 377 in women (1.5/100000) in 1997. It was originally thought that anal cancer was associated with chronic irritation from haemorrhoids, fissures, fistulae and inflammatory bowel disease. However, this is now known not to be so. The majority of anal cancers in both sexes are due to infection with human papilloma virus, particularly HPV16. There is an increased risk of anal cancer in men and women who practice anal receptive intercourse, who have had more than 10 sexual partners, or who have sexually transmitted diseases such as genital warts, gonorrhoea, or *Chlamydia trachomatis*. Other aetiological risk factors are immunosuppression, human immunodeficiency virus (HIV) infection, and smoking. Women with anal cancer have a higher incidence of vulval, vaginal, cervical and lung cancers.

Histopathology

The anal canal below the dentate or pectinate line is lined with squamous mucosa. At the level of the dentate line there is a junctional area of squamous and non-squamous mucosa. Above the dentate line there is transitional (urothelial type) or rectal glandular mucosa. Cancers arising below the dentate line are predominantly keratinising squamous cell carcinomas. Cancers arising in the junctional zone at the level of, and just above the dentate line, are termed non-keratinising squamous cell carcinomas. This group includes the previously described sub-types of basaloid cloacogenic and transitional sub-types, terms that have now been abandoned. Biological behaviour, management strategies, and prognosis of the keratinising and non-keratinising types of squamous cell carcinoma are similar.

Uncommonly, small cell carcinoma, undifferentiated carcinoma and malignant melanoma can arise within the anal canal. Cancers arising in glandular mucosa of the upper anal canal behave like, and are managed in the same way, as rectal cancers.

Patterns of tumour spread

Carcinoma of the anus is an indolent disease, which usually becomes locally extensive before distant metastases occur. The pattern of lymph node metastatic spread depends on the site of origin of the tumour within the anal canal. Above the level of the dentate line drainage is to the perirectal, internal iliac and retroperitoneal nodes. Below the dentate line, drainage is to the inguinal nodes. The TNM staging classification for anal cancer is given in *Table 10.1*. At the time of presentation, approximately 50% of patients will have a superficial mass (T1 or T2 lesion) and approximately 25% will have regional lymph node involvement.

Prognostic indicators

The tumour size and depth of penetration at presentation are the most important prognostic factors. Mobile lesions less than 2.0 cm in diameter are cured in approximately 80% of cases whereas the cure rate for lesions greater than 5.0 cm in diameter is less than 50%. Skin ulceration and nodal disease are other poor prognostic factors. The likelihood of loco-regional lymph node involvement is related to tumour size and location. Tumours at the anal verge are less likely to develop lymph node metastases than those of the anal canal, probably because of earlier clinical presentation. Women achieve better local control and longer survival than men.

Treatment

Until the 1980s, the treatment of choice for cancer arising within the anal canal was an abdomino-perineal resection (APR). In an attempt to reduce surgical failure rates, workers in the USA introduced pre-operative 5-fluorouracil (5-FU) and mitomycin, combined with radiotherapy. The first three patients treated in this way were found to have no residual tumour in the excised anus following APR. This unexpected finding led to a change in the approach to management of anal cancer. Primary treatment now employs chemoradiation, with APR reserved for patients with persistent tumour on post-radiation biopsy or those with locally recurrent disease.

Multi-centre studies in Europe (United Kingdom Coordinating Committee on Cancer Research (UKCCR) and European Organisation for Research and Treatment of Cancer (EORTC)) have confirmed the benefit of combined modality therapy over radiation therapy alone in reducing loco-regional recurrence, death from anal cancer, and producing a higher colostomy-free rate and improved progression-free survival. However, no overall survival benefit was demonstrated between the two modes of therapy. A 5-year survival rate of 67% has been achieved using combined radiotherapy, 5-FU and mitomycin. Current studies are investigating the role of cisplatin in combined modality therapy.

Table 10.1. Anal cancer staging system

Primary tumour (T)		Lymph node (N)		Distant metastasis (M)		Stage grouping			
TX	Primary tumour cannot be assessed	Nx	Regional lymph nodes cannot be assessed	Mx	Presence of distant metastasis cannot be assessed	Stage 0	Tis	N0	M0
T0	No evidence of primary tumour					Stage I	T1	N0	M0
Tis	Carcinoma *in situ*	N0	No regional lymph node metastasis			Stage II	T2	N0	M0
T1	Tumour 2.0 cm or less in greatest dimension			M0	No distant metastasis		T3	N0	M0
		N1	Metastasis in perirectal lymph node(s)	M1	Distant metastasis	Stage IIIA	T1	N1	M0
T2	Tumour more than 2.0 cm but not more than 5.0 cm in greatest dimension						T2	N1	M0
		N2	Metastasis in unilateral internal iliac and/or inguinal lymph node(s)				T3	N1	M0
T3	Tumour more than 5.0 cm in greatest dimension						T4	N0	M0
						Stage IIIB	T4	N1	M0
T4	Tumour of any size invades adjacent organ(s), e.g. vagina, urethra, bladder (involvement of sphincter muscle(s) alone is not classified as T4)	N3	Metastasis in perirectal and inguinal lymph nodes and/or bilateral internal iliac and/or inguinal lymph nodes				any T	N2	M0
							any T	N3	M0
						Stage IV	any T	any N	M1

From guidelines of the American Joint Committee on Cancer, 2002

MR IMAGING OF ANAL CANCER

Current indications

Imaging has yet to find a place in the routine evaluation of primary anal cancer. Determination of the extent and nature of lesions is currently made at examination under anaesthetic and biopsy. CT of the abdomen and pelvis is routinely used to establish lymph node or visceral metastatic disease. Transrectal sonography of cancers of the lower third of the rectum has been shown to be useful in determining the extent of longitudinal tumour spread and infiltration of the anal sphincters, with a reported accuracy of 92%. Since MRI using phased array or endoluminal coils is effective in depicting the structure of the anal canal and its diseases, MRI does have a potential role in the local staging of primary anal cancer.

The principal current indication for MRI in anal cancer is the evaluation and staging of large primary masses, particularly when the craniocaudal dimension is the maximum diameter, as endoscopy is inadequate in these cases due to the size of the mass. MRI is also useful for the evaluation of residual or recurrent tumour prior to biopsy or salvage surgery. MRI has the drawback of being poor in differentiating between tumour and post treatment fibrosis, which is usually extensive following primary chemoradiotherapy. Endo-anal MRI performed after chemoradiotherapy or local excision of anal canal tumours only had an accuracy of 50%. Therefore, biopsy confirmation of residual or recurrent tumour is required.

MRI staging accuracy

There are no published results for the staging accuracy of primary or recurrent anal cancer using MRI.

Technique

A standard technique is employed with body coil transaxial T1WI to cover the abdomen and pelvis and high-resolution thin section T2WI in the three orthogonal planes. Fat suppressed imaging can help to improve the conspicuity of the primary tumour mass. Endoluminal coil imaging suffers from near field artifact and may not be tolerated by patients with anal cancer.

Imaging features

Usually anal cancer is of intermediate to low signal intensity on T1WI and intermediate to high signal intensity on T2WI and fat suppressed imaging. Mucinous adenocarcinoma displays characteristic high signal intensity on T2WI. Tumour usually spreads circumferentially around the anal wall and may form a lobulated intra-luminal or extra-mural mass. Fistulation into adjacent organs and tissues may occur.

Nodal disease

Metastatic spread occurs to the inguinal, iliac, perirectal and retroperitoneal nodes. As with other pelvic malignancy, lymph nodes with a short axis diameter greater than 1.0 cm in the pelvis and 1.5 cm in the inguinal regions are considered pathological. Lymph nodes are not normally identified in the perirectal fat and should be regarded as pathological (hyperplastic or metastatic) when seen.

Metastatic disease

Distant metastatic spread is primarily to the liver in advanced disease.

Post treatment – chemoradiotherapy

Residual mixed, predominantly low signal intensity foci are usually seen at the site of the primary tumour. Changes in normal tissues are mainly attributable to radiotherapy. An acute reaction occurs up to 3 months following treatment and is characterised by mucosal oedema and high signal on T2WI of the anal musculature. Chronic changes develop up to 5 years following treatment and are predominantly fibrotic change with low signal on T2WI and consequent morphological distortion of the pelvic viscera and soft tissues. Affected bone marrow shows fatty change seen as high signal on T1WI.

Post treatment – surgery

Following APR there are characteristic MR appearances.

- A band of pre-sacral fibrosis occurs, seen as intermediate signal on T1WI and low signal on T2WI.
- The levator ani muscles are sutured together with a consequent irregular contour to the central pelvic floor.
- The pelvic viscera prolapse posteriorly into the void left by the excised ano-rectum.

Residual/recurrent disease

Differentiation between residual/recurrent tumour and post treatment effect can be difficult. Persistent increased signal on T2WI in the primary tumour site more than 6 months following treatment, although a nonspecific finding, is suspicious of residual disease and warrants biopsy assessment. Recurrent disease occurs at the site of the primary tumour mass, in the loco-regional lymph nodes or outside of the radiation field. It has similar signal characteristics to the original disease.

Pitfalls of MRI

Identifying the location and extent of the primary tumour can be problematical in anal cancer especially when the tumour is small.

- Reference to the clinical findings and findings at examination under anaesthetic can guide the radiologist to the site of the primary tumour.
- Fat suppressed imaging can increase tumour conspicuity.
- Describing the relationship of the tumour to the ano-rectal junction, located at the indentation of the pubo-rectalis muscle, helps differentiate between tumours of rectal and anal origin.
- Measurement of tumour volume is difficult with infiltrative anal cancers that have circumferential spread. Measurement of the radial diameter of the anal canal wall at the site of tumour is useful for comparison with subsequent examinations.

Prediction of metastatic disease in inguinal lymph nodes is particularly difficult. Inguinal nodes can normally measure up to 1.5 cm in short axis diameter. However, use of this measurement probably reduces the sensitivity for the identification of metastatic disease. Features suggestive of metastatic disease in nonenlarged and enlarged nodes are:

- round shape;
- asymmetrical clustering in the groin or on the pelvic sidewall;
- signal intensity on T2WI similar to the primary tumour mass;
- central nodal necrosis, which is a strong indicator of metastatic disease in squamous cell tumours.

FURTHER READING

1. Ryan DP, Compton CC and Mayer RJ. (2000) Carcinoma of the anal canal. *N. Engl. J. Med.* 342: 792–800. *Informative Review.*

2. Ryan DP and Mayer RJ. (2000) Anal carcinoma 'histology, staging, epidemiology and treatment.' *Curr. Opin. Oncol.* 12: 345–352. *Detailed review by same authors as above.*

3. Spratt JS. (2000) Cancer of the anus. *J. Surg. Oncol.* 74: 173–174. *Surgically orientated summary.*

4. Myerson RJ, Karnell LH and Menck HR. (1997) The national cancer database report on carcinoma of the anus. *Cancer* 80(4): 805–815 *Comprehensive epidemiological study of anal cancer in the USA.*

5. Stoker J, Rocio E, Wiersma TG and Laméris JS. (2000) Imaging of anorectal disease. *Br. J. Surg.* 87: 10–27. *Useful review of anorectal imaging but concentrating on benign disease of the anal canal and malignant disease of the rectum.*

6. Indinnimeo M, Cicchini C, Stazi A *et al.* (2000) Magnetic resonance imaging using endoanal coil in anal canal tumours after radiochemotherapy or local excision. *Int. Surg.* 85: 143–146. *Study illustrating difficulty in differentiating tumour from benign change following treatment.*

7. Grey AC, Carrington BM, Hulse PA *et al.* (2000). Magnetic resonance appearance of normal inguinal nodes. *Clin. Radiol.* 55: 124–130. *Describes 1.5cm as the upper limit of normal for inguinal lymph node size.*

8. Sugimura K, Carrington BM, Quivey JM and Hricak H. (1990) Post irradiation changes in the Pelvis: Assessment with MRI. *Radiology* 175: 805–813. *Correlates clinical and MR findings of pelvic radiation change.*

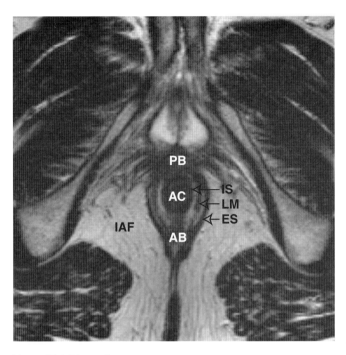

Figure 10.1. Normal anatomy.

Transaxial T2WI of male perineum showing normal anatomy of anus. Anal canal (AC), internal sphincter (IS), longitudinal muscle layer in intersphincteric space (LM), external sphincter (ES), anococcygeal body (AB), perineal body (PB), ischioanal fossa (IAF).

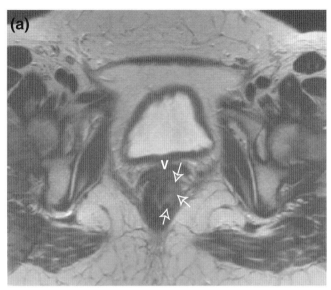

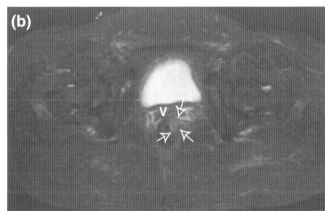

Figure 10.2. T1 anal cancer.

(a) Transaxial T2WI and (b) transaxial STIR image showing lobulated intermediate signal intensity tumour mass less than 2.0 cm maximum dimension extending through anal wall (arrows); vagina (V).

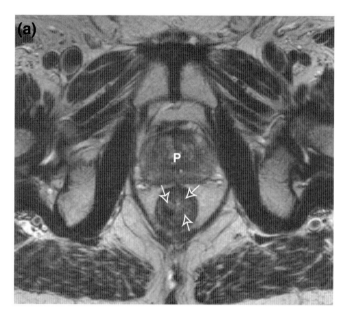

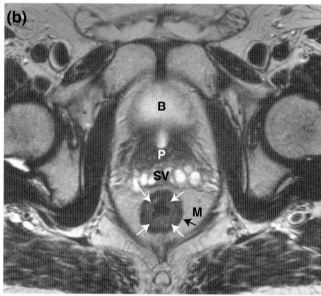

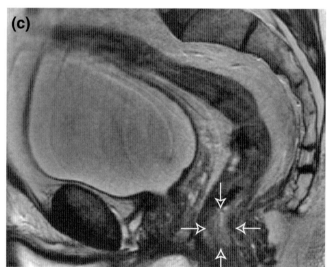

Figure 10.3. T2 anal cancer.

(a) Transaxial T2WI showing intermediate signal intensity lobulated tumour mass (arrows) between 2.0 cm and 5.0 cm maximum dimension largely filling ano-rectal lumen. **(b)** Transaxial T2WI just above (a) showing circumferential spread of tumour in lower rectum (arrows). The muscle layer remains intact. **(c)** Sagittal T2WI showing cranio-caudal extent of tumour. Differentiation between tumour stage on the basis of maximum dimension can be difficult with infiltrative tumours with circumferential spread; bladder (B); prostate (P); seminal vesicles (SV); muscle layer (M).

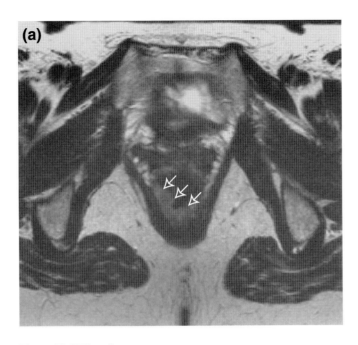
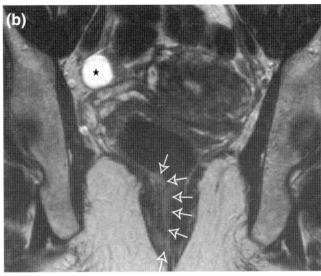

Figure 10.4. T2 anal cancer.

(a) Transaxial T2WI and (b) coronal T2WI showing intermediate signal intensity, nonlobulated tumour (arrows) between 2.0 cm and 5.0 cm maximum dimensions which extends to the anal verge. There is an incidental right adenexal cyst (asterisk).

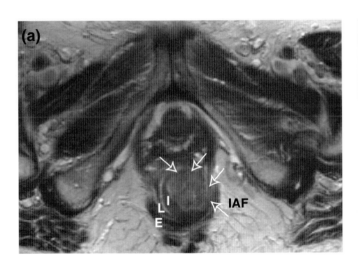

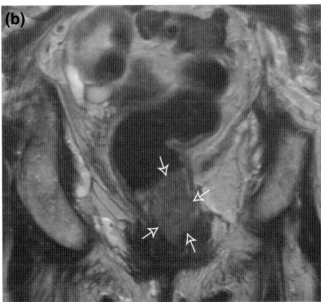

Figure 10.5. T3 anal cancer.

(a) Transaxial T2WI, (b) coronal T2WI and (c) sagittal T2WI showing intermediate signal intensity tumour (arrows) greater than 5.0 cm maximum diameter. Tumour has extended through the anal sphincter into the ischioanal fossa and extended to the anal verge. Internal sphincter (I); longitudinal muscle layer (L); external sphincter (E); ischioanal fossa (IAF).

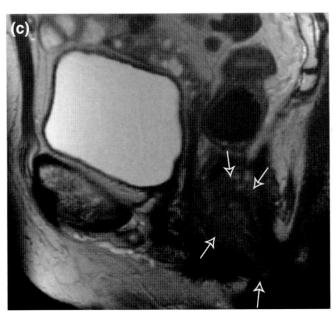

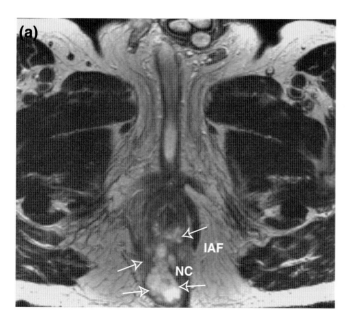

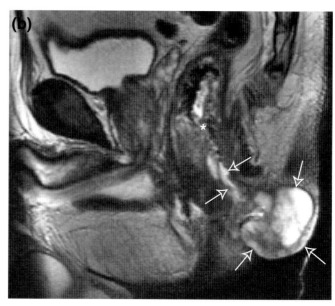

Figure 10.6. T3 anal cancer.

(a) Transaxial T2WI and **(b)** sagittal T2WI showing large lobulated high signal intensity mass (arrows) characteristic of a mucinous adenocarcinoma. Tumour has extended through the anal sphincter into the fat of the ischioanal fossa and buttock to abut onto the natal cleft, it also extends cranially into the lower rectum (asterisk). Natal cleft (NC); ischioanal fossa (IAF).

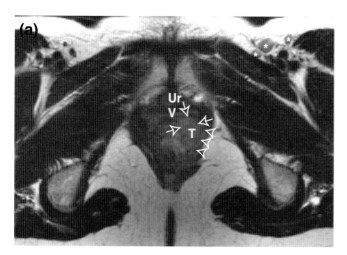

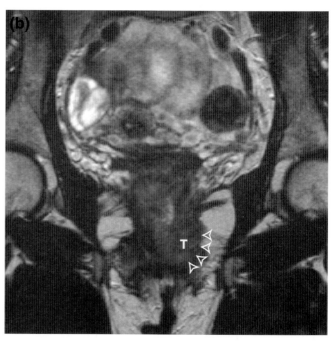

Figure 10.7. T4 anal cancer with vaginal invasion.

(a) Transaxial T2WI and **(b)** coronal T2WI showing high/intermediate signal intensity mass (T) extending anteriorly through the anal wall and recto / ano-vaginal septum to invade the left side of the vagina (arrows) and laterally to infiltrate the pelvic floor (arrowheads) but not extend into the ischioanal fossa. Note probable left inguinal lymph node metastases (asterisk) which are non-enlarged but show asymmetrical clustering and have similar signal character-istics to the primary tumour. Urethra (Ur); vagina (V).

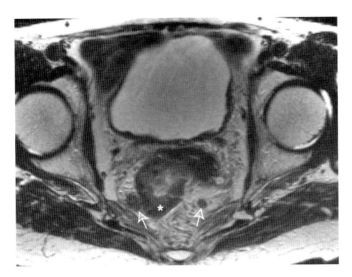

Figure 10.8. N1 anal cancer.

Transaxial T2WI showing lymph node metastases in the perirectal fat (arrows) and local spread of primary tumour to rectum (asterisk). Lymph nodes are not normally identified in the perirectal fat on MRI and should be regarded as pathological. Differentiation between malignant and hyperplastic nodes on the basis of size, is not reliable in this location. Nodes with central necrosis or a similar signal characteristic to the primary tumour, as in this case, favour malignant disease.

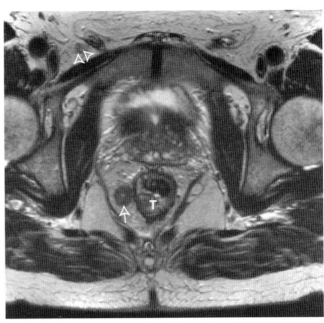

Figure 10.9. N1 anal cancer.

Transaxial T2WI of the mucinous anal cancer (T) shown in *Figure 10.6*. The perirectal lymph node (arrow) shows central high signal indicating a high probability of metastatic disease. Central lymph node high signal on T2WI occurs with metastatic mucin secreting adenocarcinoma and cystic nodal necrosis in squamous cell carcinoma. A benign right inguinal node, with fat in the hilum (arrowheads) also returns high signal on T2WI. The eccentrically located fat usually indicates its benign significance but uncertainty can be resolved with fat suppressed (STIR) sequences.

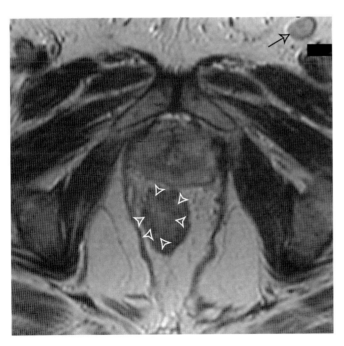

Figure 10.10. N2 anal cancer.

Transaxial T2WI showing enlarged intermediate signal intensity left inguinal lymph node (arrow). Note nodal signal intensity is slightly higher than primary tumour (arrowheads) due to its closer proximity to the surface phased array receiving coil.

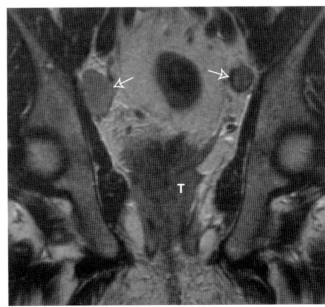

Figure 10.11. N3 anal cancer.

Coronal T2WI showing bilateral surgical obturator (internal iliac) lymph node metastases (arrows). Note infiltrating ano-rectal tumour (T).

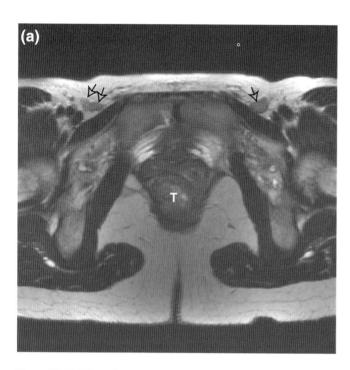

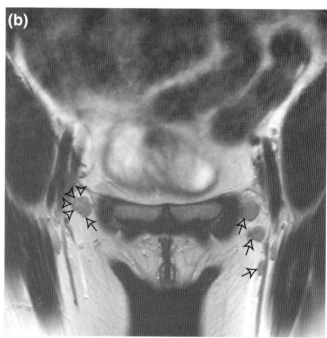

Figure 10.12. N3 anal cancer.

(a) Transaxial T2WI and **(b)** coronal T2WI showing bilateral inguinal lymph node metastases (arrows). Note intermediate signal intensity of the primary tumour (T). On the right side, the node has a ragged margin (arrowheads) indicating extra-nodal tumour extension.

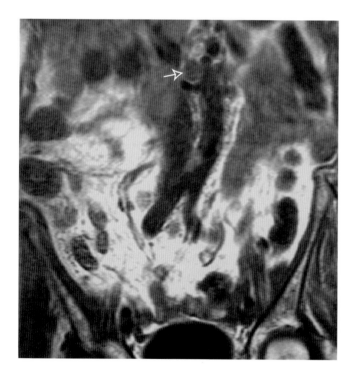

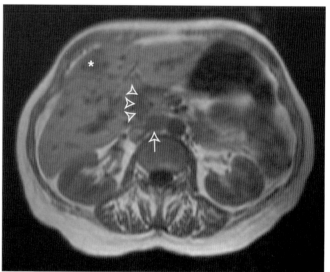

Figure 10.14. Retroperitoneal, porta hepatis lymph node and liver metastases in anal cancer.

Transaxial T1WI showing enlarged interaortocaval lymph node (arrow), porta hepatis lymph node mass (arrowheads) and liver metastasis (asterisk). Note the intrahepatic bile duct dilatation secondary to the obstructing porta hepatis mass.

Figure 10.13. Lymph node metastasis in anal cancer – retroperitoneum.

Coronal T1WI showing enlarged interaortocaval lymph node (arrow) consistent with metastatic disease. Metastases in this location are not described in the UICC staging classification but imply a poor prognosis.

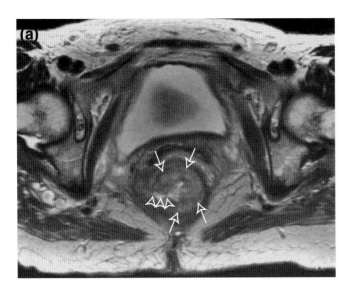

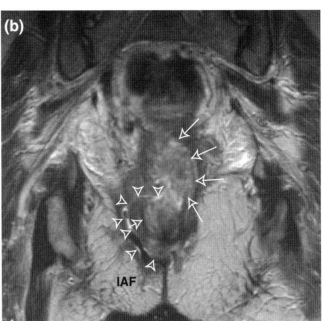

Figure 10.15. T3 anal cancer with fistula.

(a) Transaxial T2WI and (b) coronal T2WI showing circumferential spread of intermediate signal intensity tumour mass (arrows). There is transmural spread of tumour with a fluid and air-containing fistula (arrowheads) extending through the pubococcygeal portion of the levator ani muscle into the ischioanal fossa (IAF).

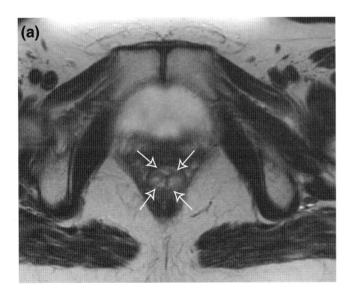

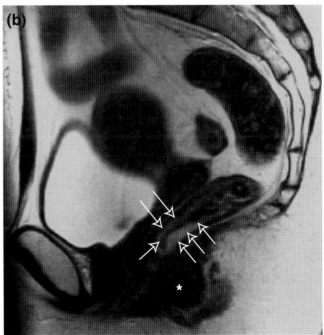

Figure 10.16. Subacute radiation reaction.

(a) Transaxial T2WI and (b) sagittal T2WI showing marked oedema and swelling of mucosa at and above the ano-rectal junction (arrows), 4 months following chemoradiotherapy for a T1 anal cancer. This has occurred at the margin of the radiation field with low signal fibrosis developing in the anal canal proper (asterisk). There is high signal in the lower sacrum due to conversion from haemopoietic to fatty bone marrow secondary to radiotherapy. A subacute radiation reaction occurs 3 to 12 months after treatment. Occasionally a chronic ano-proctitis develops.

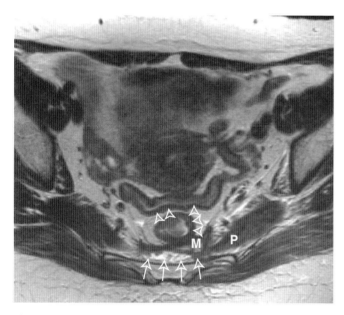

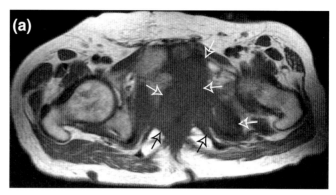

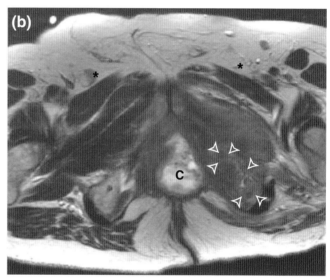

Figure 10.17. Chronic radiation reaction.

Transaxial T2WI showing changes in pelvic viscera 4 years following chemoradiotherapy for a T3 anal cancer. There is a mixed signal mass (M) fixed to the left piriformis muscle (P), stable in appearance over a 1 year period – indicating the lack of residual proliferating tumour. There is a band of pre-sacral oedema (arrows). The rectum and an adjacent loop of dependent small bowel show diffuse low signal, mural thickening, and minor serosal spiculation due to fibrosis (arrowheads). Chronic radiation reactions can develop up to 5 years following treatment and persist indefinitely.

Figure 10.18. Locally extensive recurrent anal cancer following chemoradiotherapy and abdomino-perineal resection.

(continued on next page)

(a) Transaxial T1WI showing recurrent tumour (arrows) with substantial destruction of the left ischiopubic ramus and pubic bone. T1WIs are useful for indicating the extent of bone disease. **(b)** transaxial T2WI, **(c)** coronal T2WI and **(d)** sagittal T2WI showing extent of soft tissue infiltration in the pelvis by recurrent disease. Tumour has invaded the prostate and bladder with fistulation to a complex deep pelvic / perineal cavity (C). There is circumferential thickening of the bladder wall (crossed arrows). A separate gas-containing cavity is present in the involved pelvic floor and obturator muscles (arrowheads). A suprapubic catheter is *in situ* in the bladder (SP). Note the inguinal and iliac lymph nodes (asterisk) in (b) and (c) which are equivocal for metastatic disease or hyperplasia secondary to pelvic sepsis. Multiplanar imaging is important in evaluating such complex cases and fistulae.

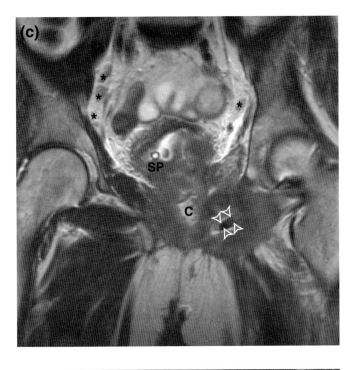

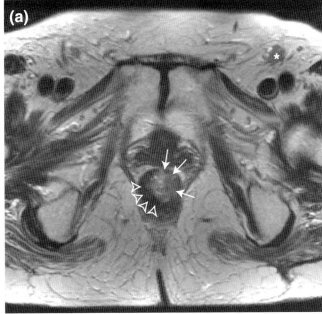

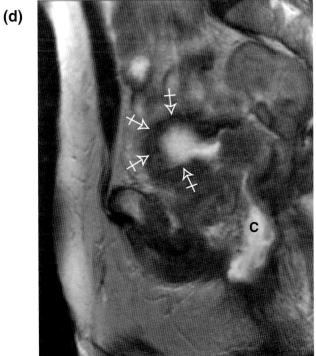

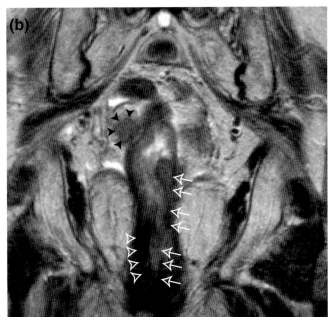

Figure 10.18. (continued)

Figure 10.19. Recurrent anal cancer following chemoradiotherapy.

(a) Transaxial T2WI and (b) coronal T2WI showing a recurrent intermediate signal intensity tumour mass in the left anal canal and rectum (arrows). The rest of the anal wall is thickened and of low signal intensity representing radiation induced fibrosis (arrowheads). Note probable inguinal lymph node metastasis (asterisk) and definite perirectal lymph node metastasis (solid arrowheads).

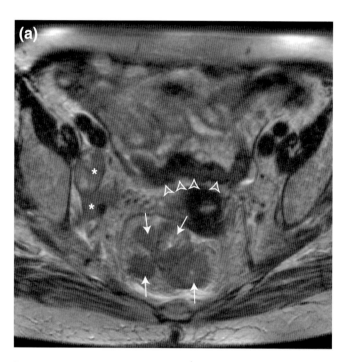
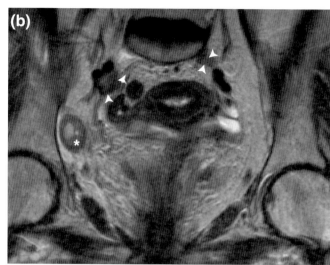

Figure 10.20. Recurrent anal cancer following chemoradiotherapy.

(a) Transaxial T2WI and **(b)** coronal T2WI showing recurrent tumour involving rectum (arrows), perirectal, right obturator and right internal iliac (asterisk) and bilateral common iliac lymph nodes (solid arrowheads). Note the dependent small bowel loop with mural thickening and mild serosal spiculation (open arrowheads) due to radiation change.

11 Bladder Cancer

Suzanne Bonington and Jeremy A.L. Lawrance

BACKGROUND INFORMATION

Epidemiology

Bladder cancer is the most common malignancy of the urinary tract, and represents 4.5% of all new malignancies. The peak incidence is in the 6th and 7th decades, although there is an increasing number of patients who present under the age of 30. The male to female ratio is 4:1. The age standardised incidence rates/100000 population for males is 19.5 in the UK and 23 in the USA. For females it is 6/100000 population both in the UK and USA.

There is an increased risk of bladder cancer with exposure to various aromatic amines, causing an occupational hazard in the chemical, rubber and paint industries. There is also an association with diesel fumes, long term phenacetin use, and smoking. Squamous cell carcinoma is associated with chronic urinary tract infections and prolonged schistosomiasis infection.

Histopathology

Bladder tumours are predominantly epithelial in origin and 90–95% of these are transitional cell type with approximately 50% arising from the lateral bladder walls and 20% from the region of the trigone. Squamous cell, or mixed transitional cell and squamous cell carcinoma, accounts for 5–10% of malignancies. Adenocarcinomas, which account for 2–3% of malignancies, are more prevalent in patients with a patent urachus and thus usually occur in the urachal remnant. Other cell types such as small cell are extremely rare, accounting for less than 1% of cases. At presentation about one third of tumours are multifocal in origin. Approximately two thirds of bladder tumours are superficial and are usually papillary. One third show infiltration into or beyond the bladder wall.

Patterns of tumour spread

Direct spread of tumour occurs into the perivesical fat, pelvic organs and to the pelvic sidewalls. Lymph node metastases are rare in superficial tumours, but occur in 30% of patients when the deep muscle layer of the bladder is involved and in 60% of cases where there is extravesical tumour spread. The first lymph nodes involved are the anterior and lateral paravesical nodes and the pre-sacral nodes. Subsequent nodal spread is to the internal iliac, obturator and external iliac nodes and finally the common iliac and para-aortic nodes. Common iliac and para-aortic nodes are considered as distant metastases (M1) in the TNM staging system. Occasionally, metastatic lymph nodes may be identified above the diaphragm. Distant metastases to the bones, lungs, brain and liver are late features of bladder cancer.

Two main classifications for bladder cancer exist – the TNM system and the Jewett-Strong-Marshall (JSM) system. The TNM system is now the system in general use as it provides greater detail about superficial lesions and also defines extravesical spread more clearly. A summary of the TNM system is seen in *Table 11.1*, and illustrated in Diagram 1.

Table 11.1. TNM (2002) staging of bladder cancer		
TNM	**JSM**	**Histopathological findings**
Tis		Carcinoma *in situ*
Ta	0	Papillary tumour confined to the epithelium (mucosa)
T1	A	Tumour invades subepithelial connective tissue (lamina propria)
T2		Tumour invades muscle
T2a	B1	Tumour invades superficial muscle (inner half)
T2b	B2	Tumour invades deep muscle (outer half)
T3	C	Tumour invades perivesical tissue
T3a		Tumour invades perivesical fat microscopically
T3b		Tumour invades perivesical fat macroscopically
T4a	D1	Tumour invades surrounding organs – prostate, uterus or vagina
T4b		Tumour invades pelvic or abdominal wall
N0		No regional lymph node metastases
N1	D1	Metastasis in a single lymph node ≤ 2.0 cm in greatest dimension
N2	D1	Metastasis in a single lymph node >2.0 cm but ≤ 5.0 cm in greatest dimension, or multiple nodes
N3	D1	Metastasis in a lymph node >5.0 cm in greatest dimension
M0		No distant metastasis
M1	D2	Distant metastasis

Prognostic indicators

- Tumour stage. Five-year survival decreases from approximately 70% for T1 disease to 5–10% for T4 disease. A major adverse feature is the presence of any lymph node metastases.

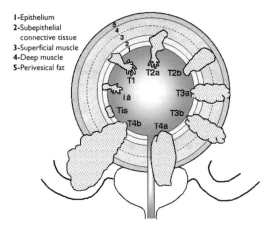

1-Epithelium
2-Subepithelial connective tissue
3-Superficial muscle
4-Deep muscle
5-Perivesical fat

Diagram 1: T Staging of Bladder Cancer

- Tumour grade. High histological grade tumours are more likely to become infiltrative and to metastasise, irrespective of tumour stage at presentation.

- Multiple lesions. Multifocal tumour adversely affects survival.

- Other factors. The following have been identified as adverse features: hydronephrosis, anaemia, tumour size, expression of blood group substances, expression of epidermal growth factor receptors, mutation of p53, up-regulation of Rb and other oncogene expression.

Treatment

Patients with superficial bladder tumours are treated with regular local endoscopic resection and intravesical chemotherapy or immunomodulators. Patients with frequent recurrences or high-grade disease are often treated with a radical cystectomy. Stage 2a-3a disease, with muscle invasion but minimal perivesical spread, is most commonly treated by radical cystectomy and lymph node resection, or with radiotherapy after chemotherapy. Such patients can be treated with radical radiotherapy, although this is decreasing in popularity. Advanced disease is palliated with either mitomycin-based chemotherapy or radiotherapy.

MR IMAGING OF BLADDER CANCER

Technique

The bladder should be moderately full to separate the walls, but not too distended as to cause degradation of the images by motion artifact due to patient restlessness. This can usually be achieved by asking the patient to micturate 2 hours before the examination. Respiratory motion is limited by putting a band across the patient's abdomen. In practice this is achieved with the phased-array pelvic coil. Many centres use either hyoscine butylbromide or glucagon to reduce artifact from bowel motion.

A standard technique using T1 and high resolution turbo fast spin echo T2 sequences is used for staging.

The use of orthogonal planes frequently gives valuable additional information. Sagittal and coronal planes are particularly useful for assessing tumours at the dome and trigone of the bladder.

Fat saturated / STIR sequences with intravenous contrast are sometimes used and studies suggest a 9–14% improvement in staging accuracy with contrast-enhanced imaging. Enhancement should appear earlier and be greater in the tumour compared to the normal bladder wall. Fast dynamic MR imaging, using one image every 2 seconds, can be useful in differentiating tumour which enhances earlier at approximately 6 seconds, from post biopsy change which enhances after approximately 10 seconds, or from radiation effects.

Other modifications in technique include the use of endorectal coils. These provide excellent detail of the dorsal bladder wall, but have the drawback that the entire bladder and rest of the pelvis cannot be assessed.

If intravenous contrast has been given during the examination a breath-hold T1-weighted MR angiographic sequence can produce a contrast urogram which may be helpful to view the upper renal tracts, where synchronous tumours may be seen in 0.5% of patients.

Current indications

Cystoscopic examination and biopsy remain the basis for evaluation of superficial tumours. With invasive disease, clinical evaluation with bimanual palpation and assessment of adherence to local structures is only 50–75% accurate, so that MR imaging may be helpful in this circumstance.

Staging accuracy

MRI has been shown to be superior to clinical staging for patients treated with radiotherapy in that MR stage correlated better with risk of treatment failure and cancer-specific survival.

The accuracy of MR in staging of bladder cancer varies between 73 and 96%. This is 10–30% higher than achieved with CT. The improvement in accuracy is due to better visualisation of the dome and trigone of the bladder and superior assessment of adjacent organ invasion. MR staging accuracy is less for low stage tumours due to the difficulty in differentiating between superficial and deep muscle invasion, and early extra-vesical spread. In this tumour group, it remains superior to CT due to the ability of MR to identify the layers of the bladder wall.

Imaging features

Primary tumour

On T1W sequences, the perivesical fat appears high signal, the normal bladder wall intermediate signal and urine in the bladder low signal. In general, the individual muscle layers of the bladder wall are not discriminated. This sequence is most useful for assessing extra-vesical spread of tumour into the perivesical fat as either a mass or an intermediate signal stranding of the fat. T1W sequences are also useful for assessing the skeleton for bone metastases.

On T2W images the bladder muscle layer is of low signal intensity and tumour is of intermediate signal intensity, slightly higher than that of the bladder wall. This sequence is therefore used to assess bladder wall invasion and is useful for evaluating tumour extension into the prostate, uterus or vagina, since intra-organ anatomy is best delineated on this sequence.

Nodal disease

Features suggestive of nodal ;involvement include nodal size, round shape and the presence of asymmetrical clusters of nodes. Nodes are considered enlarged if they measure more than 8.0 mm in short axis if round, and 10.0 mm if oval shaped. Note that in bladder cancer the long axis measurement of a nodal mass is the N stage determinant.

Post treatment and recurrence

After cystectomy, the bladder bed may demonstrate low signal intensity fibrosis and bowel often prolapses into it or becomes adherent to the fibrotic tissue. The ileal loop diversion may be visualised, usually in the right iliac fossa. Neobladder formation is performed only occasionally in patients with small tumours localised to the bladder dome. Local tumour recurrence post cystectomy is usually evident as a solid mass of intermediate to high signal in the bladder bed.

Radiation therapy usually results in low signal fibrous change, but it can also cause generalised or focal bladder wall thickening of intermediate to high signal intensity on T2 images for up to 4 years after treatment making differentiation from tumour difficult. Dynamic contrast enhanced scans have been shown to be useful in differentiating recurrent tumour from post treatment effects.

Pitfalls of MRI

- Differentiation between T1, T2a, T2b and T3a tumours. It can be difficult on MRI to differentiate between the superficial and deep muscle layers of the bladder wall and to identify small volume extra-vesical extension. Whilst this differentiation affects prognosis, it does not affect management and is usually determined histologically.

- Over- or under-distension of the bladder. If the bladder is too full, images may be degraded by motion artifact. If the bladder is poorly distended, the tumour and bladder wall may not be well

visualised. Motion artifact can also degrade images at the dome of the bladder. Care in patient preparation and administration of smooth muscle relaxants may prevent these problems.

- Recent cystoscopic biopsy causing post-operative oedema and inflammatory reaction can result in over-staging. It is therefore imperative to have accurate information regarding the dates and depths of biopsies. In some circumstances, it may be necessary to rescan the patient at a later date.

- Chemical shift artifact can potentially impair staging by affecting the perception of tumour depth of invasion. This is overcome using orthogonal planes and adjusting machine parameters.

- Differentiation between late fibrosis, granulation tissue and residual/recurrent tumour may be difficult. Tumour is more likely if there is a new or enlarging mass, or new disease outside the treated area. Dynamic contrast-enhanced sequences may be helpful when tumour should enhance earlier than fibrosis.

FURTHER READING

1. Husband JES. (1998) Bladder cancer. In: *Imaging in Oncology*. (eds Husband JES and Reznek R). Isis Medical Media Ltd, Oxford, UK pp. 215–238. *Good overview of bladder cancer.*

2. Urinary Bladder. (2002) In: *AJCC Cancer Staging Manual*. 6th edition. (eds Greene FL, Page DL, Fleming ID et al.). Springer-Verlay, New York, USA pp. 335–340. *Current TNM staging of Bladder cancer. Succinct summary of prognostic indicators.*

3. Barentsz JO, Jager GJ and Witjes JA. (2000) MR imaging of the urinary bladder. Oncologic MR imaging. *Magn. Reson. Imaging Clin. N.Am.* 8(4): 853–867. *Good description of technique.*

5. MacVicar AD. (2000) Bladder Cancer staging. *BJU* 86 Suppl 1: 111–122. *Compares the use of MR and CT in staging bladder cancer.*

6. Hall RR and Prout GR. (1990) Staging of bladder cancer: is the tumour, node, metastasis system adequate? *Semin. Oncol.* 17(5): 517–523. *Discusses the problems with the TNM staging system for the bladder and underlines the key areas which significantly alter clinical management.*

7. Robinson P, Collins CD, Ryder WD *et al.* (2000) Relationship of MRI and clinical staging to outcome in invasive bladder carcinoma treated with radiotherapy. *Clin. Radiol.* 55(4): 301–306. *Identifies the most important findings on MR that alter prognosis.*

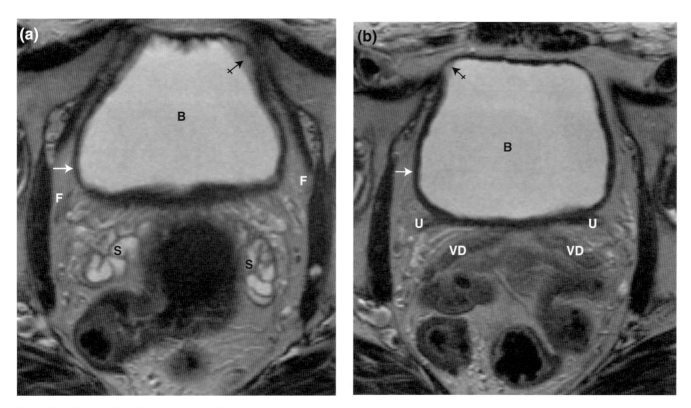

Figure 11.1. Normal bladder – moderate distension.

(a) and **(b)** Transaxial T2WI of the bladder. The normal bladder muscle layer demonstrates low signal intensity (arrow), the mucosa intermediate signal (crossed arrow) with high signal urine within the bladder (B) and intermediate signal perivesical fat (F). In (a), the normal high signal return from the seminal vesicles (S) is seen. In (b), a more cranial section, the distal ureters (U) are seen as they enter the bladder (B). The vas deferens (VD) is also clearly seen.

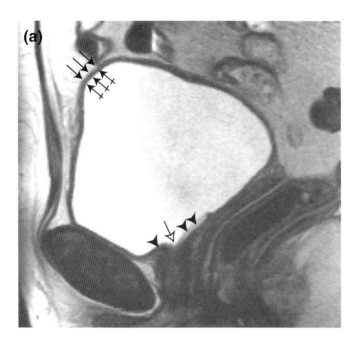

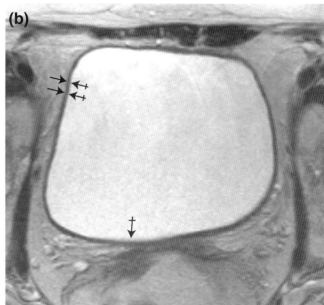

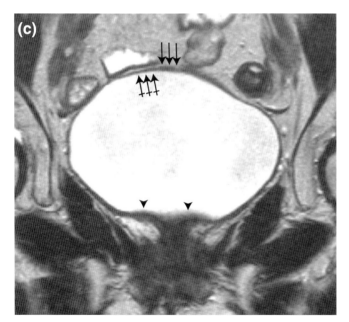

Figure 11.2. Normal bladder – extreme distension.

(a) Midline sagittal T2WI, **(b)** transaxial T2WI and **(c)** coronal T2WI through the bladder, following an injection of 20 mg hyoscine butylbromide. The normal bladder muscle is seen as a thin band of low signal intensity (arrows), the mucosa is a fine line of intermediate signal on the inner aspect of the muscle layer (crossed arrows) with high signal urine within the bladder. Urethral meatus (open arrow), bladder trigone (arrowheads).

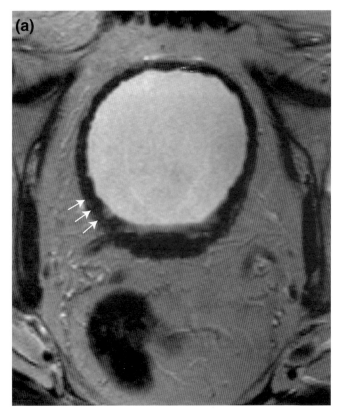

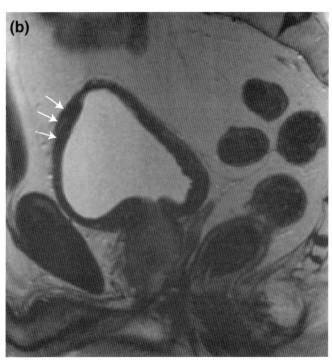

Figure 11.3. Bladder wall trabeculation.

(a) Transaxial T2WI and (b) sagittal T2WI through the bladder.
These images demonstrate circumferential low signal thickening of the bladder wall (arrows) in keeping with detrusor muscle hypertrophy due to chronic bladder outlet obstruction.

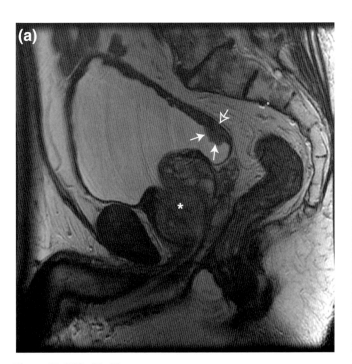

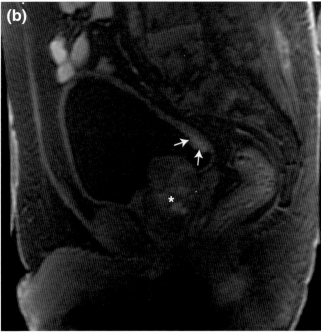

Figure 11.4. T2a Bladder cancer

(a) Sagittal T2WI and (b) fat saturation contrast-enhanced T1WI demonstrating an enhancing tumour invading the superficial bladder muscle (arrows). The intact outer bladder wall is demonstrated (open arrow). The patient has benign prostatic hypertrophy (asterisk). (Courtesy of Dr. M. Haider, Princess Margaret Hospital, Toronto.)

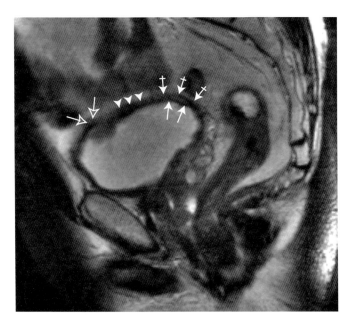

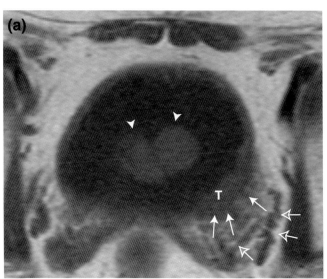

Figure 11.5. Multifocal bladder cancer, with areas showing T2a, T2b and T3b tumour.

Sagittal T2WI through the bladder. There are multiple nodules of intermediate signal tumour involving the superficial bladder muscle (arrows). These areas show an intact outer low signal bladder wall (crossed arrows). Lying adjacent to this is abnormal intermediate signal that has extended across the full thickness of the bladder wall (arrowheads) indicating T2b tumour. One of the focal areas of tumour shows a deficit of the low signal bladder wall with intermediate signal extending across the whole thickness of the bladder wall, with subtle extension into the perivesical tissues (open arrow), this area is therefore radiologically a T3b tumour.

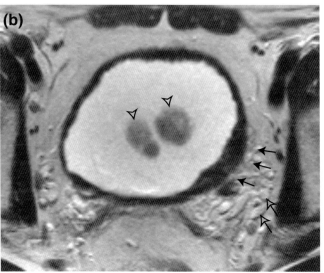

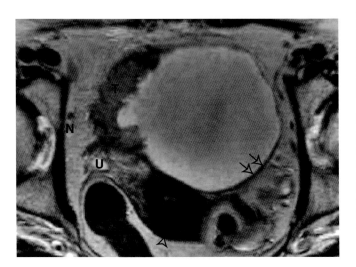

Figure 11.6. T3b Bladder cancer.

(a) Transaxial T1WI and **(b)** transaxial T2WI of a male patient with transitional cell carcinoma (T) of the bladder demonstrating transmural extension with stranding within the perivesical fat (arrows). There are also multiple serpiginous structures (open arrows) in the perivesical fat immediately adjacent to the tumour, which are of intermediate signal on T1 and high signal on T2. These are perivesical vessels and could be confused with extra-vesical tumour if only the T1W sequence was assessed. The filling defect within the bladder represents benign prostatic hypertrophy (arrowheads).

Figure 11.7. T3b Bladder cancer.

Transaxial T2WI demonstrating extension of tumour into the perivesical fat. Note the normal bladder wall demonstrates low signal intensity (open arrows) while the tumour demonstrates intermediate-to-high signal intensity (T), outlined by high signal urine and intermediate to high signal intensity perivesical fat. The tumour is involving the right ureteric orifice and causing a right-sided hydroureter (U). Right external iliac lymph node (N). Uterus (arrowhead). Rectum (R).

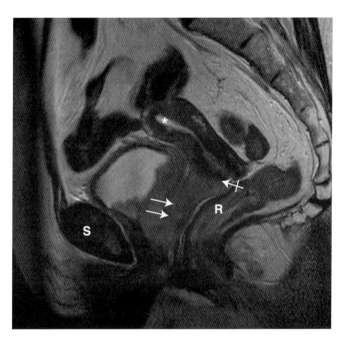

Figure 11.8.T4a Bladder cancer.

Sagittal T2WI. There is a large bladder tumour arising from the base of the bladder and extending along the postero-superior bladder wall. The tumour is extending through the posterior bladder wall and perivesical fat and is invading the vagina (arrows) and lower cervix (crossed arrow). Uterus (asterisk), rectum (R), symphysis pubis (S).

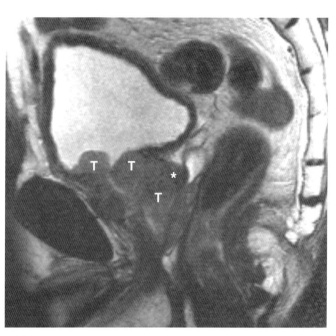

Figure 11.9.T4a Bladder cancer.

Sagittal T2WI lobulated tumour (T) is invading the prostate and inferior aspect of the seminal vesicle (asterisk).

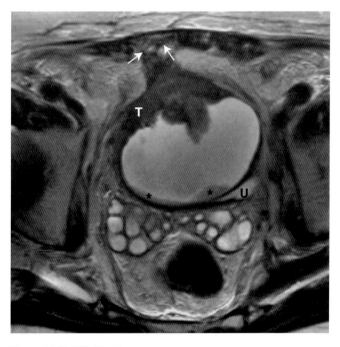

Figure 11.10.T4b Bladder cancer.

Transaxial T2WI of the bladder. There is a large bladder tumour (T) extending to the rectus sheath anteriorly (arrows). There is also tumour arising in the posterior bladder (asterisks) which is not invading muscle (T2 or less) but is obstructing the left ureter(U).

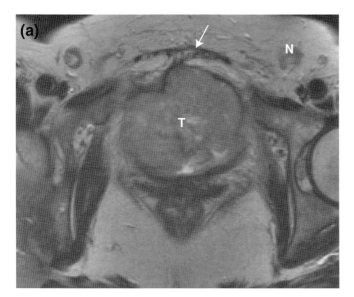

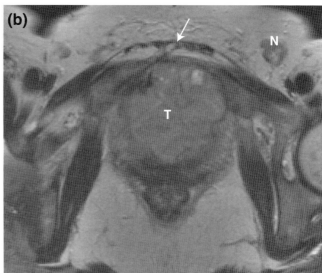

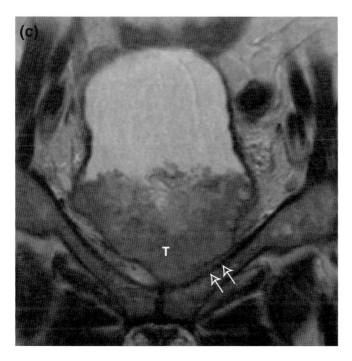

Figure 11.11.T4b Bladder cancer.

(a) and **(b)** transaxial T2WI and **(c)** coronal T2WI demonstrating a large bladder tumour (T) extending to the rectus sheath anteriorly (arrows) and to the left pubic bone inferiorly (open arrows). The cortex appears slightly irregular and thinner than the adjacent and contra-lateral pubic arch, with a long area of contact between tumour and bone. An inguinal node (N) is noted, which has the same signal intensity as the primary tumour and is therefore likely to be metastatic. This is an unusual site for nodal disease from a bladder tumour but is likely to be secondary to the tumour extension into the pubic bone.

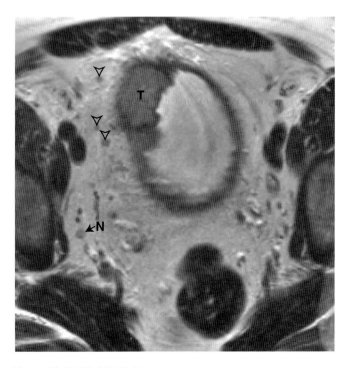

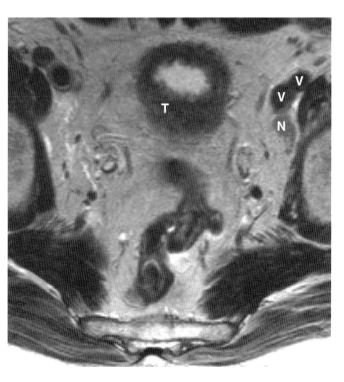

Figure 11.12.T3b N1 Bladder cancer.

Transaxial T2WI of the bladder. There is a large intermediate signal tumour (T) involving the right antero-lateral bladder wall, extending into the perivesical fat. Multiple small perivesical nodes are seen (arrowheads). These are noted to be of a similar signal intensity to the main bladder tumour. A right internal iliac node (N) is seen with similar signal intensity to the tumour proper making it more likely to be metastatic.

Figure 11.13. N1 Bladder cancer.

Transaxial T2WI demonstrating a single intermediate signal left obturator node ≤ 2.0 cm in long axis diameter (N) and an intermediate to low signal bladder tumour (T). Left external iliac vessels (V).

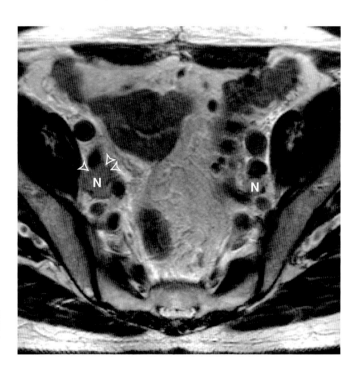

Figure 11.14. N2 Bladder cancer.

Transaxial T2WI showing bilateral metastatic obturator nodes (N). The right obturator node measures between 2.0 and 5.0 cm in greatest dimension, and has an irregular margin anteriorly (arrowheads) indicating extra-capsular extension.

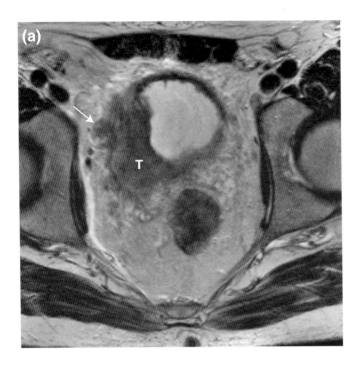

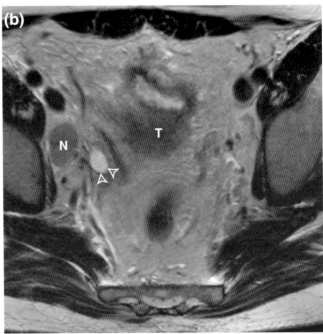

Figure 11.15. T3b N2 Bladder cancer.

(a) and (b) Transaxial T2WI and (c) coronal T2WI. A bladder tumour (T) is extending into the perivesical fat (arrows) and obstructing the right ureter (arrowheads). There is a right obturator lymph node metastasis (N) with a maximum diameter between 2.0 and 5.0 cm.

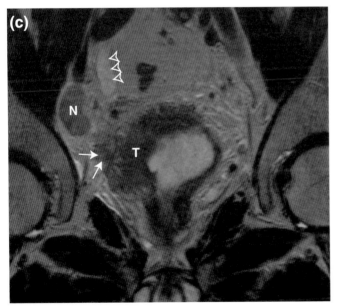

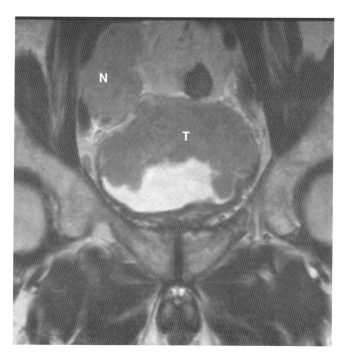

Figure 11.16. T3b N3 Bladder cancer.

Coronal T2WI showing a large bladder tumour (T) extending into the perivesical fat. There is a right external iliac node (N), >5.0 cm in longest dimension and of identical signal intensity to the primary tumour.

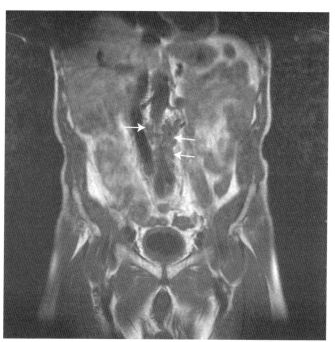

Figure 11.17. M1 Bladder cancer.

Coronal T1WI showing multiple para-aortic (arrows) and aortocaval (open arrow) lymph node metastases. Common iliac and retroperitoneal nodes are considered to be distant metastases (M1) in the TNM staging of bladder cancer.

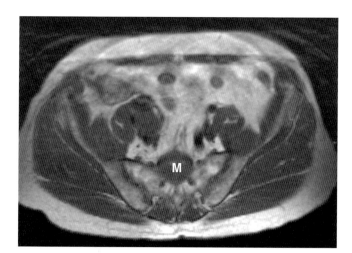

Figure 11.18. M1 Bladder cancer – bone metastasis.

Transaxial T1WI through the pelvis showing an intermediate signal mass (M) in the body of the sacrum due to a bone metastasis from the patient's transitional cell bladder tumour.

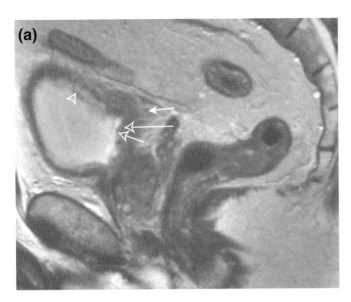
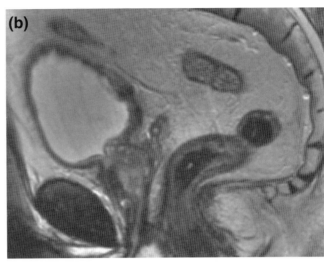

Figure 11.19. Post biopsy effect.

(a) and **(b)** Sagittal T2WI through the bladder. In (a) there is extensive abnormality of the bladder wall with intermediate signal thickening (open arrows), predominantly posteriorly with associated stranding of the perivesical fat (arrow), suggesting a T3b tumour. Thickening and irregularity of the bladder mucosa (arrowhead) is also noted. (b) Three months later these appearances have virtually resolved with no intervention and were due to biopsy-induced inflammation and oedema.

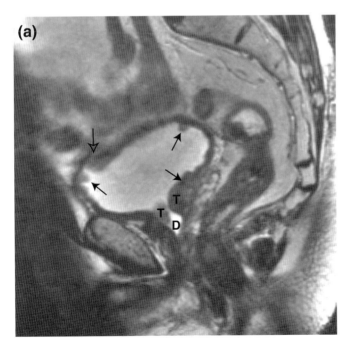
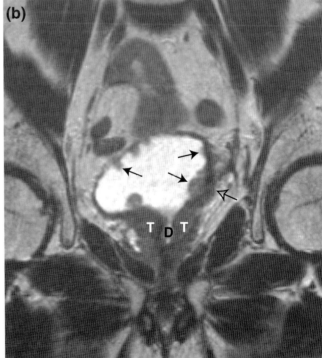

Figure 11.20. Multifocal bladder cancer.

(a) Sagittal T2WI and **(b)** coronal T2WI. There are multiple nodules of intermediate signal tumour involving the superficial bladder muscle (arrows). Some lesions show extension through the deep muscle layers (open arrow). Tumour (T) is also noted to extend into the defect (D) from a transurethral resection of the prostate for benign prostatic hypertrophy.

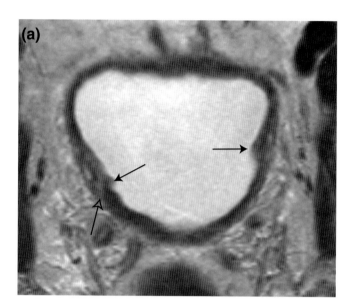

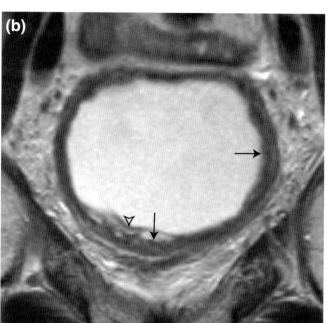

Figure 11.21. Multifocal bladder cancer.

(a) Transaxial T2WI and **(b)** coronal T2WI showing multiple areas of intermediate signal intensity tumour, involving the superficial bladder muscle (arrows). Some lesions show extension through the deep muscle layer (open arrow). There is also evidence of bladder mucosal oedema (arrowhead), which appears as superficial high signal.

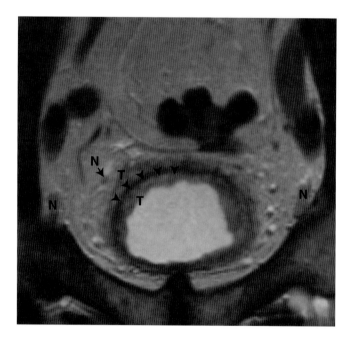

Figure 11.22. Diffuse bladder cancer with layering.

Transaxial T2WI through the bladder. Extensive tumour (T) is seen spreading circumferentially around the bladder wall with components superficial and deep to the muscle layer, which appears intact between them (arrowheads). This is therefore T3b disease. Small perivesical and pelvic sidewall nodes (N) are noted.

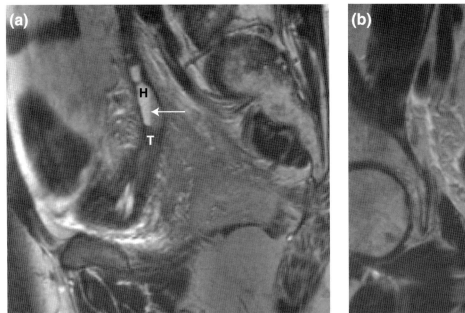
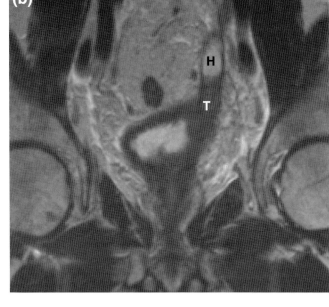

Figure 11.23.T3b Bladder cancer with tumour extending into the left ureter.

(a) Sagittal T2WI and (b) coronal T2WI through the bladder demonstrate a T3b tumour (T) involving the left bladder wall and base and extending into the lower left ureter. There is a left sided hydroureter (H) with layering of urine and debris or haemorrhage seen in the ureter (arrow). Hydronephrosis and/or tumour extension into the ureter do not alter the tumour stage but are associated with a worse prognosis.

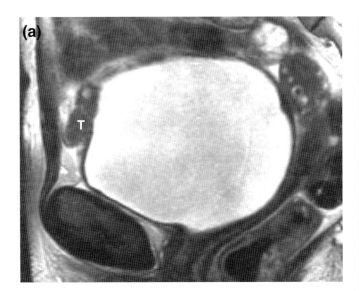
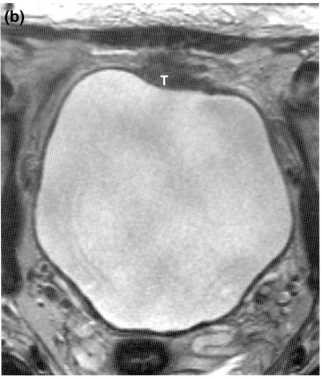

Figure 11.24. Urachal cancer.

(a) Sagittal T2WI and (b) transaxial T2WI showing tumour (T) centred on the obliterated urachus (median umbilical ligament), adjacent to the anterior bladder wall. The epicentre is extra-luminal, but knowledge of this anatomy allows the correct diagnosis of a urachal tumour, most commonly an adeno-carcinoma.

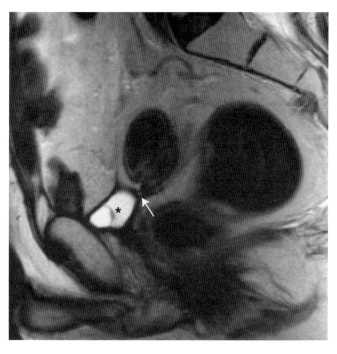

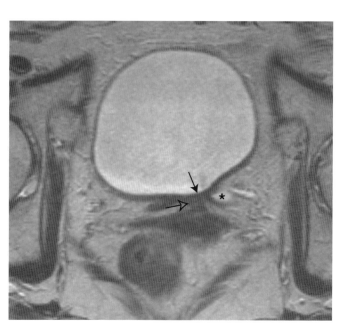

Figure 11.26. Treatment related change following localised radiotherapy.

Transaxial T2WI showing low signal thickening of the left postero-lateral bladder wall (arrow) due to fibrosis and resulting in left-sided hydronephrosis (asterisk). The bladder is tethered to the anterior vagina (open arrow).

Figure 11.25. Treatment related change following cystectomy and radiotherapy.

Sagittal T2WI. A small post-operative fluid collection (asterisk) is seen in the bladder bed and there are low signal fibrotic bands causing tethering of the sigmoid colon (arrow).

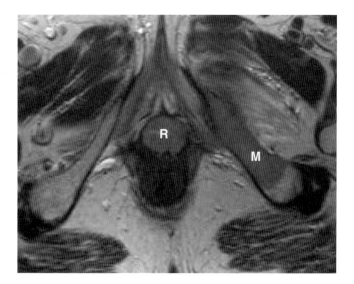

Figure 11.27. Tumour recurrence post cystectomy.

Transaxial T2WI in a patient who had a previous cystectomy for bladder cancer demonstrating an intermediate signal tumour recurrence (R) in the urethral bed and a bone metastasis in the left inferior pubic ramus (M).

12   Prostate Cancer

Rhidian Bramley

BACKGROUND INFORMATION

Epidemiology

Worldwide, prostate cancer is commonest among black American and Scandinavian populations. The incidence is rising in the USA and UK, and prostate cancer is now the second leading cause of male cancer deaths in these countries. Incidence statistics may be misleading, however, due to the high prevalence of occult disease. Approximately 30% of men in their 50s are said to harbour microscopic foci of prostate cancer, but most never progress. Age is the most important risk factor, clinical disease being rare in men below 50.

Histopathology

Nearly all prostate cancers are adenocarcinomas. Rare tumours include squamous and transitional cell carcinomas, and sarcomas. The most widely used classification system is the Gleason score. This is calculated as the sum of the two predominant cell types within the resected tumour tissue. The combined score can be further subgrouped into grades 2 to 4 (well differentiated), 5 to 7 (moderately differentiated) and 8 to 10 (poorly differentiated).

Approximately 75% of tumours arise in the peripheral zone of the gland, 15% in the transitional zone and 10% in the central zone.

Patterns of tumour spread

The outer prostatic 'capsule' is strictly a pseudocapsule of fibromuscular tissue inseparable from the prostatic tissue. Prostate cancer spreads locally through the pseudocapsule to involve the periprostatic connective tissues, seminal vesicles, bladder base and pelvic floor. The rectum is usually spared, as Denonvilliers' fascia forms a barrier to direct tumour extension. Lymphatic spread occurs most frequently to the obturator nodes, with the pararectal, pre-sacral and internal iliac nodal groups also commonly involved. Haematogenous spread arises through the periprostatic venous plexus, producing bone metastases particularly in the spine and pelvic girdle. Other common sites for metastatic disease are the liver and lung.

Table 12.1. Prostate cancer: TNM (2002) staging classification

Tx	Primary tumour cannot be assessed
T0	No evidence of primary tumour
Tis	Carcinoma *in situ*
T1	Tumour identified on histology but not apparent clinically or radiologically
	T1a Tumour is an incidental finding in <5% resected tissue
	T1b Tumour is an incidental finding in >5% resected tissue
	T1c Tumour identified only on needle biopsy
T2	Tumour palpable or visible on imaging confined to the prostate
	T2a Tumour involves less than one half of one lobe
	T2b Tumour involves more than one half of one lobe
	T2c Tumour involves both lobes
T3	Tumour extends beyond the prostatic pseudocapsule
	T3a Extra-capsular extension
	T3b Invading seminal vesicles
T4	Tumour fixed or invading adjacent structures, bladder neck, external sphincter, rectum, levator muscles, pelvic sidewall
N0	No lymph nodes involved
N1	Regional nodal metastases
M0	No metastases
M1	Non-regional lymph nodes and distant metastases
	M1a Non-regional lymph nodes
	M1b Bone involvement
	M1c Other sites involved

Prognostic indicators

TNM stage is the most important prognostic variable. The 5-year disease specific survival for patients with metastatic disease (M1) is approximately 30%.

The Gleason score is an independent prognostic indicator correlating with progression to metastatic disease and survival. The 10-year disease specific survival for clinically localised disease (managed conservatively) is 87% for well and moderately differentiated tumours, dropping to 34% for poorly differentiated tumours.

Prostate specific antigen (PSA) is primarily used in diagnosis and in detection of disease recurrence. High levels correlate with advanced TNM stage at diagnosis, and a rising PSA post treatment is indicative of tumour relapse. Overlaps in PSA ranges however limit staging accuracy for individual patients. Newly diagnosed asymptomatic patients with a PSA <10 ng ml^{-1} have a very low risk of skeletal metastases, and routine radionuclide bone scanning is not considered necessary.

Tumour volume and the number of positive biopsies on transrectal ultrasound (TRUS) are other prognostic variables. Tumour neovascularisation and molecular tumour-cell specific markers are the subject of ongoing research.

Treatment

The management of prostate cancer continues to be the subject of much debate. Watchful waiting (surveillance) with deferred treatment is a valid option, especially for well-differentiated localised tumours in elderly patients, with a normal life expectancy less than 10 years. This has to be weighed against an increased risk of interval disease progression and the potential complications of other treatments.

Radical prostatectomy is a curative treatment option for patients with localised (T1–2N0M0) prostate cancer. Some centres restrict surgery to patients with a Gleason score <7 and PSA <20 ng ml^{-1} due to increased risk of occult extra-capsular disease at higher levels. The main advantages of surgery are that definitive staging is possible, PSA levels are reliably suppressed following treatment and radiotherapy remains an option for locally recurrent disease.

External beam radiotherapy (EBRT), including conformal radiotherapy, may also be offered with curative intent. Radical radiotherapy is suitable for patients with clinically localised disease (T1–2N0M0) and locally advanced tumours (T3N0M0) after 'down-sizing' with hormonal therapy. Radiotherapy has similar results to surgery and it can be administered on an outpatient basis without the need for a major operation.

Brachytherapy, the implantation of radioactive seeds into the prostate, is gaining popularity, but is only available in specialist centres. This technique delivers a high dose to the prostate gland with relative sparing of the surrounding tissues. Criteria are more stringent than for EBRT and currently only small volume T2N0M0 tumours are considered.

Metastatic disease is managed by a combination of hormone therapy and palliative radiotherapy. Radioactive strontium can be effective for diffuse bone metastases. Chemotherapy for hormone refractory disease is the subject of ongoing clinical trials.

MR IMAGING OF PROSTATE CANCER

Technique

MRI evaluation of the prostate requires optimal technique using phased array pelvic surface coils. Endo-rectal coils (ERCs) used either alone or in combination with pelvic phased array coils have been shown to improve staging accuracy by better depiction of pseudocapsular penetration. ERCs have the drawbacks of causing patient discomfort and therefore possible movement artifact, and producing near field artifact although the latest scanners have software to overcome this problem.

Thin section T2-weighted turbo spin echo sequences are essential for differentiating normal internal zonal prostatic anatomy and pathology. The prostate and seminal vesicles must be covered in their entirety. Off-axis imaging, parallel to the prostate, can be helpful in evaluating extra-prostatic extension.

T1-weighted spin echo images are useful for detecting enlarged pelvic lymph nodes, bone metastases, and in distinguishing tumour from post biopsy haemorrhage. Fat suppressed imaging has no staging benefit over conventional T1- and T2-weighted spin echo sequences. Dynamic Gd-enhanced imaging can improve tumour recognition and staging accuracy, but is not widely used.

Magnetic resonance spectroscopy is currently under evaluation in prostate cancer. Initial findings indicate that there is increase in the ratio of choline plus creatine to citrate in prostate tumour tissue. This has been used to determine the presence and localisation of tumour within the prostate and to improve the assessment of extra-glandular extension.

Current indications

The indications for MRI are controversial and depend on local surgical and oncological practice, the availability of MRI and local radiological expertise. Many centres do not perform routine MRI, instead relying on clinical assessment (digital rectal examination (DRE)) combined with PSA level and Gleason grade to predict tumour stage.

MRI can provide additional useful information in assessing for extra-capsular tumour and seminal vesicle invasion. Decision analysis studies indicate MRI is most helpful in patients with an intermediate clinical risk of extra-capsular extension (clinically localised at DRE, PSA level ≥ 10–20 ng ml^{-1}, Gleason score of 5–7). In these circumstances, MRI signs of extra-capsular disease can stratify patients into low and high-risk groups for disease progression, based on PSA levels at 3 years post treatment. This information may influence the choice of treatment modality and the decision to offer adjuvant hormonal therapy.

MRI is useful in the selection of patients for brachytherapy. Accurate staging information is essential, as disease must be contained within the prostatic pseudocapsule (T1–2 N0 M0). Despite the low positive predictive value of MRI, features suggestive of extra-capsular extension are usually taken as a contraindication to treatment. MRI can also give an accurate assessment of prostatic volume, which should be <50 cm^3.

MRI may assist radiotherapy planning for locally advanced disease. The greater soft tissue contrast and multiplanar capabilities of MRI provide a more accurate assessment of disease extent and involvement of adjacent organs. Fusion imaging systems are in development to facilitate radiotherapy planning using MRI data.

MRI may also be useful in evaluating patients with a rising PSA following radical prostatectomy. Locally recurrent tumours or isolated lymph nodes may be suitable for salvage radiotherapy in the absence of more widespread disease.

Imaging features

Prostate cancer occurs in the peripheral zone in 75% of patients and usually has low signal intensity compared to the normal high signal of the peripheral zone on T2-weighted turbo spin echo images. Tumours in the central gland may be indistinguishable from normal tissue or benign prostatic hyperplasia. The prostatic pseudocapsule is seen as a thin band of low signal between the peripheral zone and periprostatic connective tissue. Features suggestive of capsular penetration are extra-capsular tumour, capsular retraction, focal capsular bulging, periprostatic stranding, capsular thickening and tumour contiguity with the pseudocapsule >12.0 mm.

Following radiotherapy the prostate gland shrinks and the peripheral zone becomes intermediate signal intensity on T2-weighted imaging. After radical prostatectomy, residual fibrosis in the prostatic bed has low signal intensity on all sequences. This may be differentiated from the intermediate signal intensity of recurrent tumour on T2-weighted images.

Staging accuracy

MRI offers the single most accurate imaging assessment of local disease and regional metastatic spread. The integration of MRI findings with standard clinical diagnostic tests has also been shown to improve the overall accuracy of prostate cancer staging. A meta-analysis of studies evaluating MRI staging accuracy in patients with clinically localised prostate cancer produced a maximum combined sensitivity and specificity on the receiver operating characteristic (ROC) curve of 74%, using pathological stage as the gold standard. At a specificity of 80% on the ROC curve, sensitivity was 69%.

As with any diagnostic test, however, the positive and negative predictive values will vary according to the prevalence in the population studied. Most published results give positive predictive values below 50%, indicating MRI usually overcalls extra-capsular disease extension prior to radical prostatectomy. It is recognised that pathological stage is an imperfect gold standard, however, and selected sections may miss extra-capsular disease extension if the gross specimen is not evaluated throughout.

Pitfalls of MRI

- Signal changes within the prostate should be interpreted with caution as other pathological processes may mimic prostate cancer. Infection, inflammation and haemorrhage will all produce low signal changes within the peripheral zone on T2-weighted imaging. The normal fibromuscular bands of the peripheral zone may also appear thickened as a normal variant, and should not be confused with tumour.

- Staging accuracy is reduced following transrectal ultrasound (TRUS) guided biopsy. Evaluation of extra-capsular extension is particularly difficult if the pseudocapsule or seminal vesicles have been multiply biopsied in an attempt to gain pathological evidence of locally advanced disease. Signal characteristics may be helpful as, unlike tumour, methaemoglobin within haemorrhage is high signal on T1-weighted imaging. If equivocal findings are present, radical treatment can be deferred and the MRI repeated, as post biopsy changes will resolve with time.

- Similarly, signal changes within and around the seminal vesicles can be misinterpreted on MR imaging. Haemorrhage, inflammatory scarring, stones and amyloid can all produce focal abnormalities and tubular thickening. Normal fibrous tissue around the ejaculatory ducts and infero-medial tips of the seminal vesicles can also be misdiagnosed as tumour. Some published reports have disregarded signal changes in the seminal vesicles unless there is evidence of tumour within the adjacent prostate on TRUS biopsy.

FURTHER READING

1. DeVita VT, Hellman S, Rosenberg SA (Eds) (2001) Carroll PR, Lee RL, Foks ZY, et al. In: Cancer Principles and Practice of Oncology, 6th Edition. Lippincott Williams and Wilkins, Philadelphia, USA, pp. 1418–1469. *The leading oncology reference text provides a comprehensive review of the management of prostate cancer.*

2. Husband J, Resnick H (Eds) (1998) Jages G and Basentz J. Prostate Cancer In: Imaging in Oncology. Isis Medical Media Ltd, Oxford, UK, pp. 239–257. *Aimed at the clinical radiologist, this textbook has a detailed chapter reviewing prostate cancer imaging.*

3. Kirby RS et al. (1998) Fast Facts; Prostate cancer. Health Press. *Concise easily readable overview of the diagnosis and management of prostate cancer.*

4. Royal College of Radiologists Clinical Oncology Information Network & British Association of Urological Surgeons (1999) Guidelines on the management of prostate cancer. Clinical Oncology 11: 55–81. *Also known as the UK COIN guidelines.*

5. Partin AW, Kattan MW, Subong EN et al. (1997) Combination of prostate-specific antigen, clinical stage and Gleason score to predict pathological stage of localised prostate cancer. A multi-institutional update. JAMA 277: 1445–1451. *Partin's tables may be used to predict the probability of extra-capsular disease extension.*

6. Chodak GW, Thisted RA, Gerber GS et al. (1994) Results of conservative management of clinically localized prostate cancer. N. Engl. J. Med. 330: 242–248. *Data showing the 10-year disease specific survival for clinically localized disease (managed conservatively) is 87% for well and moderately differentiated tumours, dropping to 34% for poorly differentiated tumours.*

7. Outwater EK, Petersen RO, Siegelman ES, et al. (1994) Prostate carcinoma: assessment of diagnostic criteria for capsular penetration on endorectal coil MR images. Radiology 193: 333–339. *Results from 30 patients who underwent MR imaging and prostatectomy. Diagnostic criteria of extra-capsular extension are presented although it is concluded that the sensitivity and specificity are generally low.*

8. D'Amico AV, Whittington R, Schnall M et al. (1995) The impact of the inclusion of endorectal coil magnetic resonance imaging in a multivariate analysis to predict clinically unsuspected extraprostatic cancer. *Cancer* 75: 2368–2372. *Study showing a positive MRI stratified patients with an intermediate clinical risk of locally advanced prostate cancer into groups with a 78% versus 21% 3-year rate of actuarial freedom from PSA failure.*

9. Getty DJ, Seltzer SE, Tempany CMC, et al. (1997) Prostate cancer: relative effects of demographic, clinical, histologic, and MR imaging variables on the accuracy of staging. *Radiology* 204: 471–479. *Optimal merging of diagnostic test results yielded an improvement in the overall accuracy of prostate cancer staging.*

10. Sonnad SS, Langlotz CP and Schwartz JS. (2001) Accuracy of MR imaging for staging prostate cancer: a meta-analysis to examine the effect of technologic change. *Acad. Radiol.* 8(2):149–157. *Meta-analysis of 27 studies comparing MRI with a pathological standard in clinically localised prostate cancer. A summary receiver operating characteristic curve for all studies had a maximum joint sensitivity and specificity of 74%. At a specificity of 80% on this curve, sensitivity was 69%.*

11. Jager GJ, Severens JL, Thornbury JR et al. (2000) Prostate Cancer Staging: Should MR Imaging Be Used?-A Decision Analytic Approach. *Radiology* 215: 445–451. *Concluded that it is not yet conclusively determined whether preoperative MRI staging is appropriate, but results of decision analysis suggest that MRI staging is cost-effective for men with moderate or high prior probability of extra-capsular disease.*

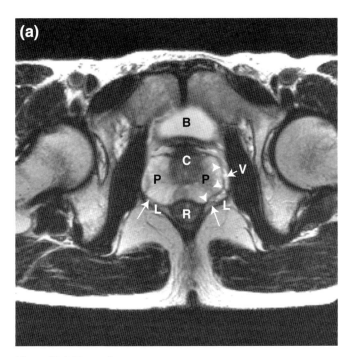

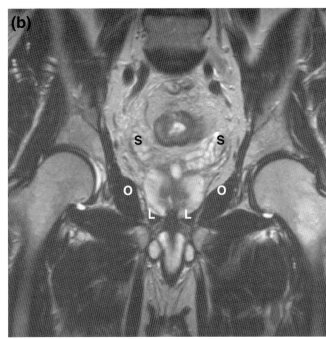

Figure 12.1. Normal prostate anatomy.

(a) Transaxial T2WI. The normal zonal anatomy of the prostate is well demonstrated on T2WI. The central gland (C) is comprised of central and transitional zones, and encloses the urethra. These zones are low signal on T2WI and may thus mask any low signal tumour within. Fortunately, 75% of tumours arise in the peripheral zone (P) of the gland, and are usually well demarcated from the high signal glandular stroma. The pseudocapsule is seen as a thin surrounding low signal band (arrowheads). Lateral to the pseudocapsule, the high signal periprostatic venous plexus (V) can sometimes cause confusion as to the true margin of the gland. The neurovascular bundles supplying the corpora cavernosa are positioned at the 5 and 7 o'clock positions, just outside the pseudocapsule (arrows). The rectum (R) is closely applied to the prostate separated by the thin low signal Denonvilliers' fascia. The bladder (B) may be seen anteriorly on transaxial sections. **(b)** Coronal T2WI. The seminal vesicles (S) are high signal with regular thin-walled tubules. The prostate sits within the levator sling (L). Laterally, the obturator internus muscles (O) form the pelvic sidewalls.

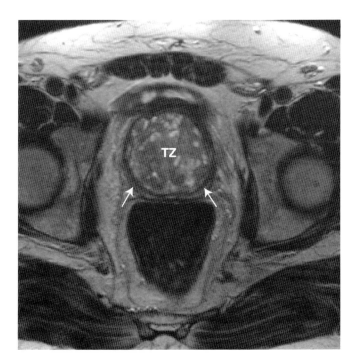

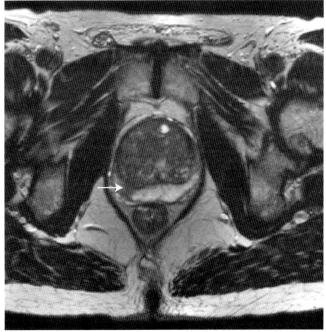

Figure 12.2. Benign prostatic hypertrophy (BPH).

Transaxial T2WI. BPH results in enlargement of the transitional zone of the gland. The peripheral zone is thinned (short arrows), and the normal high signal intensity may diminish, although not usually to the extent seen with tumour infiltration. The hypertrophied transitional zone (TZ) has heterogeneous signal on T2WI.

Figure 12.3. Stage T2a prostate cancer.

Transaxial T2WI. Low signal tumour is seen within the peripheral zone of the right lobe of the prostate (arrow). Changes of BPH are noted. The tumour occupies less than one half of one lobe indicating stage T2a disease. There is no evidence of extension beyond the pseudocapsule.

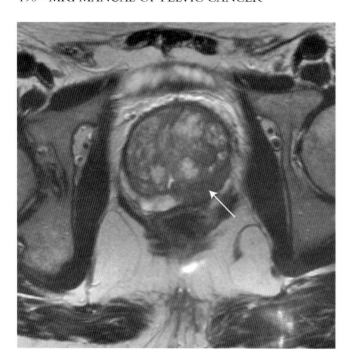

Figure 12.4. Stage T2b prostate cancer.

Transaxial T2WI. Tumour involving more than one half of one lobe is classified as T2b (arrow). The low signal is contiguous with the pseudocapsule for >12.0 mm, which increases the probability of microscopic extra-capsular disease. This may influence patient selection for brachytherapy or other radical treatments.

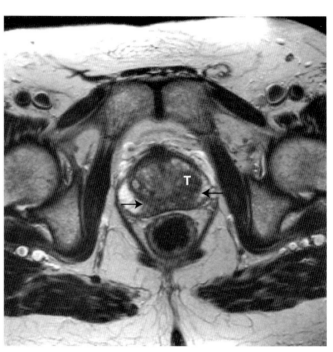

Figure 12.5. Stage T2c prostate cancer.

Transaxial T2WI. Tumour (arrows) involves both lobes, crossing the midline. Tumour is also seen within the central gland (T). There is no extra-capsular extension.

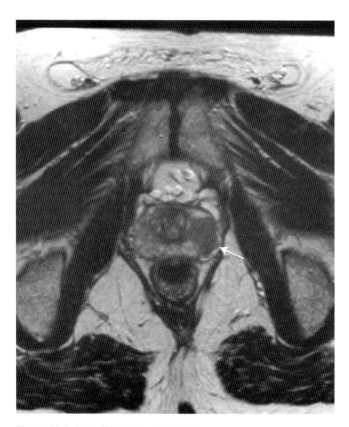

Figure 12.6. Stage T3a prostate cancer.

Transaxial T2WI. Extra-capsular extension is most commonly seen from the posterior and lateral aspects of the prostate, often in the region of the neuro-vascular bundle. Here, small volume low signal tumour breaches the prostatic pseudocapsule on the left (arrow), indicating stage 3a disease.

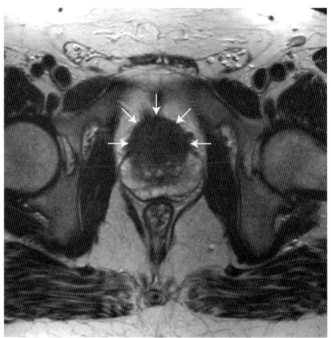

Figure 12.7. Stage 3a prostate cancer.

Transaxial T2WI. Tumour in the central gland can breach the anterior pseudo-capsule extending into the fat deep to the symphysis pubis (arrows). Anterior extra-capsular extension is usually not detectable clinically.

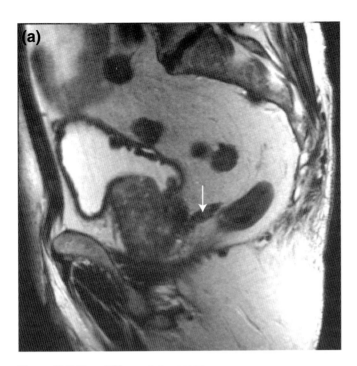

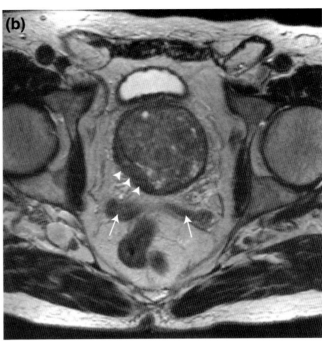

Figure 12.8. Stage T3b prostate cancer.

(a) Sagittal T2WI and (b) transaxial T2WI. The prostate is enlarged due to BPH. Low signal is seen in the right peripheral zone in keeping with tumour. There are indirect signs of extra-capsular disease as the pseudocapsule is retracted and thickened (arrowheads), and there is contiguity with the tumour over a prolonged distance (>12.0 mm). Both seminal vesicles and ejaculatory ducts (arrows) are replaced with material of similar signal intensity indicating T3b disease.

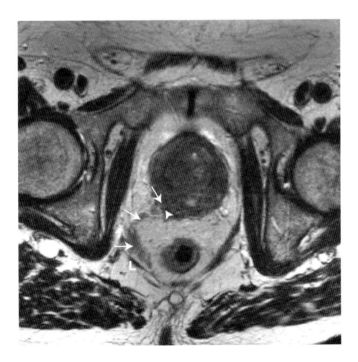

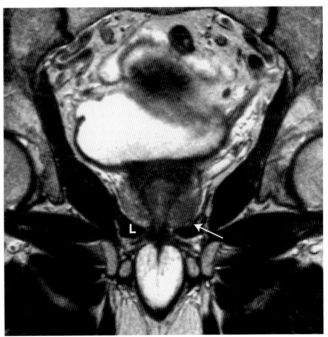

Figure 12.9. Stage T3a/T4 prostate cancer.

Transaxial T2WI. There is extra-capsular tumour extension (arrows) into the right neurovascular bundle (arrowhead), and posteriorly to the right levator muscle (L). MR staging is equivocal and clinical correlation may be required to distinguish between stage T3a and stage T4 disease. In stage T4 disease the tumour is 'fixed' to the pelvic sidewall.

Figure 12.10. Stage T4 prostate cancer.

Coronal T2WI. There is extra-capsular extension of tumour on the left (arrow) with tumour bulging into the left levator muscle (L). This would be stage T3a were it not for the muscular invasion.

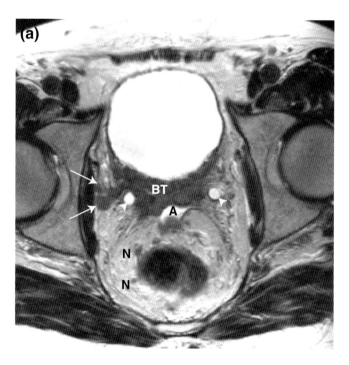

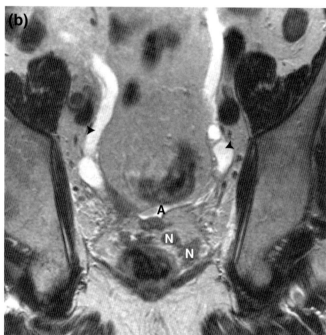

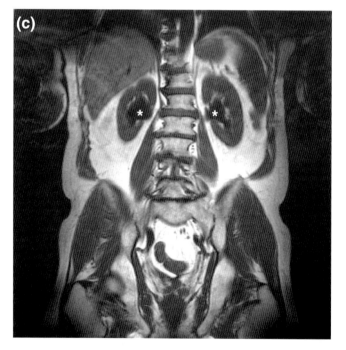

Figure 12.11. Stage T4 prostate cancer.

(a) Transaxial T2WI, (b) coronal T2WI and (c) coronal T1WI. Tumour extends to the right pelvic sidewall (arrows). Bilateral hydroureter (arrowheads) is present due to invasion of the bladder trigone (BT). A trace of ascites (A) is seen in the rectovesical pouch. Several small perirectal nodes (N) are noted. Bilateral hydronephrosis (asterisks) is confirmed on the T1-weighted images.

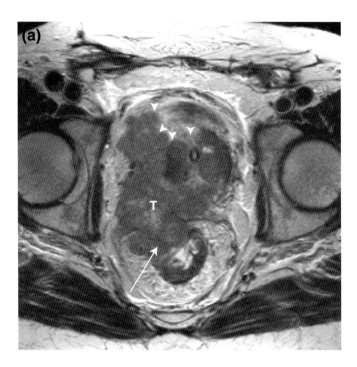

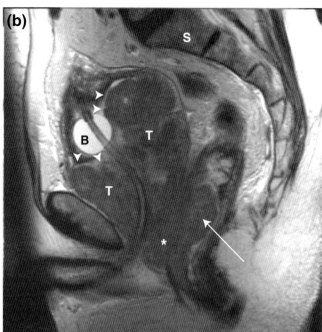

Figure 12.12. Stage T4 prostate cancer.

(a) Transaxial T2WI and **(b)** sagittal T2WI. There is an extensive tumour (T) infiltrating the bladder (arrowheads) and rectum (arrow). A balloon catheter (B) is *in situ*. Inferiorly, disease extends through the pelvic floor into the perineum (asterisk). Marrow hyperplasia due to anaemia accounts for the signal change in the sacrum (S).

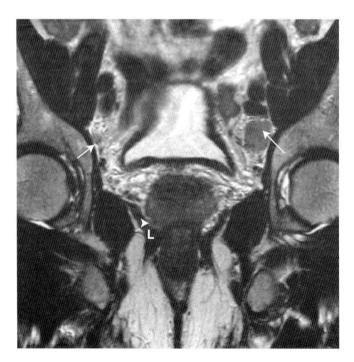

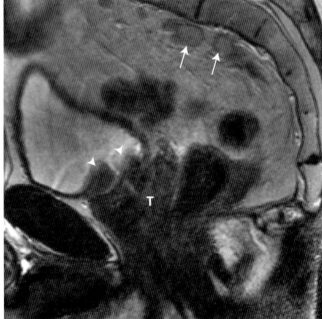

Figure 12.13. Stage N1 prostate cancer.

Coronal T2WI. The obturator and iliac nodes are most commonly involved in prostate cancer. Here, there is a large left external iliac nodal metastasis (long arrow). A small right external iliac node has similar signal intensity and is likely to be involved (short arrow). Local extra-capsular tumour extension is seen from the right side of the prostate (arrowhead) abutting the levator ani muscle (L).

Figure 12.14. Stage N1 prostate cancer.

Sagittal T2WI. Multiple pre-sacral nodes (arrows) in a patient with a T4 prostatic tumour (T) involving the bladder base (arrowheads).

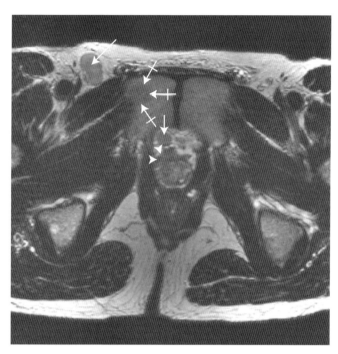

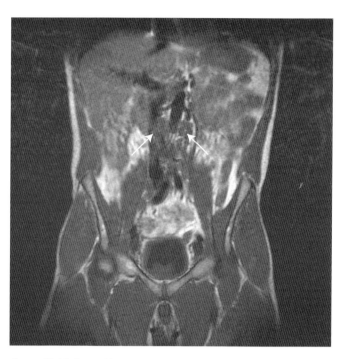

Figure 12.15. Stage N1 M1b prostate cancer.

Transaxial T2WI. Metastasis in a right inguinal node (long arrow). There is extracapsular tumour extension anteriorly at the prostatic apex (arrowheads). Note also a smaller node in between the prostatic apex and the pubic symphysis (short arrow). There is a bone metastasis in the right pubic bone (crossed arrows).

Figure 12.16. Stage M1a prostate cancer.

Coronal T1WI. Multiple interaortocaval and paraaortic retroperitoneal lymph nodes are present (arrows), indicating stage M1a disease. A transaxial upper T1W block of images may assist in equivocal cases.

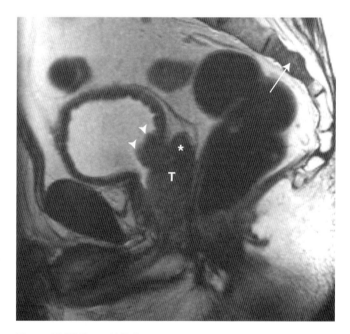

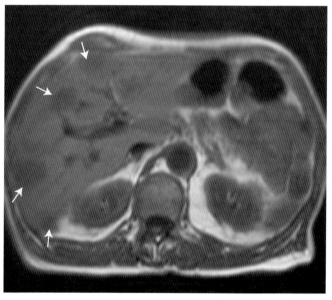

Figure 12.17. Stage M1b Prostate cancer

Sagittal T2WI. A bone metastasis is present in the third sacral segment (arrow) indicating stage M1b disease. The local staging is T4 disease as there is direct invasion of the bladder base (arrowheads) from a large prostate tumour (T), which is also engulfing the seminal vesicles (asterisk).

Figure 12.18. Stage M1c prostate cancer.

Transaxial T1WI. There are multiple hepatic metastases (arrows). Extra-skeletal non-lymph node metastases are classified as stage M1c disease.

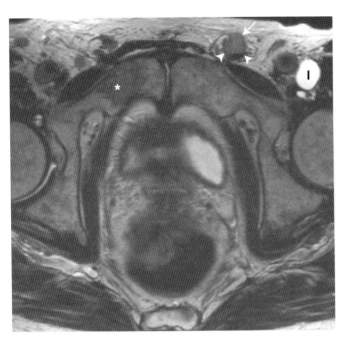

Figure 12.19. Stage M1c prostate cancer.

Transaxial T2WI. An unusual metastasis is seen within the left spermatic cord (arrow). The metastasis is differentiated from an inguinal lymph node by its medial position, similar to the uninvolved right spermatic cord, and the compressed left spermatic cord structures (arrowheads) seen posteriorly. Note a metastasis (asterisk) in the right pubic bone and other smaller bone metastases throughout the pelvis. Iliopsoas bursa (I).

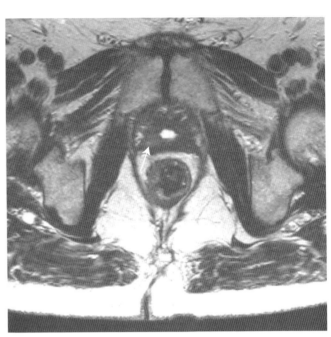

Figure 12.20. Post prostatectomy tumour recurrence.

Transaxial T2WI. Following radical prostatectomy, there is normally a ring of low signal representing post-operative fibrosis in the prostatic bed. Recurrent tumour usually shows as an area of intermediate signal intensity within the fibrotic tissue or adjacent periprostatic fat. In this example the recurrent tumour (arrow) is present between the 7 o'clock and 9 o'clock positions within the fibrous ring.

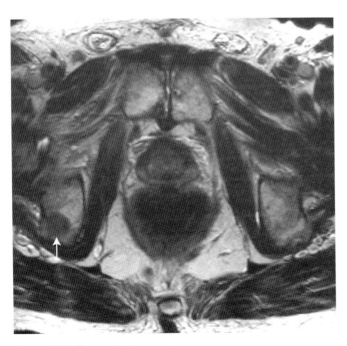

Figure 12.21. Post radiotherapy tumour recurrence.

Transaxial T2WI. Following radiotherapy, the prostate gland reduces in size and signal intensity decreases on T2WI, most obviously in the peripheral zone. Local tumour recurrence is usually heralded by a rise in PSA. This patient with a rising PSA had developed a bone metastasis (arrow) in the right ischium.

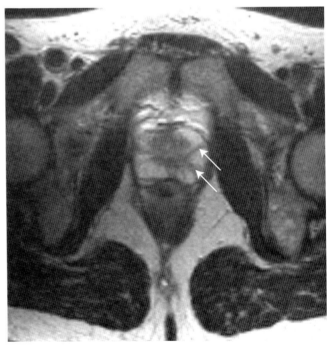

Figure 12.22. Fibromuscular bands.

Transaxial T2WI. The fibromuscular bands traversing the peripheral zone may appear prominent, as a normal variant (arrows). These linear radial bands should be easily distinguished from the more amorphous mass-like low signal change representing tumour infiltration.

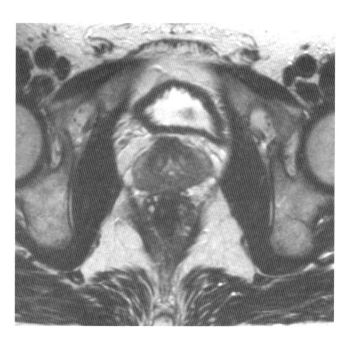

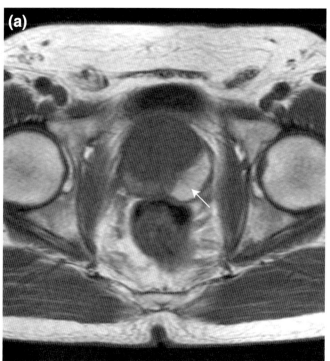

Figure 12.23. Prostatitis.

Transaxial T2WI. This patient had prostatitis producing diffuse low signal change throughout the peripheral zone. Tumour and inflammation may be indistinguishable on MR imaging and prostatic biopsy is required to diagnose tumour in the absence of widespread metastatic disease.

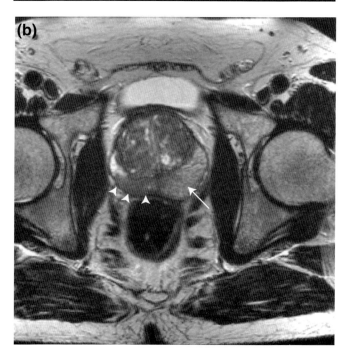

Figure 12.24. Post biopsy haemorrhage.

(a) Transaxial T1WI and (b) transaxial T2WI. There is post biopsy haemorrhage producing an asymmetrical left-sided bulge to the prostate peripheral zone. Methaemoglobin accounts for the high signal on the T1 and T2WI (arrows). Low signal (arrowheads) in the right peripheral zone of the prostate is consistent with tumour. The signal changes associated with haemorrhage evolve over several weeks and, depending on the stage of evolution, haemorrhage may either mask or simulate tumours in the peripheral zone on T2WI. Repeat imaging can help in equivocal cases, but, in our experience, changes can persist up to three months.

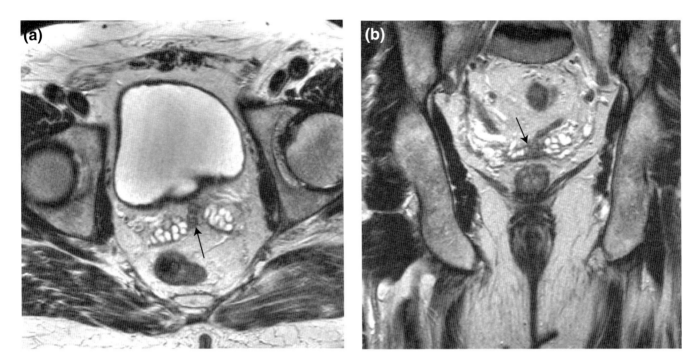

Figure 12.25. False positive seminal vesicle invasion.

(a) Transaxial T2WI and **(b)** coronal T2WI. A localised increase in fibrous tissue is normally found around the insertion of the vas deferens and origin of the ejaculatory ducts, which may encompass the medial tips of the seminal vesicles (arrows). This should not be interpreted as tumour invasion (Stage T3b) unless there is contiguous tumour extending from the adjacent prostate.

13   Pelvic Metastases

Fenella J. Moulding and Bernadette M. Carrington

INTRODUCTION

Pelvic metastatic disease may be **lymphatic, osseous** or **visceral**. MRI offers the most accurate cross-sectional assessment of potential metastatic sites in the pelvis.

LYMPH NODE METASTASES

Since lymphatic tumour spread is common in pelvic malignancy, it is important to identify the anatomical location of all the pelvic nodal groups and to be aware of the usual pathway of lymphatic drainage for each organ involved.

Normal lymph node sites

There are **perivisceral nodes** in the meso-rectal fat, parametrium, and paravesical fat. While meso-rectal lymph node metastases are often identified in rectal cancer, the other perivisceral nodes are only rarely seen.

Nodal metastases are most frequently identified in the **pelvic sidewall chains**, which are the **external iliac, internal iliac and common iliac** nodal groups, each named after the artery it accompanies.

- **External iliac lymph nodes** are composed of medial, anterior and lateral chains. **Intermediate nodes** lie just posterior to the external iliac vein and medial to the obturator internus. These are known as the '**surgical obturator**' group, since they are adjacent to the obturator vessels. Some authorities consider this group to be part of the internal iliac nodes. The **medial** chain lies between the external iliac artery and vein. The **lateral** chain is lateral to the external iliac artery. The external iliac lymph nodes drain to the middle and lateral common iliac chains.
- **Internal iliac lymph nodes** accompany the internal iliac vessels and drain to the common iliac chain. This group also includes two outlying nodal sites, the **sacral nodes** and the '**anatomical obturator**' nodes. The former accompany the median and lateral sacral vessels and may drain directly into the lumbar lymphatics. The latter lie in the obturator foramen but are identified in less than 10% of the population.
- **Common iliac lymph nodes** are composed of medial, middle and lateral nodes. The **medial** chain lies between both common iliac arteries and includes nodes anterior to the sacral promon-

tory. The **lateral** chain lies lateral to the common iliac artery. The **middle (posterior)** chain lies posterior to the common iliac vessels, between the psoas muscle and the spine. Enlargement of this chain produces the filled-in fat sign at the pelvic brim. The common iliac lymph nodes drain to the left and right lateral aortic chains, which are part of the lumbar (upper retroperitoneal) nodal chain.

The other local nodal group of relevance in pelvic cancer is the **inguinal chain** composed of superficial and deep subgroups. The superficial inguinal nodes lie immediately below the inguinal ligament and drain to the external iliac chain. The deep inguinal nodes lie medial to the femoral vein and also drain to the external iliac chain.

The usual pathways of lymphatic drainage for each of the pelvic organs are listed in *Table 13.1*. However certain tumour types may skip nodal stations, giving rise to non-contiguous nodal spread. For example, in cervical carcinoma the pelvic nodes may appear normal on imaging but retroperitoneal and supra-clavicular lymph node enlargement may be identified. Also, surgery can radically alter lymphatic drainage, which is relevant in the assessment of nodal metastases in recurrent disease.

Prognostic significance of lymph node metastases

Pelvic metastatic lymph node involvement alters tumour staging, treatment options and prognosis. For example, the 5-year survival of women with FIGO stage IB node-positive cervical cancer has been reported as 45–55%, compared to 85–95% for stage IB node-negative tumours. In bladder cancer, 5-year survival for T1N1 tumours is 15% but is 85% for T1N0 tumours.

Accuracy of imaging in the detection of lymph node metastases

Ultrasound, CT and MRI rely on morphological features, mainly lymph node size, to suggest the presence of lymph node metastases. Ultrasound is of little value in lymph node staging of pelvic malignancy as it has a relatively poor sensitivity for the detection of retroperitoneal and pelvic nodes. Assessing the relative accuracy of CT and MRI is difficult despite the numerous published studies because they vary in the criteria adopted for malignant infiltration and in the scan technique employed. Overall, the range of accuracies quoted for detection of lymph node metastases with MRI and CT are 85–93%

Table 13.1. Normal sites of lymphatic drainage for the pelvic organs

Organ	Lymph drainage
Ovary	• **Para-aortic** via lymphatic chain accompanying the ovarian vessels, on the left to the renal vein and on the right to the IVC at L1
	• **External and common iliac, obturator** via the broad ligament
	• **Superficial inguinal** via round ligament
Uterus	• Fundus – **Para-aortic** via lymph chain accompanying the ovarian vessels
	• Body – **External and internal iliac** → **common iliac**
	• Region of Fallopian tube – **Superficial inguinal** via round ligament
Cervix	• **Parametrial, obturator and pre-sacral** (via the utero-sacral ligament) initially
	• **External iliac, internal iliac** → **common iliac**
Vagina	• Upper $\frac{1}{3}$ – **Internal and external iliac** accompanying uterine artery
	• Middle $\frac{1}{3}$ – **Internal iliac** accompanying vaginal artery
	• Lower $\frac{1}{3}$ – **Superficial inguinal**
Prostate	• **Obturator** most frequently
	• **Internal and external iliac** → **common iliac**
	• **Pre-sacral**
Bladder	• **Anterior / lateral paravesical and pre-sacral** initially, followed by
	• **Obturator and external iliac** → **common iliac**
Rectal	• **Pararectal / meso-rectal** initially
	• Upper $\frac{1}{2}$ – **Pararectal** at origin of inferior mesenteric artery via the lymph chain accompanying the superior rectal artery
	• Lower $\frac{1}{2}$ – **Internal iliac** via lymph chain accompanying the middle rectal artery
Anus	• Above dentate line – **Perirectal, internal iliac**
	• Below dentate line – **Superficial inguinal**

and 65–80%, respectively. The sensitivities of MRI and CT range from 50–73% and 44–86%, respectively with specificities of 83–98% and 78–97%, respectively. CT and MRI are therefore equivalent in the detection of lymph node metastases.

There has been some work on the use of an ultra-small super-paramagnetic iron oxide (SPIO) contrast agent in lymph node assessment. This is taken up by the reticulo-endothelial system and acts to shorten T1, T2 and T2* resulting in decreased signal intensity on T2- or T2*-weighted images. In metastatic lymph nodes, the normal reticulo-endothelial system macrophages are replaced by tumour cells, which do not take up SPIO and show no signal drop post SPIO injection. Using this agent there have been some encouraging results in differentiating benign from malignant lymph nodes.

[18]Fluorodeoxyglucose positron emission tomography (FDG PET) is a functional imaging modality relying on increased glucose metabolism in cancer cells. In the detection of lymph node metastases, FDG PET sensitivities range from 24 to 91% and specificities from 77 to 100%. While many studies demonstrate increased staging accuracy of FDG PET compared to cross-sectional imaging, its availability is limited and CT and MRI remain the primary imaging modalities in lymph node assessment.

MR imaging technique for lymph node assessment

The body coil is used to obtain images of the upper retroperitoneal nodal stations and a pelvic phased array coil should be used to assess the pelvic lymph node stations if possible. Intravenous hyoscine butylbromide (Buscopan) may be given to reduce artifacts caused by bowel peristalsis, and improve image quality. T1-weighted sequences enable identification of lymph nodes against the high signal intensity of the pelvic fat. T2-weighted sequences allow the signal intensity characteristics of the nodes to be compared with those of the primary tumour. A fat suppressed sequence may make pelvic lymph nodes more conspicuous. Intravenous MRI contrast agents and specific lymphatic contrast agents such as SPIOs are not routinely indicated.

Normal lymph node appearances

Normal pelvic lymph nodes may appear homogenous or have a central fatty hilum. They are best detected on T1-weighted images, where they appear of homogenous low/intermediate signal contrasting well with the surrounding high signal fat, or have a high signal hilum consistent with intra-nodal fat, surrounded by an intermediate signal rim giving a characteristic target appearance. On T2-weighted images lymph nodes may be less conspicuous due to reduced contrast between their intermediate/high signal and the high signal of the surrounding fat. On a fat suppressed short tau inversion recovery (STIR) sequence lymph nodes tend to be well seen as high signal structures. The STIR sequence is particularly helpful for differentiating between hilar fat and central nodal necrosis.

Imaging features of lymph node metastases

When differentiating benign from metastatic nodes on CT and MRI, lymph node size is the only imaging criterion widely accepted to be useful. However, there are other helpful imaging features including shape, site, clustering and asymmetry, contour and signal intensity, which should also be considered when deciding if a node is involved by metastatic disease.

Size

When assessing lymph node size it is important to measure the maximum short axis diameter (MSAD), since that remains relatively constant irrespective of nodal orientation in the plane of the scan. Moreover diseased nodes are known to expand by becoming rounder before they become longer. Currently there is no universally agreed normal pelvic lymph node size in the imaging literature and the range varies between 6.0 mm and 15.0 mm with the most frequently used upper limit of normal short axis diameter being 10.0 mm. This is because studies have been performed on a mix of patient groups, such as normal controls or patients with early stage cancers who were eligible for surgical correlation. In these groups, normal lymph nodes often have a small short axis diameter (5.0 mm or less). However, in later stage larger tumours, which are often necrotic and infected, the regional lymph nodes are more likely to undergo reactive hyperplasia and there may be a need for a higher size threshold.

Nodal site influences normal size limits. United Kingdom guidelines quote normal short axis diameter lymph node size as 9.0 mm in the common iliac chain, 7.0 mm in the internal iliac chain, 10.0 mm in the external iliac chain, 8.0 mm in the obturator chain and 15.0 mm in the inguinal region.

Shape

Normal lymph nodes are kidney bean shaped or oval. Round nodes should be regarded with suspicion.

Site

The normal lymph drainage pathway of the pelvic organs should be considered when assessing a lymph node for metastatic involvement. If a node is detected in a recognised drainage site, although borderline on size criteria, it should be considered with caution. For example, the presence of a prominent obturator node in a patient with bladder, prostate or cervical cancer should be considered suspicious for disease involvement.

Clustering, asymmetry and contour

Asymmetry of normal lymph nodes can be seen in up to 10% of patients and therefore this feature cannot be solely relied upon. However, clustering of numerous small nodes is a suspicious finding. In the absence of local acute inflammation, a node with irregular margins suggests extra-capsular spread of tumour. In such cases over 75% of nodes are already enlarged and will have been considered abnormal on size criteria.

Signal intensity

If the nodal tissue is of similar signal to the primary tumour on T2-weighted images then one should be suspicious of metastatic involvement. Likewise, central nodal necrosis is a good predictor of metastases in patients with squamous cell carcinoma or teratoma. This appears as central high signal on T2-weighted images and low signal on T1-weighted images but is best appreciated on contrast-enhanced T1-weighted images, when the nonenhancing necrotic centre of the node contrasts well against the enhancing periphery.

Pitfalls of MRI

- **Lymph node hyperplasia** can be confused with metastatic lymph node enlargement. In many cases, no clear differentiation can be made but if the node is enlarged and does not have a signal intensity similar to the primary tumour, then reactive nodal hyperplasia should be considered.

- **Normal anatomical structures** may be mistaken for lymph nodes on MR imaging. These include the ovaries, bowel, tortuous vessels, ureters and prominent iliopsoas bursae. A helpful landmark in identification of the ovary is the round ligament. This extends from the groin into the pelvis, passing medial to the external iliac vessels, and links to the ipsilateral adnexa. The ovarian follicles may be clearly visible on T2-weighted scans in premenopausal women. Bowel, tortuous blood vessels, vessels with slow flow and the ureters may be differentiated from lymph nodes by scrolling through the images to confirm they are tubular structures. In addition, fast flowing blood produces a flow void particularly in arteries. A ureter may have high signal urine within the lumen on T2-weighted images. An enlarged iliopsoas bursa is low signal on T1-weighted images and high signal on T2-weighted images, smoothly demarcated and characteristically positioned posterolateral to the iliofemoral vessels.

- **Post-surgical complications** such as haematomas or lymphocoeles may mimic enlarged lymph nodes. Haematomas may demonstrate the concentric ring sign on T1-weighted images. Lymphocoeles form in less than 5% of patients post-operatively. They are collections of lymph fluid, which typically lie adjacent to the pelvic sidewall and are invested by parietal peritoneum. They return low signal on T1-weighted images and high signal on T2-weighted images.

BONE METASTASES

Malignant bone infiltration occurs due to direct tumour invasion or from haematogenous spread. Direct invasion may be due to erosion by the primary tumour, as in rectal cancer involvement of the sacrum, or due to extra-capsular lymph node infiltration, as in cervical cancer. Bone metastases due to haematogenous spread can occur with any pelvic tumour, most commonly in prostate cancer and rarely in ovarian cancer.

Accuracy and use of MRI in detection of bone metastases

Compared to bone scintigraphy, MRI is known to be more sensitive in detecting metastases with a sensitivity of 82–91% compared with 71–84%. This is because MRI detects metastases by altered signal at sites of early marrow involvement before osteoblastic stimulation (the cause of the radionuclide avidity) occurs. During a routine pelvic staging MRI examination, the pelvis, proximal femora and lumbar spine are imaged. As this coverage includes a large number of common metastatic bone sites, the majority of bone metastases should be detected.

MR imaging technique for assessment of bone metastases

T1-weighted and fat suppressing STIR sequences are the most useful sequences for identifying lesions. T2*-weighted gradient echo images, though less sensitive than T1 and STIR sequences, may show lesions by their loss of susceptibility artifact, due to disruption of the trabeculae, and may help identify fractures and osteoblastic healing in osteoporosis. T2-weighted spin echo sequences are of limited use. Intravenous contrast may be helpful as the metastatic tumour will enhance, though this is not routinely used.

In the specific case of suspected vertebral metastases, the whole spine should be imaged to detect all metastatic deposits. Parasagittal sections should be performed with axial sections through areas of concern. In addition to T1-weighted, STIR images and T2*-gradient echo images, diffusion-weighted images may also be helpful. T2-weighted spin echo sequences will help to evaluate concomitant degenerative disc disease.

Imaging features

Normal marrow appearances

Normal bone marrow may be haemopoietically active, containing myeloid elements and known as 'red marrow', or haemopoietically inactive containing mainly fat cells and known as 'yellow marrow'. At birth, virtually the whole skeleton contains red marrow. During normal aging, this is converted to yellow marrow in a uniformly predictable manner, starting from the extremities and moving proximally. In adults the only remaining red marrow is in the axial skeleton and most proximal appendicular skeleton. There is a mix of red and yellow marrow in some portions of the skeleton.

Red and yellow marrow have different imaging characteristics. Because of its fat content, yellow marrow tends to be relatively high signal on T1- and T2-weighted images and to suppress on STIR sequences resulting in low signal. Red marrow is intermediate signal on T1-weighted images and higher signal on T2-weighted images and STIR sequences. When there is a mix of red and yellow marrow, the overall result is to increase the signal intensity of the marrow on T1-weighted images so that the islands of red marrow are often poorly demarcated intermediate areas within the marrow.

Bone metastases

Metastases show as discrete intermediate to low signal areas contrasting well with the predominantly higher signal fatty marrow on T1-weighted images. On STIR sequences, metastases are usually high signal. In prostate cancer, sclerotic metastases appear as low signal on both sequences.

Pitfalls of MRI

- **Normal retraction of red marrow**, which partially affects a particular bone, can be a problem, particularly in the femoral head and ilium where patchy signal may be detected. This is often relatively symmetrical within the skeleton, and the red marrow appears band like or ill-defined enabling differentiation from bone metastases.

- **Bone marrow reconversion** may occur in times of increased demand for haemopoiesis, for example in chronic anaemic states, and as a result of haemopoietic growth factor therapy. Yellow fatty marrow converts back to red haemopoietic marrow starting centrally and spreading more peripherally. T1-weighted images will show areas of intermediate signal, whereas T2-weighted images and STIR sequences will show variable, high signal, though not as high signal as in metastatic disease. The reconversion is relatively symmetrical with uniform involvement of the marrow spaces. While diffuse malignant infiltration from lymphoma, myeloma or leukaemia could be confused with bone marrow reconversion, the pattern is dissimilar to solid tumour bone metastases.

- **Radiotherapy effect** tends to cause fatty change within the marrow, with high signal on T1-weighted and T2-weighted images and suppression of marrow signal on STIR sequences. It can be readily identified as it is usually very uniform with a sharp demarcation, which corresponds to the boundary of the radiotherapy field.

  Other effects of radiotherapy include insufficiency fractures, which occur in bone weakened by radiation osteitis, particularly the sacrum. They manifest as bands of low signal on T1-weighted images, which are high signal on STIR images and within which the fracture line itself may be observed centrally as a fine low signal intensity line. When the sacrum is affected, bilateral vertical sacral fractures may occur with a bridging horizontal fracture producing the classical H pattern or 'Honda' sign. MR scans are the most sensitive imaging modality for detection of insufficiency fractures but CT scans may define the fracture line more readily, therefore increasing diagnostic confidence.

  Abnormalities in bone marrow adjacent to the sacroiliac joints have also been demonstrated on MRI in patients treated by radiotherapy with no demonstrable fracture seen on other radiological modalities. These lesions are ill-defined low signal on T1-weighted images and high signal on T2-weighted images. Biopsy in such cases has shown evidence of peritrabecular fibrosis and inflammatory infiltration.

- **Osteoporotic vertebral collapse**, when chronic, can usually be distinguished from metastases by the relatively normal signal of the collapsed vertebra, the lack of an associated perivertebral soft tissue mass and lack of enhancement after intravenous contrast medium injection. Acute osteoporotic fracture and collapse may be difficult to differentiate from metastatic disease because of abnormal vertebral signal due to haemorrhage and oedema, enhancement after intravenous contrast medium, and perivertebral haemorrhage into the soft tissues.

  On diffusion-weighted images pathological compression fractures are hyperintense, whereas benign vertebral compression fractures are hypo- or isointense compared to adjacent normal vertebral bodies. T2*-weighted images may help by demonstrating the osteoporotic fracture site and reactive trabecular sclerosis producing increased susceptibility low signal intensity.

- **Haemangiomas** tend to be focal areas with signal varying from intermediate to high on T1-weighted, T2-weighted and STIR images, depending on the relative proportions of their fat and soft tissue vascular components, as well as any interstitial oedema. Accentuated vertical trabeculation may be seen within larger lesions. They are most commonly seen in the vertebrae, particularly the lower thoracic and upper lumbar spine and are rarely seen in the flat and long bones. They typically occur in females in the 4th and 5th decades.

- **Benign bone islands** are composed of compact bone within the medullary canal and exhibit low signal on all image sequences. Their small size and lack of cortical involvement or periosteal reaction may help differentiate them from sclerotic metastases.

- **Subchondral cysts** in degenerative joint disease are of low signal on T1-weighted images and high signal on T2-weighted and STIR images. Their typical subchondral location and associated features of loss of joint space, osteophyte formation and low signal subchondral sclerosis should help in their diagnosis.

- **Nutrient foramina** may be seen in all bones extending from the cortical margin into the medulla. They are small, low signal, well-defined lesions which appear linear when scrolling through the images. They are bilateral, virtually symmetrical and found in typical anatomical locations(e.g. the medial aspect of the ilium).

- **Paget's disease** occurs most commonly in middle aged males. It may be solitary or multifocal, thereby simulating metastases. MRI features are nonspecific. The affected bone may appear enlarged, and of heterogenous signal with low signal cortical thickening. The cortex may occasionally be of higher signal due to remodelling of the cortical bone. Correlation should be made with plain radiographs, which have much more characteristic and specific appearances.

METASTASES TO PELVIC VISCERA

Rarely, extra-pelvic tumours may metastasise to the pelvic viscera and diagnosis depends on a known history of extra-pelvic primary malignancy with biopsy of the pelvic mass where appropriate. The commonest organ to harbour metastases is the ovary. Krukenberg tumours are bilateral ovarian metastases from a gastrointestinal tract tumour, most commonly gastric cancer. They occur in 2% of the female population with gastric carcinoma and may precede diagnosis of the primary tumour in up to 20% of patients. On MRI, the only described imaging feature differentiating between Krukenberg and primary ovarian tumours is that primary tumours are more frequently multilocular.

Breast carcinoma can metastasise to any organ. The lobular subtype is prone to spread to unusual sites including the gastrointestinal tract, peritoneum and adnexae, which are affected in up to 20% of patients. At autopsy, 50% of patients with breast cancer will have ovarian metastases. Uterine metastases also occur in breast cancer. In our experience, metastases to the uterus from breast cancer have produced an enlarged uterus with the myometrium demonstrating low signal intensity on T2-weighted images, similar to diffuse adenomyosis.

Malignant melanoma may also metastasise to the pelvic viscera or subcutaneous soft tissues. Typically lesions are of intermediate or high signal on T1-weighted images. The high signal is due to the paramagnetic effect of intra-lesional melanin. Lesions may be of mixed high and intermediate signal on T2-weighted images. Large lesions may undergo central necrosis.

FURTHER READING

1. Williams AD, Cousins C, Souffer WP et al. (2001) Detection of pelvic lymph node metastases in gynaecological malignancy: A comparison of CT, MR imaging and positron emission tomography. *AJR* 177: 343–348. *Assesses the relative values of CT, MRI and PET, with histological correlation, in the detection of pelvic lymph node metastases.*

2. Vinicombe SJ, Norman AR, Nicolson V and Husband JE. (1995) Normal pelvic lymph nodes: Evaluation with CT after bipedal lymphangiography. *Radiology* 194: 349–355. *Normal lymph node size assessed on CT with lymphangiogram correlation.*

3. Kim SH, Kim SC, Choi BI and Han MC. (1994) Uterine cervical carcinoma: evaluation of pelvic lymph node metastases with MR imaging. *Radiology* 190(3): 807–811. *Assesses the accuracy of MRI in the detection of lymph node metastases and confirms that the short axis diameter is more accurate than long axis diameter.*

4. Bellin MF, Roy C, Kinkel K et al. (1998) Lymph node metastases: safety and effectiveness of MR imaging with ultrasmall superparamagnetic iron oxide particles- initial clinical experience. *Radiology* 207: 799–808. *Confirms safety and usefulness of SPIO particles in differentiating metastatic from benign lymph nodes.*

5. McCauley TR, Rifkin MD and Ledet CA. (2002) Pelvic lymph node visualization with MR imaging using local administration of ultrasmall superparamagnetic iron oxide contrast. *J. Magn. Reson. Imaging* 15: 492–497. *Demonstrates the increased number of lymph nodes detected with local interstitial injection in comparison with intravenous injection.*

6. Carrington B. (1998) Lymph nodes. In: *Imaging in Oncology* (eds Janet ES Husband and Rodney Rezneck). Isis Medical Media Ltd, Oxford, pp. 729–748. *Good overview of lymph node metastases and a variety of imaging techniques.*

7. Daldrup-Link HE, Franzius C, Link TM et al. (2001) Whole-body MR imaging for detection of bone metastases in children and young adults. *AJR* 177: 229–236. *Good comparison of MR, skeletal scintigraphy and PET scanning for the detection of bone metastases.*

8. Taoka T, Mayr NA, Lee HJ et al. (2001) Factors influencing visualization of vertebral metastases on MR imaging versus bone scintigraphy. *AJR* 176: 1525–1530. *Demonstrates that cortical involvement is the likely cause of positive findings on bone scans whereas MR scans may detect very early small intramedullary metastases.*

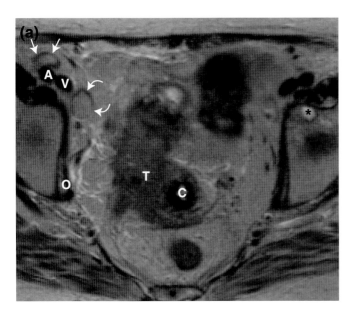 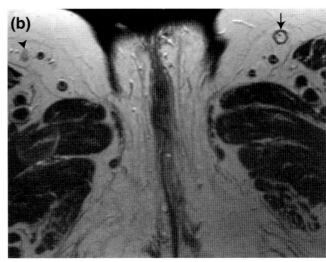

Figure 13.1. Normal lymph nodes.

(a) Transaxial T2WI showing two lymph nodes in the right lateral external iliac (straight arrows) and surgical obturator regions (curved arrows), both with a high signal intensity fatty central hilum and an intermediate signal intensity margin. The patient has a large bladder tumour (T) extending to involve the cervix (C). An incidental bone cyst (asterisk) is present in the left acetabulum. External iliac artery (A); external iliac vein (V); obturator internus muscle (O).

(b) Transaxial T1WI showing a nonenlarged lymph node in the left inguinal region (straight arrow). This has an intermediate signal intensity centre with a rim of fatty high signal and an intermediate signal intensity margin, which gives it a typical 'target' appearance. Nodes with this appearance are less likely to be infiltrated with tumour. Note a small right inguinal lymph node (arrowhead) of more uniform intermediate to high signal intensity.

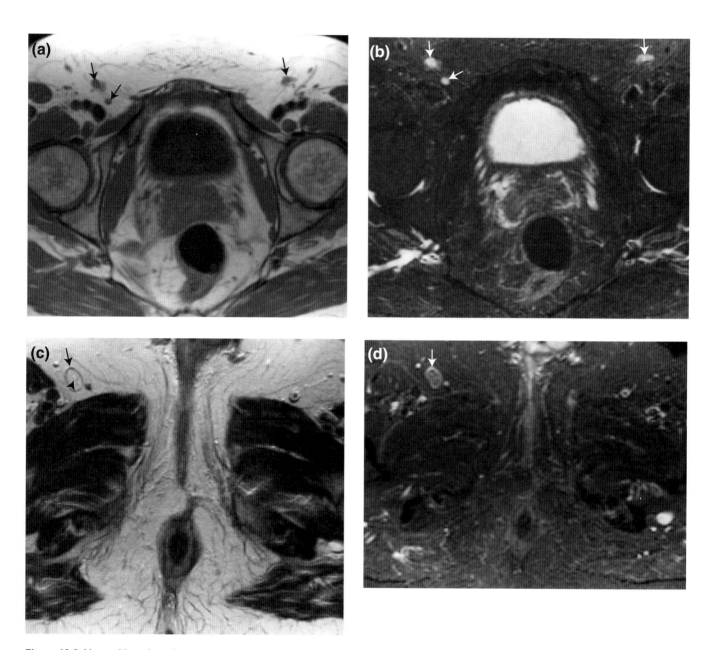

Figure 13.2. Normal lymph node appearances on STIR sequences.

(a) Transaxial T1W and (b) STIR images demonstrating small bilateral inguinal lymph nodes (arrows) which demonstrate high signal on STIR. (c) Transaxial T2W and (d) STIR images in a different patient demonstrating a right inguinal lymph node (arrows) which is predominantly of fat signal but with some internal structure as shown by chemical shift artifact within the node in (c) (arrowhead). On the STIR image the capsule of the node increases in signal, the fat within the node suppresses and the soft tissue structure becomes evident as small foci of high signal.

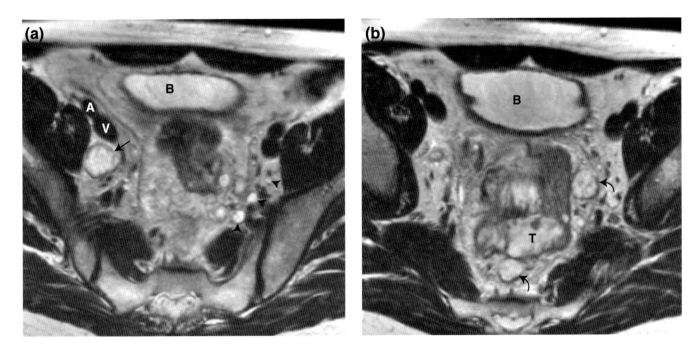

Figure 13.3. Mucinous rectal carcinoma with perirectal, internal iliac and obturator lymph nodes.

(a) and **(b)** Transaxial T2WI showing an enlarged right surgical obturator lymph node (straight arrow in (a)) and perirectal lymph nodes (curved arrows in (b)) which are the same high signal as the primary mucinous rectal tumour (T). This is due to the presence of mucin in the lymph node metastases. There is also a cluster of left internal iliac lymph nodes (arrowheads) of small size but similar signal to the primary tumour making them likely to be metastatic. External iliac artery (A); external iliac vein (V); bladder (B).

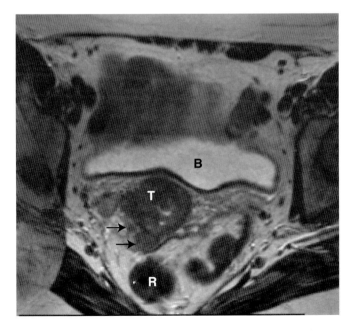

Figure 13.4. Paracervical metastatic lymph node in cervical cancer.

Transaxial T2WI of the cervix. There are two paracervical lymph nodes (arrows), which should not normally be visualised. They are of similar signal intensity to the cervical primary tumour (T). Bladder (B); rectum (R).

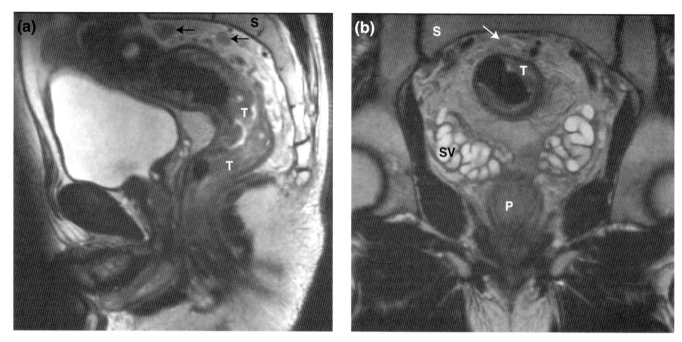

Figure 13.5. Pre-sacral lymph nodes in rectal carcinoma.

(a) Sagittal and **(b)** coronal T2WI demonstrating pre-sacral lymph nodes (straight arrows) which are of abnormal signal similar to that of the primary rectal tumour (T). Pre-sacral nodes are not normally seen therefore their presence, however small, raises the suspicion of metastatic lymph node disease. Sacrum (S); seminal vesicles (SV); prostate (P).

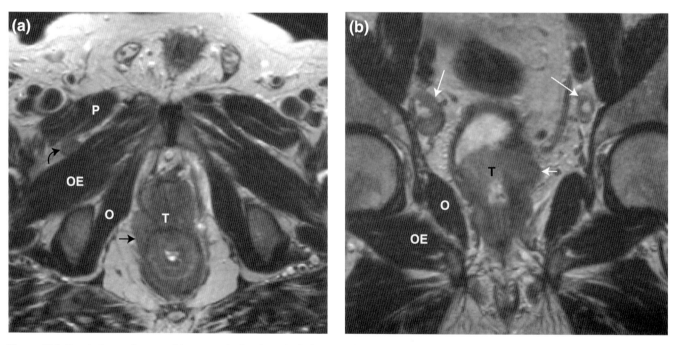

Figure 13.6. Prostatic carcinoma with anatomical and surgical obturator lymph nodes.

(a) Transaxial and **(b)** coronal T2WI demonstrating a prostate tumour (T) with extra-capsular spread (short arrow). There is a right-sided anatomical obturator lymph node (curved arrow in (a)) which is of similar signal to the primary prostatic tumour (T). There are bilateral enlarged right surgical obturator nodes (long arrows in (b)) which have a high signal centre, greater than fat, indicating central necrosis. Obturator internus muscle (O); obturator externus muscle (OE); pectineus muscle (P).

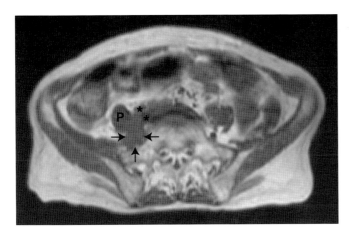

Figure 13.7. Common iliac lymph nodes – 'filled in fat' sign.

Transaxial TIWI through the proximal common iliac vessels demonstrates enlarged middle/posterior common iliac lymph nodes (arrows) situated behind the iliac vessels filling in the fat and eroding into the sacrum. Compare with the normal left side. Psoas muscle (P); iliac vessels (asterisk).

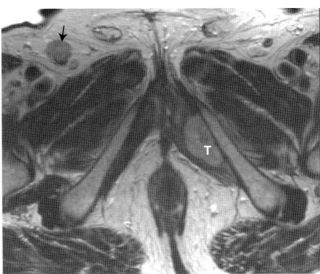

Figure 13.8. Alteration in pattern of lymph node metastases after surgery for bladder cancer.

Transaxial T2WI showing an enlarged right inguinal lymph node (straight arrow) which is as the same signal as the pelvic recurrence of the patient's bladder tumour (T). The usual pattern of lymph node spread from bladder carcinoma is to the paravesical, obturator and external iliac nodes. After cystectomy, altered lymphatic drainage has resulted in the left pelvic recurrence spreading to the right inguinal region.

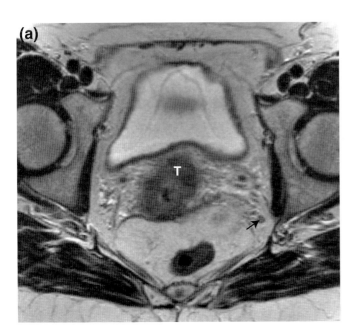

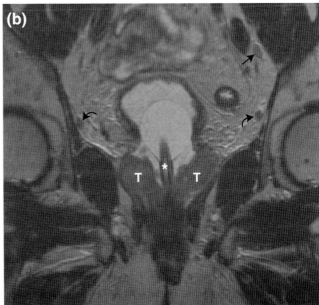

Figure 13.9. Metastatic lymph nodes which are nonenlarged but in the recognised drainage pathway of the primary tumour.

(a) Transaxial T2WI in a patient with cervical cancer demonstrating a nonenlarged left internal iliac lymph node (straight arrow). This is of similar signal intensity to the primary cervical tumour (T) and is highly suspicious of metastatic involvement. (b) Coronal T2WI in a patient with prostate cancer with nonenlarged lymph nodes in the proximal left external iliac (straight arrow) and both obturator regions (curved arrows). Again, these are of similar signal to the primary prostatic tumour (T). Bladder catheter (asterisk).

In these patients, lymph nodes are located in the known drainage pathway of the primary tumour and their signal intensity mirrors the signal intensity of the primary tumour increasing the likelihood of metastatic involvement despite their small size.

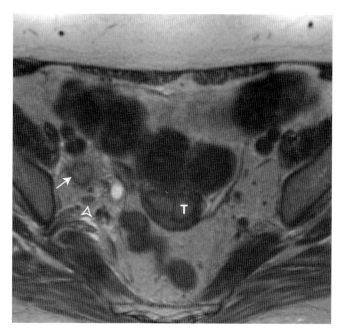

Figure 13.10. Metastatic lymph nodes – extra-capsular extension of tumour.

Transaxial T2WI showing an enlarged right obturator lymph node (straight arrow), which has an irregular wall indicating likely extra-capsular spread. The signal intensity is also abnormal and similar to that of the primary tumour (T) involving the uterus. A small but asymmetrically prominent right internal iliac lymph node (arrowhead) is also noted.

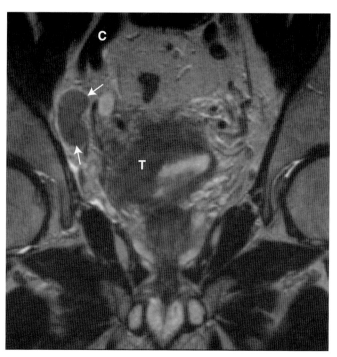

Figure 13.11. Metastatic lymph node – tumour signal.

Coronal T2WI demonstrating an enlarged right obturator node (straight arrows), which has an abnormal signal intensity similar to that of the primary bladder tumour (T). Common iliac artery and vein (C).

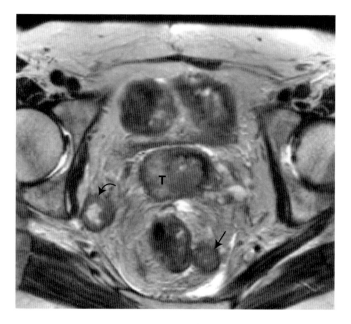

Figure 13.12. Perirectal and right external iliac nodal metastases with central nodal necrosis.

Transaxial T2WI in a patient with a squamous cell tumour (T) of the cervix showing an enlarged abnormal perirectal lymph node (straight arrow). It is of similar signal intensity to the cervical tumour. There is also an enlarged right internal iliac lymph node (curved arrow). It has an irregular medial contour indicating extra-capsular tumour spread. There is a high signal central area in keeping with central nodal necrosis, though a preserved central fatty hilum may also have a similar appearance. These can be differentiated using STIR or fat suppressed images.

The finding of central nodal necrosis is consistent with metastatic disease in patients with squamous cell carcinoma, irrespective of the size of the lymph node.

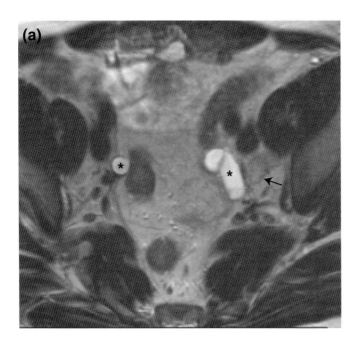

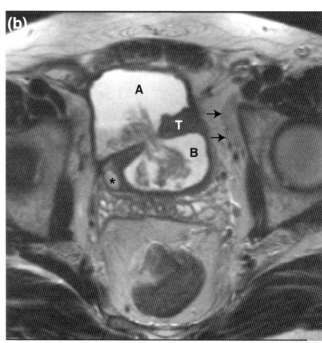

Figure 13.13. Lymph node pitfall – reactive lymph node hyperplasia.

(a) and (b) Transaxial T2WI demonstrating enlarged left obturator and external iliac lymph nodes (straight arrows) due to infection resulting from a bladder tumour perforation with abscess formation (A). The primary tumour (T) is of different signal intensity to the hyperplastic lymph nodes. There are bilateral hydroureters (asterisk). Bladder (B).

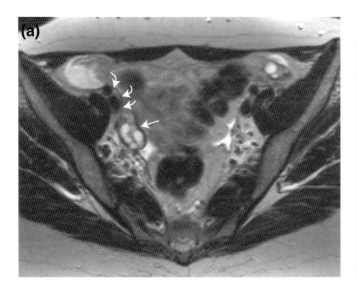

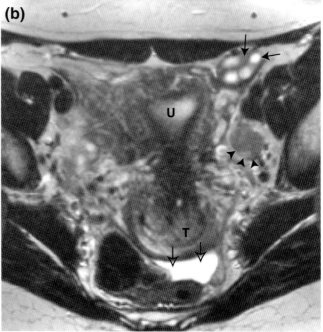

Figure 13.14. Lymph node pitfall – normal ovary.

(a) and (b) Transaxial T2WI showing normal ovaries (straight arrows) containing high signal follicles. The round ligament is identified on the right (curved arrows in (a)) as it extends towards the right ovary. There is a left obturator lymph node metastasis (arrowheads (b)). This is of abnormal signal similar to that of the primary cervical tumour (T). Of incidental note is free fluid within the Pouch of Douglas (open arrows). This could be physiological or pathological. Uterus (U).

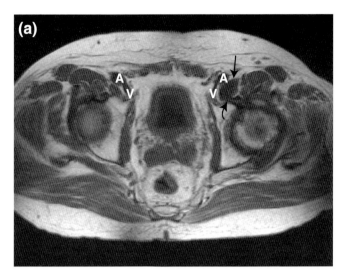

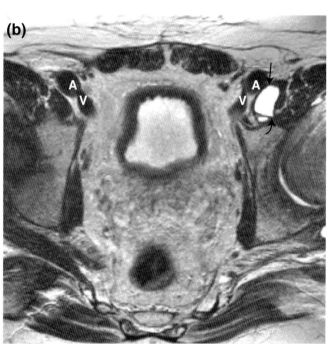

Figure 13.15. Lymph node pitfall – iliopsoas bursa.

(a) Transaxial T1WI and **(b)** transaxial T2WI demonstrate a well-defined iliopsoas bursa on the left (straight arrow). The signal intensity characteristics of the bursa are in keeping with fluid content and it has a typical location posterolateral to the distal external iliac vessels. There is a beak of tissue extending from the bursa (curved arrow) towards the left hip joint, which represents the bursa's communication with the hip joint. External iliac artery (A); external iliac vein (V).

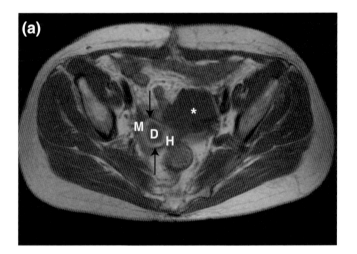

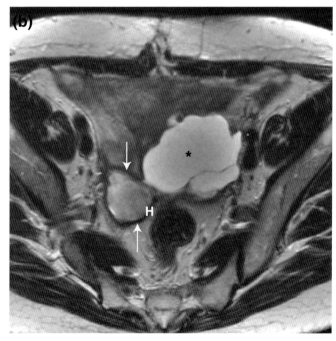

Figure 13.16. Lymph node pitfall – post surgical haematoma.

(a) Transaxial T1WI and **(b)** transaxial T2WI demonstrating a right pelvic haematoma (straight arrow) abutting a fluid collection (asterisk). On T1WI this is of central intermediate signal due to the presence of deoxyhaemoglobin (D) with a high signal rim due to extra-cellular methaemoglobin (M), which shortens the T1. The most peripheral rim is of low signal due to the presence of haemosiderin (H). In (b) the haematoma centre is of more uniform high signal intensity with improved visualisation of the haemosiderin ring.

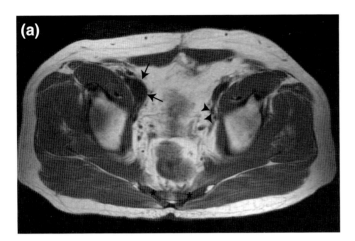

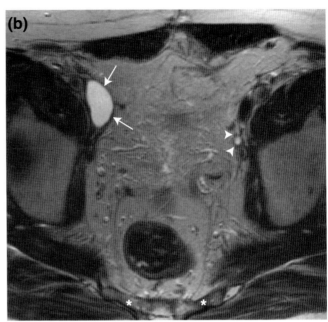

Figure 13.17. Lymph node pitfall – right pelvic sidewall lympho-coele.

(a) Transaxial T1WI and (b) transaxial T2WI showing a well-defined lymphocoele on the right pelvic sidewall (arrows). This is of homogeneous low signal on T1WI and homogeneous high signal on T2WI, demonstrating its fluid content. A smaller left-sided lymphocoele is also seen (arrowheads). The patient had undergone cystectomy and pelvic lymph node resection for bladder cancer. There is also metastatic infiltration of the sacrum (asterisk).

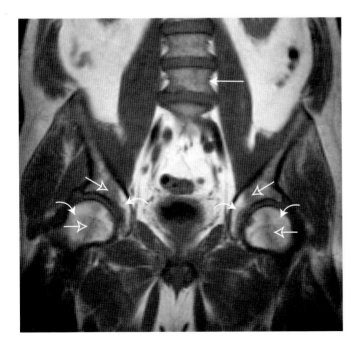

Figure 13.18. Normal bone marrow – transition zone between red and yellow marrow.

Coronal T1WI showing haemopoietic red marrow in the axial skeleton, which is intermediate signal on T1WI (straight arrow). The zone of transition to fatty yellow marrow in the proximal appendicular skeleton shows the characteristic high signal yellow marrow (curved arrows) with interposing islands of poorly demarcated intermediate signal red marrow (open arrows). Comparing left to right, this is a fairly symmetrical process and is easily differentiated from bone metastases, which would be well defined and asymmetrical.

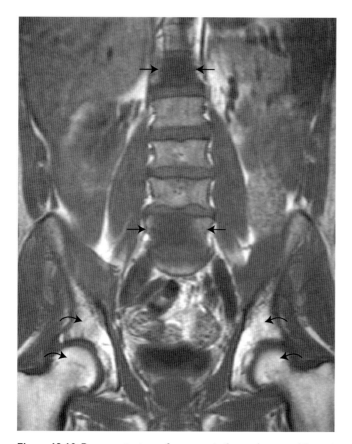

Figure 13.19. Bone metastases from prostatic carcinoma with post treatment radiotherapy change seen within the pelvis.

Coronal T1WI of the lumbar spine and pelvis. There are multiple well-defined areas of low signal seen within the lumbar vertebrae (straight arrows), which represent bone metastases from prostatic carcinoma. These contrast well with the intermediate to high signal of the normal adjacent vertebral bone marrow. Homogeneous high signal due to radiation induced fatty marrow replacement is seen in the pelvis and femora (curved arrows).

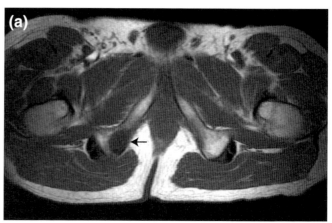

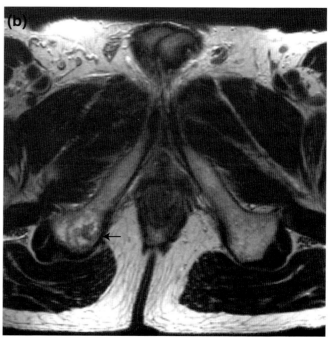

Figure 13.20. Bone metastasis from rectal cancer.

(a) Transaxial T1WI and **(b)** transaxial T2WI showing a metastasis in the right ischial tuberosity (straight arrow) in a patient with rectal cancer. The lesion appears of low signal compared to the surrounding fatty bone marrow on T1WI in (a) and high signal on T2WI in (b) due to the higher relative water content of the metastasis in comparison to the normal marrow.

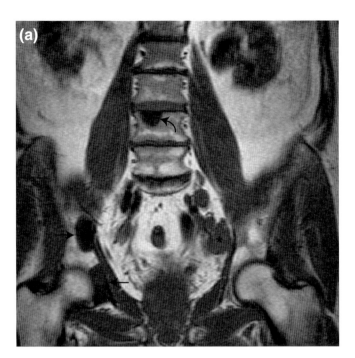

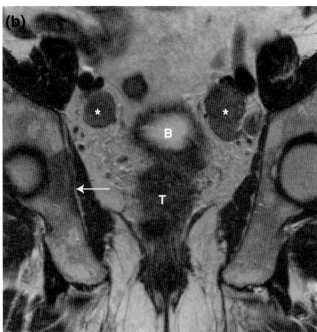

Figure 13.21. Sclerotic bone metastases in prostatic carcinoma.

(a) Coronal T1WI and (b) coronal T2WI showing sclerotic metastases in the right hemi pelvis which are low signal on T1 and maintain reduced signal on T2WI (straight arrows). There is a further sclerotic metastasis in the L3 vertebral body (curved arrow in (a)). Benign bone islands may have similar appearances, but these are smaller, well-defined and very low signal on both sequences. Also note the enlarged metastatic iliac lymph nodes (asterisks). Bladder (B); primary tumour (T).

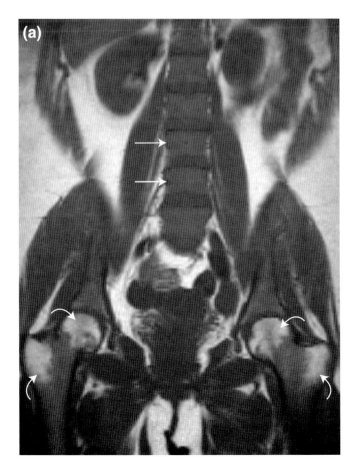

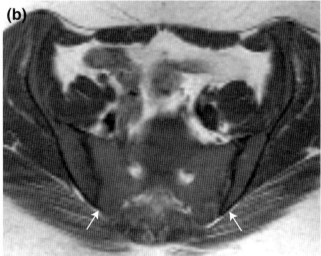

Figure 13.22. Bone metastases pitfall – hyperaemic marrow.

(a) Coronal and (b) transaxial T1WI demonstrate homogeneous intermediate-to-low signal intensity within the vertebral marrow (straight arrows) in keeping with haemopoietic transformation of the marrow secondary to anaemia. The transformation starts within the axial skeleton and progresses peripherally but this may be patchy as in the femoral heads and greater trochanters (curved arrows) where there is still some normal high signal fatty yellow marrow. The appearances in the vertebrae may be misinterpreted as metastases, which also result in low signal on T1WI, but solid tumour metastases are usually nonuniform, discrete, asymmetrical lesions.

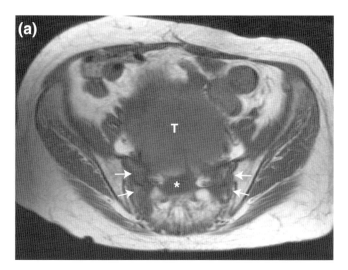

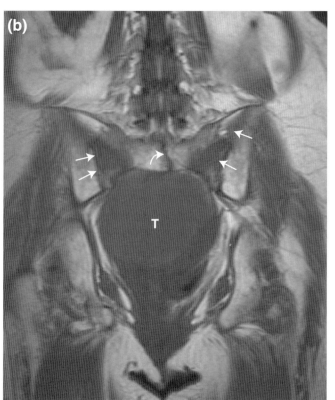

Figure 13.23. Sacral insufficiency fractures post radiotherapy.

(a) Transaxial and (b) coronal T1WI showing classical low signal vertical bands (straight arrows) through both sacral alae with an additional central sacral vertical band (curved arrow in (b)) and a transverse low signal intensity region at S1–2 level (asterisk in (a)). There is a large ovarian tumour recurrence (T). Sacral insufficiency fractures are usually vertically orientated through the sacral alae with a horizontal bridging fracture, often through the junction between 2 sacral vertebrae. This produces the 'H' or Honda sign on radionuclide imaging. The central vertical fracture is unusual and may have occurred because of the pressure effect exerted on the irradiated bone by the large pelvic tumours.

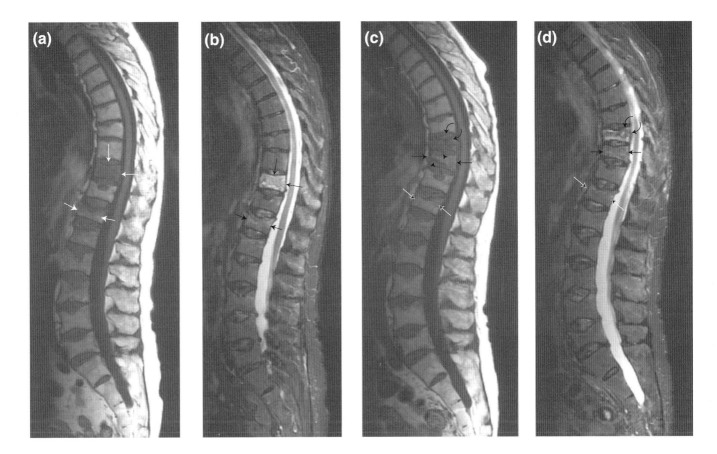

Figure 13.24. Bone metastasis pitfall- osteoporotic vertebral collapse.

(a) Sagittal T1WI and (b) sagittal STIR images demonstrate diffuse low signal throughout the T10 vertebral body on T1WI which is high signal on STIR image (straight arrows). (c) Sagittal T1WI and (d) sagittal STIR images 4 months later. There has been progression with collapse of the T10 vertebra which is now of more normal signal. A fracture through the vertebral body is apparent (arrowheads in (c)). T9 has sustained a new fracture and collapse with altered signal (curved arrows in (c) and (d)). (a) and (b) demonstrate the early features of haemorrhage and oedema in T10 followed by resolution of the marrow signal intensity abnormality but persistence of the vertebral collapse and visualisation of the fracture line, likely due to incomplete healing in (c) and (d). Also note other vertebrae at different stages of vertebral collapse, for example T12 (open arrows).

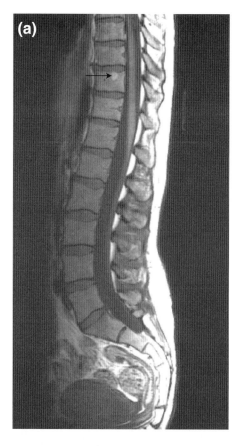

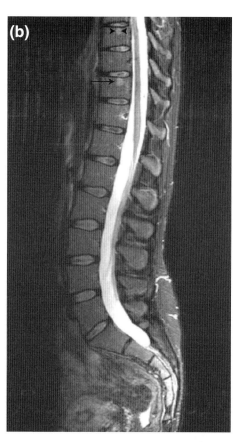

Figure 13.25. Bone metastasis pitfall – haemangioma.

(a) Sagittal T1WI and **(b)** sagittal STIR images demonstrate a small well-defined lesion in the T10 vertebral body, which is high signal on T1W and STIR images (straight arrows). A further lesion is seen in the T8 vertebral body on the STIR image (arrowheads) also in keeping with a haemangioma. The signal on T1WI and STIR imaging depends on the relative fat and soft tissue constituents of each lesion.

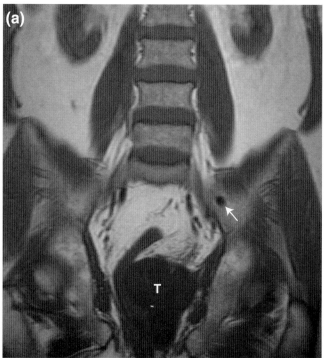

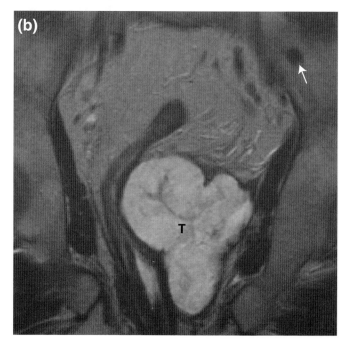

Figure 13.26. Bone metastasis pitfall – benign bone island.

(a) Coronal T1WI and **(b)** coronal T2WI showing a well-defined rounded lesion in the left iliac bone, which is low signal on both T1WI and T2WI (straight arrow). This can usually be differentiated from a non-sclerotic bone metastasis, which would be intermediate signal on T2WI, however a sclerotic metastasis may be of similar appearance. The lesion does not change over time. Note the pararectal recurrent tumour (T).

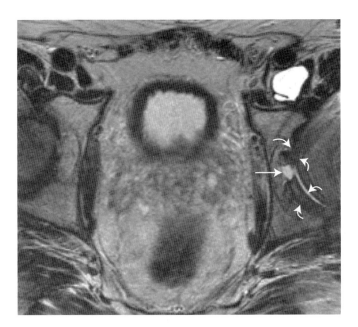

Figure 13.27. Bone metastasis pitfall – subchondral cyst in degenerative joint disease.

Transaxial T2WI showing a well-defined subchondral cyst in the left acetabulum (straight arrow). This is of high signal on T2WI indicating its fluid content. The associated subchondral sclerosis (curved arrows) and reduction in joint space all indicate degenerative joint disease. Also, note the prominent iliopsoas bursa on the left (same patient as *Figure 13.15*).

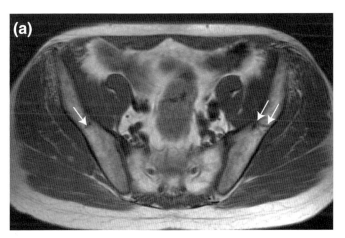

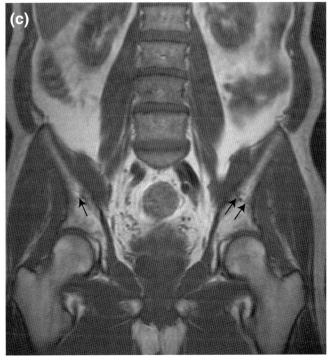

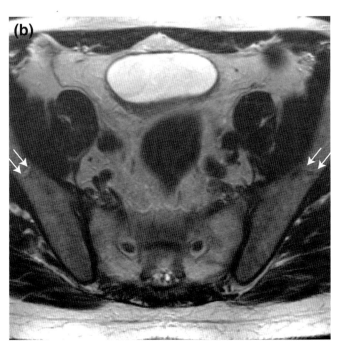

Figure 13.28. Bone metastasis pitfall – normal nutrient foramina.

(a) Transaxial T1WI, **(b)** transaxial T2WI and **(c)** coronal T1WI showing well defined linear or tubular structures (arrows) within both iliac wings. These extend centrally from the cortical surface, are bilaterally symmetrical and occur in this typical location within the ilium.

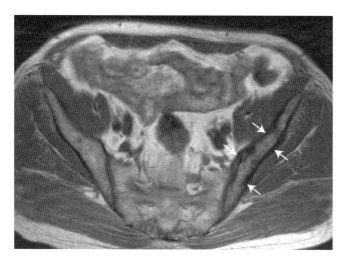

Figure 13.29. Bone metastasis pitfall – Paget's disease.

Transaxial T1WI demonstrating diffuse low signal cortical thickening (straight arrows) of the left iliac bone in comparison with the right. The medulla is of slightly lower signal intensity due to a combination of trabecular thickening and marrow change. The latter is due to increased fibrovascular tissue which replaces yellow marrow in more active disease.

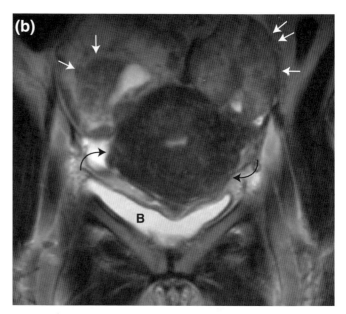

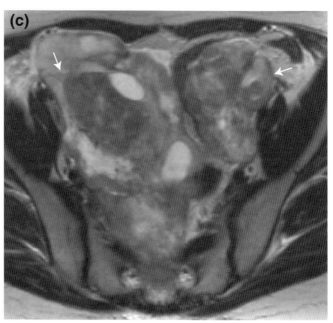

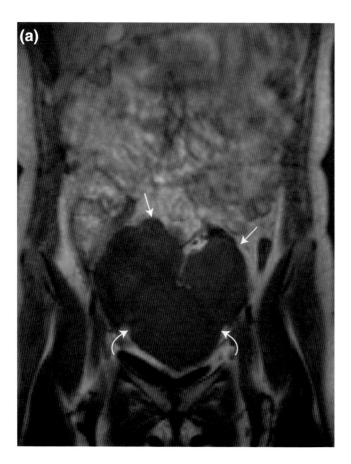

Figure 13.30. Krukenberg tumours – ovarian metastases from colonic carcinoma.

(a) Coronal T1WI, **(b)** coronal T2WI and **(c)** transaxial T2WI show bulky heterogeneous metastatic tumour masses arising from both ovaries (straight arrows). These are intermediate signal on T1WI and intermediate/high signal on T2WI. Signet ring cell tumours arising from the gastrointestinal tract, particularly the stomach but also from the colon as in this case, may metastasise to the ovaries and are known as Krukenberg tumours. Note also the tumour infiltration of the uterus (curved arrows in (a) and (b)) producing abnormal low signal on T2WI, increased size and irregular margins. Bladder (B).

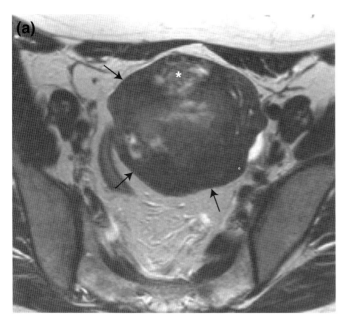

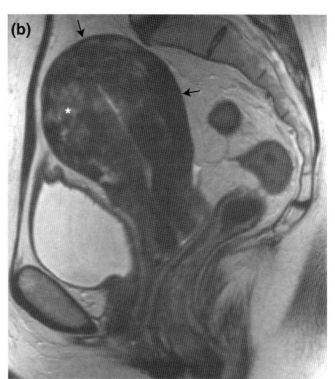

Figure 13.31. Uterine metastases from breast carcinoma.

(a) Transaxial and (b) sagittal T2WI showing an enlarged, bulky low signal uterus (straight arrows), with foci of high signal metastatic tumour (asterisk) within the myometrium. Note the normal, preserved, high signal endometrial stripe.

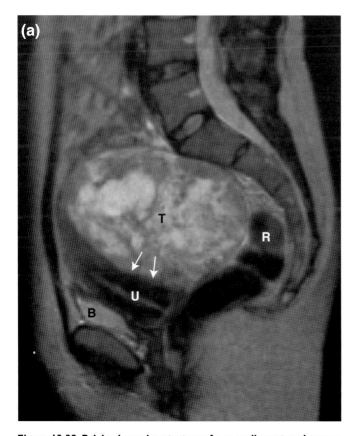

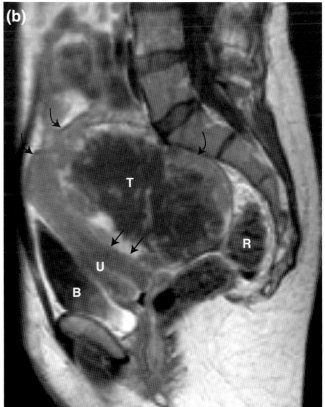

Figure 13.32. Pelvic visceral metastases from malignant melanoma.

(a) Sagittal T2WI and (b) post-Gd T1WI showing a large heterogenous metastatic tumour (T), arising from the left adnexa and lying in the Pouch of Douglas pushing the bladder and uterus forwards (straight arrows). After intravenous contrast medium injection, there is enhancement of the mass periphery (curved arrows) but the centre does not enhance due to central necrosis. Uterus (U); bladder (B); rectum (R).

14 MR Imaging of Residual and Recurrent Tumour Before Pelvic Clearance Surgery

Bernadette M. Carrington

INTRODUCTION

Magnetic resonance imaging has a key role in assessing local disease extent in patients with primary or treated pelvic cancer. In patients with primary cancers, the information provided influences clinical treatment decisions, for example patient eligibility for surgery and the type of surgery required. In treated cancer patients MR imaging is used to identify residual or recurrent tumour as well as to determine the feasibility and extent of salvage surgery. In both primary and residual or recurrent cancer, pelvic clearance (exenteration) is an important treatment option.

RESIDUAL AND RECURRENT TUMOUR

Residual tumour is defined as tumour which persists after initial treatment. It is diagnosed clinically by nonregression of the tumour mass and radiologically by a persisting tumour mass, incomplete restoration of organ zonal anatomy or nondevelopment of expected treatment effects.

Tumour recurrence is locoregional tumour detected more than 6 months after initial therapy when there has been a documented treatment response. Recurrence can be diagnosed clinically by physical examination or rising biochemical tumour markers. It may be diagnosed radiologically by the identification of a new mass, increasing size of an existing mass or new abnormal signal intensity within an organ. Infiltrative recurrence may be difficult to detect and relies upon the identification of more subtle changes such as thickening of fascial planes.

When residual or recurrent tumour is detected, biopsy confirmation should be obtained before further treatment is started. For pelvic cancers the treatment given to the patient with residual or recurrent disease depends on the primary tumour site and type, the previous therapy received, and the current clinical findings. In this situation, pelvic clearance should be considered.

PELVIC CLEARANCE (EXENTERATION)

Pelvic clearance is the removal of most or all of the pelvic viscera when pelvic tumours are large and locally extensive. It is divided into three types. **Anterior** pelvic clearance is the removal of the bladder, urethra and male or female sex organs with the formation of a urinary diversion via an ileal conduit. **Posterior** pelvic clearance involves resection of the rectum and the male or female pelvic sex organs with a bowel anastomosis or formation of an end colostomy. In male patients the bladder is reanastomosed to the membranous urethra. **Total** pelvic clearance is when the entire contents of the extra-peritoneal pelvic cavity are resected. In these procedures, the vagina is usually partially resected and the remnant oversewn to form a foreshortened vagina. Occasionally the vagina is totally resected. Pelvic lymph node resection is performed in those patients undergoing primary surgery or in those with recurrence who have not already had lymph node dissection.

More extensive pelvic clearance may require resection of the pelvic floor if the tumour is invading any part of it. Historically, tumour involvement of blood vessels or the sacrum rendered the patient ineligible for pelvic clearance. Recent improvements in surgical techniques, and in perioperative support, mean that vascular resection and grafting can be contemplated and sacral resection below S2–3 level is now feasible.

Indications for pelvic clearance

The commonest tumour treated by pelvic clearance is recurrent cervical cancer in the central pelvis. Other gynaecological malignancies which recur here may also be suitable for pelvic clearance. Because ovarian cancer metastasises widely within the abdomen and pelvis, it is not usually considered amenable to exenteration, unless it can be shown that the pelvic tumour mass is an isolated finding.

Locally advanced and recurrent rectal cancers and, less frequently recurrent bladder cancer, can be treated by exenteration. The results of exenteration for advanced prostate cancer are poor and patients with this condition are considered ineligible. Rare pelvic tumours such as sarcoma are also potentially curable by exenteration.

Outcome after pelvic clearance

In carefully selected patients the outcome of pelvic clearance is 95% survival in the immediate post-operative period with a 20–60% survival at 5 years. When exenteration is performed for gynaecological cancers, 5-year survival is 40–60% but it is approximately 20% less when performed for colorectal cancer. Patients in whom exenteration is performed as a primary treatment have a better 5-year survival compared to those operated on for recurrence, and those with primary tumours which are node negative have a high 5-year survival of 80%. When patients relapse after pelvic clearance nearly all will have local recurrence and approximately half will have systemic metastases.

THE ROLE OF MRI IN TUMOUR RECURRENCE AND PELVIC CLEARANCE

MRI has a role in the identification of recurrent carcinomas of the cervix, vagina and vulva as well as the bladder and ano-rectum. In patients who have undergone radical prostatectomy and who then develop a rising prostate specific antigen, MRI may be used to identify tumour recurrence in the surgical bed. For ovarian cancers, CT is often more appropriate for the identification of abdomino-pelvic tumour recurrence.

PATIENT EVALUATION BEFORE PELVIC CLEARANCE

MRI has a recognised role in patients being considered for pelvic clearance. Its superior contrast resolution, multiplanar imaging facility and excellent spatial resolution (with a pelvic phased array coil) permit detailed evaluation of the pelvis.

Before a patient undergoes pelvic clearance, an intensive work-up is required, involving clinical and radiological assessment.

Clinical evaluation

This includes examination under anaesthesia when there is palpation of the tumour mass to determine its mobility within the pelvis under conditions of optimal patient muscle relaxation. The surgeon assesses central visceral involvement by palpation and by cystoscopy, recto-sigmoidoscopy and vaginoscopy with biopsy where appropriate. Tumour fixity to the pelvic sidewall and floor is sought. Laparoscopy may be performed to assess the abdominal cavity in patients with primary disease, but treatment-related adhesions make laparoscopy hazardous in patients with recurrence.

Radiological evaluation

Relevant clinical information which should be available to the radiologist includes:

- the histological type and stage of the primary tumour;
- the treatments the patient has received, and when they were administered;
- current clinical symptoms;

- any recent biopsy procedure performed, including the date of the biopsy, the number and sites of biopsy and the histological or cytological findings;
- the proposed management.

It is necessary to have the patient's previous cross-sectional imaging available for comparison with the current examination.

Radiological investigation has three purposes:

1. To confirm the presence of an abnormality which is likely to be tumour, and to identify sites suitable for clinical or image-guided biopsy. Tumour is more easily identified when it appears as a well-defined mass. Infiltrative disease is much more difficult to diagnose and to differentiate from the effects of previous treatment, particularly radiotherapy. Interpretation relies on scrutiny of the images and careful comparison with previous cross-sectional examinations.

2. To delineate local tumour extent, the presence of additional pelvic tumour deposits separate from the main tumour mass and the presence of enlarged pelvic lymph nodes. Structures to be assessed are the **central pelvic organs**, the **pelvic sidewall**, the **pelvic floor** and the **sacrum**, including the exiting **sacral nerve roots**. In addition, involvement of **small bowel loops**, the **caecum**, the **sigmoid mesocolon** or **small bowel mesentery** by the superior-most extent of the tumour mass should be documented. Evaluation of the **ureters** must include their course and any displacement or obstruction produced by the mass. Disease involving the **anterior abdominal wall** should be identified. **Major blood vessel** involvement must be documented, particularly of the common and external iliac vessels. Imaging evidence of a hypervascular tumour mass should be recorded and is shown by the presence of multiple collateral vessels. Tumour extension to involve major nerves such as the **sciatic nerve** or **femoral nerve** should be sought and any extension of tumour through the **sciatic notch** identified. Invasion of the **lumbar spine** rules out curative exenteration. If ascites is present then the peritoneum should be assessed for possible implants, as should pelvic bowel loops.

3. To identify metastatic disease outside the pelvis. Metastatic abdominal tumour may be identified on MRI but this often requires long scan times and intravenous contrast medium administration. In most cases a CT scan is required to permit evaluation of the lungs and liver, and can identify metastatic tumour within the abdomen or disease involving the abdominal wall.

The imaging contributes to multidisciplinary evaluation regarding feasibility of exenterative surgery, and whether it is likely to be curative or palliative. Radiological findings which are an absolute contraindication to pelvic clearance are extension to the pelvic sidewall, invasion of the lumbar spine or sacrum above S3, involvement of the lumbo-sacral plexus or sciatic nerve, extension of tumour through the sciatic notch and involvement of the small bowel mesentery.

Relative contraindications are major vessel involvement and metastatic disease. The former increases the complexity of surgery and the latter renders exenteration palliative though it may still be required to improve the patient's quality of life.

When pelvic clearance is to be performed, an appropriately skilled surgical team is constituted to enable a safe and effective procedure, and the patient is counseled about the extent of surgery required and the likelihood for one or multiple stomata.

MRI technique

Patients should be scanned with a phased array pelvic surface coil and high-resolution thin sections performed to optimise spatial resolution. The entire tumour should be imaged and this may necessitate two contiguous sequences in some planes. T1-weighted images are obtained in the transaxial plane to assess the tumour for haemorrhage and the pelvis and retroperitoneum for lymph node enlargement. Turbo spin echo T2-weighted pelvic sequences are required in all three planes to adequately assess tumour extent and to examine the signal intensity characteristics of any enlarged lymph nodes.

ACCURACY OF MRI IN RECURRENCE

The accuracy of MRI in diagnosing recurrent disease varies depending on the tumour type and morphological appearance of the recurrence. In locally recurrent prostate cancer the sensitivity and specificity of MRI can be up to 100% when typical signal intensity appearances are seen in a palpable tumour nodule (usually intermediate to high T2-weighted signal for recurrences). However, in rectal cancer, the effects of surgery and radiotherapy make recurrence more difficult to identify and this is often compounded by the infiltrative nature of the disease process. The recurrences may be high, intermediate or low signal intensity on T2-weighted images. High signal intensity inflammation, oedema, and acute or subacute radiotherapy effect may mimic tumour, and low signal established radiation fibrosis may be indistinguishable from tumours with a high fibrotic component. Accuracy of diagnosis of recurrent rectal cancer is 75% using conventional sequences. Dynamic contrast enhanced MRI results in greater enhancement of rectal tumour recurrence than treatment effect and hence improved sensitivity and specificity. In cervical cancer recurrence, accuracy of diagnosis is 74% employing T2-weighted images, with sensitivities and specificities of 90% and 38%. Using dynamic contrast-enhanced MRI and pharmacokinetic analysis accuracy of diagnosing cervical cancer recurrence rises to over 90%. However, this technique requires more sophisticated image analysis.

ACCURACY OF MRI BEFORE PELVIC CLEARANCE

There are few published papers reporting the use of MRI in patients prior to pelvic clearance. In one study of 23 patients MRI has been shown to be accurate in selection of appropriate patients for exenteration, exceeding 80% when MRI and laparotomy findings were compared. In this study MRI had high negative predictive values for tumour extension to the pelvic sidewall and lymph node metastases. In 27 patients with recurrent pelvic bowel cancer MRI was more accurate than EUA by approximately 15% in determining tumour involvement of the anterior, lateral and posterior pelvis, with an overall MRI accuracy of 90%. The negative predictive values for organ and sidewall involvement were high in this study exceeding 90%.

PITFALLS OF MRI

Infiltrative recurrence may be difficult to distinguish from treatment effect, particularly after radiotherapy. The difficulty increases if the tumour is of low or intermediate signal on T2-weighted images. It is important to compare sequential examinations, to assess the patient for disease outside the treatment field and to consider multiple biopsies. Positron emission tomography may be of use in these patients if available. In some cases, it may be necessary to consider exploratory laparotomy.

Pelvic organ involvement may be difficult to exclude when there are large masses, which compress and displace the pelvic viscera simulating infiltration. It is necessary to assess the interface between the tumour and the viscera on all images and look for definite tumour signal intensity in the organ wall or lumen.

Small volume peritoneal, omental or mesenteric deposits can be difficult to identify separate from abdominal structures unless technique is meticulous. Optimal assessment includes fat suppressed, contrast-enhanced MRI which is not routine in many centres. Antiperistaltic agents may be administered to improve image quality. If there is uncertainty then CT may be required.

Lymph node enlargement may occur secondary to sepsis in patients with extensive pelvic tumours, particularly when there is formation of a fistula or an abscess, but also if the tumour is necrotic. A helpful indication of metastatic lymph node enlargement is when the T2-weighted signal of the node is similar to the tumour T2-weighted signal. If necessary, image guided biopsy can be performed.

FURTHER READING

1. Crowe PJ, Temple WJ, Lopez MJ and Ketcham AS. (1999) Pelvic exenteration for advanced pelvic malignancy. *Semin. Surg. Oncol.* 17: 152–160. *Good review of exenteration.*

2. Silverman JM and Krebs TL. (1997) MR imaging evaluation with a transrectal surface coil of local recurrence of prostatic cancer in men who have undergone radical prostatectomy. *AJR* 168(2): 379–385. *Useful paper discussing the power of MRI to identify local recurrence in this population.*

3. Kinkel K, Tardivon AA *et al.* (1996) Dynamic contrast-enhanced subtraction versus T2-weighted spin-echo MR imaging in the follow-up of colorectal neoplasm: a prospective study of 41 patients. *Radiology* 200(2): 453–458. *This paper discusses the advantages of dynamic MR imaging in recurrence.*

4. Müller-Schimpfle M, Brix G, Layer G *et al* (1993) Recurrent rectal cancer: Diagnosis with dynamic MR imaging. *Radiology* 189: 881–889. *One of the original papers reporting the reliability of MR dynamic contrast enhancement in differentiating tumour recurrence from fibrosis and comparing it to standard T2-weighted imaging.*

5. Hawighorst H, Knapstein PG *et al.* (1996). Pelvic lesions in patients with treated cervical carcinoma: efficacy of pharmacokinetic analysis of dynamic MR images in distinguishing recurrent tumours from benign conditions. *AJR* 166(2): 401–408. *In this paper, sophisticated analysis of dynamic contrast enhanced MRI improved the evaluation of treated cervical cancer patients with suspected recurrence.*

6. Popovich MJ, Hricak H *et al.* (1993) The role of MR imaging in determining surgical eligibility for pelvic exenteration. *AJR* 160(3): 525–531. *One of the original papers covering this subject.*

7. Robinson P, Carrington BM, Swindell R, Shanks JH and O'Dwyer ST (2002). Accuracy of MRI in determining extent of recurrent pelvic bowel cancer prior to salvage surgery. *Clin. Radiol.* 57: 514–522. *A comparison of EUA and MRI assessment before attempted exenteration.*

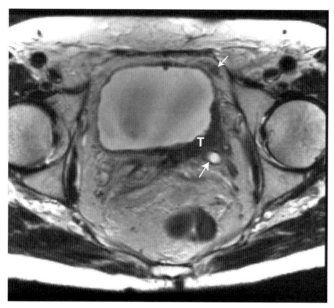

Figure 14.1. Residual tumour mass post radiotherapy.

Transaxial T2WI demonstrating a residual bladder tumour (T) obstructing the left ureter (arrow) and associated with a left antero-lateral paravesical lymph node (small arrow).

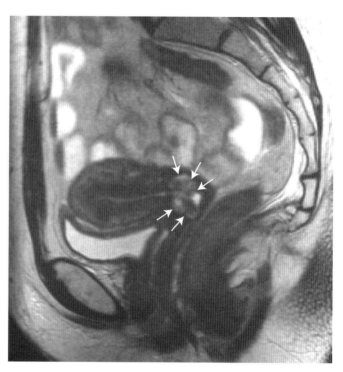

Figure 14.2. Failure to develop normal post treatment appearances.

Sagittal T2WI of a patient who was treated for cervical cancer with radiotherapy. Six months after treatment the cervix still demonstrates heterogeneous signal intensity (arrows) instead of the uniform low signal intensity post treatment appearance. The patient went on to have salvage surgery after biopsy confirmation of residual tumour.

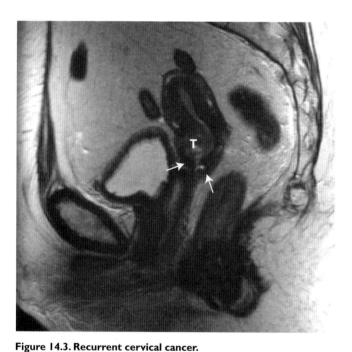

Figure 14.3. Recurrent cervical cancer.

Sagittal T2WI demonstrating a recurrent tumour mass (T) in the anterior lip of the cervix, two years after finishing radiation therapy. Note the signal voids (arrows) from the metallic marker seeds placed in the vagina and the low signal intensity of the treated uterus, posterior lip of the cervix and upper vaginal canal.

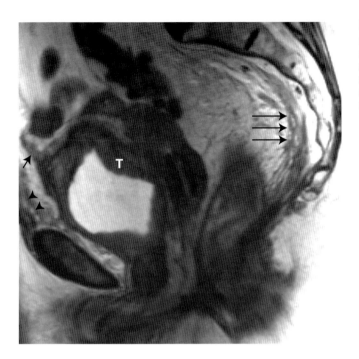

Figure 14.4. Infiltrative bladder cancer recurrence.

Sagittal T2WI demonstrating diffuse low signal intensity tumour (T) of the bladder wall with extension into the distal portion of the urachus (short arrow) and further diffuse soft tissue band-like stranding of the peritoneum anteriorly (arrowheads) and pre-sacral fascia (long arrows). The symmetrical nature of the abnormalities makes differentiation from radiotherapy treatment effect difficult.

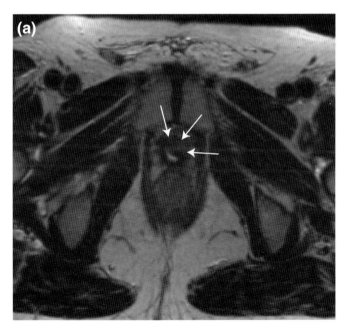

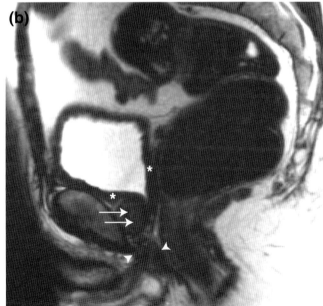

Figure 14.5. Recurrent tumour in prostate bed after radical prostatectomy.

(a) Transaxial and (b) sagittal T2WI demonstrating a small soft tissue mass (arrows) immediately above the anastomosis and adjacent to the bladder neck. Note that this mass is of low intermediate signal intensity, higher in signal than the bladder muscle layer (asterisks), anastomotic site (arrowheads) and muscle of the pelvic floor.

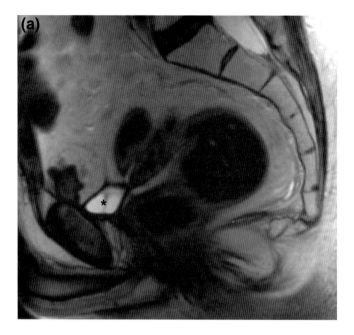

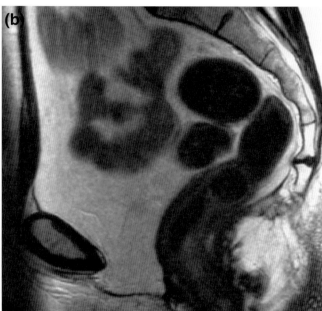

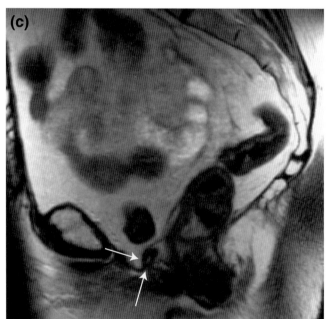

Figure 14.6. Anterior pelvic clearance.

Sagittal T2WI in **(a)** a male, **(b)** a female patient and **(c)** a female patient. In (a) the bladder, prostate and seminal vesicles have been resected. A small post-surgical collection is seen (asterisk) in the bladder bed. Note the tethering of the recto-sigmoid to the posterior margin of the collection. In (b) the bladder, urethra, uterus and vagina have been resected. Fat fills the surgical bed. This can be due to surgical placement of the omentum to prevent small bowel loops extending into the true pelvis. In (c) the patient has undergone anterior pelvic clearance but with preservation of the distal third of the vagina (arrows).

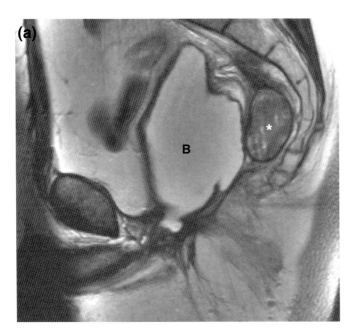

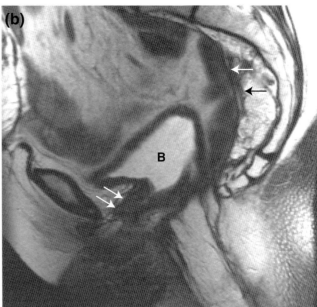

Figure 14.7. Posterior pelvic clearance.

Sagittal T2WI in **(a)** a male and **(b)** a female. In (a) the patient has undergone an abdomino-perineal resection with removal of the prostate and seminal vesicles and reanastomosis of the bladder (B) to the membranous urethra. In this patient note an incidental post-surgical haematoma (asterisk) in the pre-sacral space. In (b) the patient has undergone abdomino-perineal resection with removal of the uterus and vagina. Note the extensive band-like post-operative change in the pre-sacral space (arrows). The bladder and urethra demonstrate slight posterior prolapse with an increased angle between the symphysis pubis and the urethra (arrows).

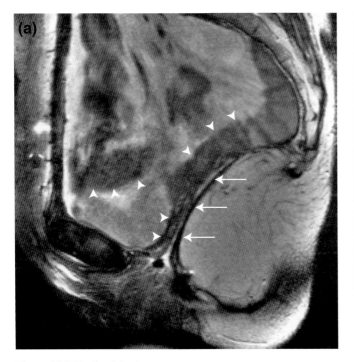

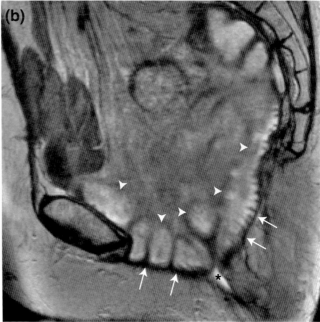

Figure 14.8. Total pelvic clearance.

(a) Sagittal T2WI demonstrating total pelvic clearance with preservation of the pelvic floor (arrows). Small bowel has entered the pelvic cavity (arrowheads). **(b)** Sagittal T2WI in a patient who has undergone total pelvic clearance with resection of the pelvic floor muscles. Note multiple dependent loops of small bowel (arrowheads) within the true pelvis with minor herniation of small bowel into the perineum (arrows). There is a small post-surgical collection (asterisk). When the pelvic floor is resected, patients may develop large and troublesome perineal hernias post-operatively.

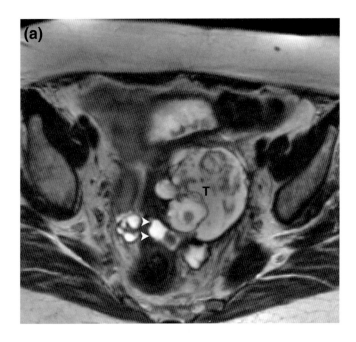

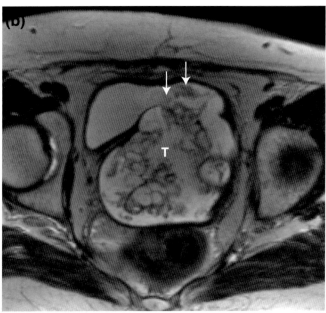

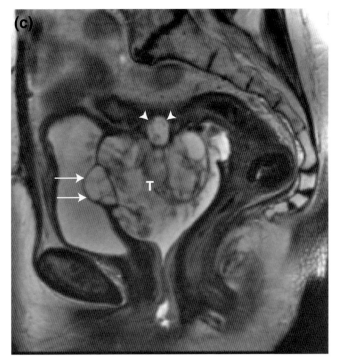

Figure 14.9. Tumour involving the bladder and sigmoid colon.

(a) and (b) Transaxial and (c) sagittal T2WI demonstrating a tumour mass (T) arising at the vaginal vault in a patient with recurrent ovarian cancer. The tumour has infiltrated through the posterior wall of the bladder and lobulated tumour is identifiable within the bladder lumen (arrrows), the superior-most portion of disease is infiltrating into the sigmoid colon with the tumour mass reaching the lumen (arrowheads). An apparent separate nodule in the right pelvis in (a) is a lobular extension of disease underneath the recto-sigmoid junction. Note that the mid- and distal rectum are displaced by the tumour mass but there is no evidence of infiltration. Surgery required by MRI criteria: anterior exenteration and sigmoid colectomy.

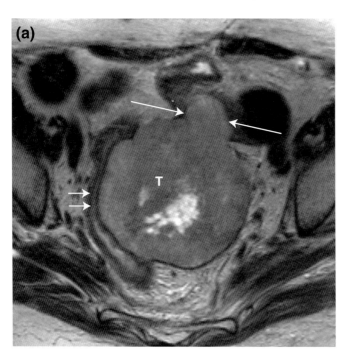

Figure 14.10. Tumour mass involving the sigmoid and left ureter.

(a) Transaxial and (b) coronal T2WI in a patient with a pelvic soft tissue sarcoma tumour (T) which is displacing the recto-sigmoid colon to the right of the midline (small arrows in (a)) with infiltration of the proximal sigmoid colon (long arrows in (a)) and with obstruction of the left ureter at the pelvic brim (asterisk in (b)). The bladder and recto-anal canal are clear of disease. Extent of surgery by MRI criteria: resection of the mass, sigmoid colectomy and left ureteric reimplantation. A psoas hitch of the bladder or a Boari bladder flap will be required to bridge the gap between the shortened ureter and the bladder.

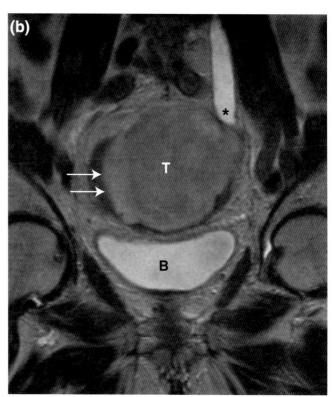

Figure 14.11. Tumour recurrence involving the rectum, anal canal and vagina.

Sagittal T2WI demonstrating a substantial tumour mass (T) involving the rectum and anal canal (arrows) with tumour extending into the vagina and involving the posterior wall superiorly (arrowheads) and both the anterior and posterior wall inferiorly. There is an air-containing fistula (asterisk) between the vault of the vagina and the rectum. The bladder is not involved but tumour is extending to the urethral meatus (small open arrow). Note that the tumour does not extend to the pre-sacral fascia (curved arrows) or sacrum proper. There is one small pre-sacral node (N) which is of concern for an early metastasis. Surgery required by MRI criteria: total exenteration. If the pre-sacral lymph node is positive then this would be a palliative exenteration performed to alleviate the disabling symptoms of pain, bleeding and discharge.

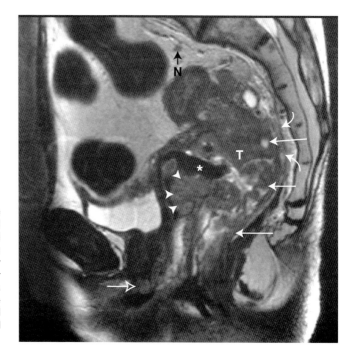

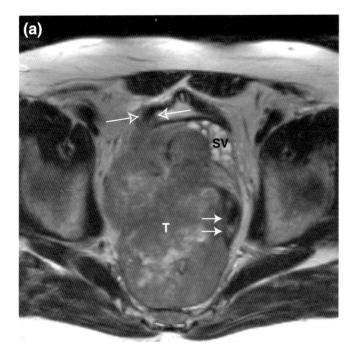

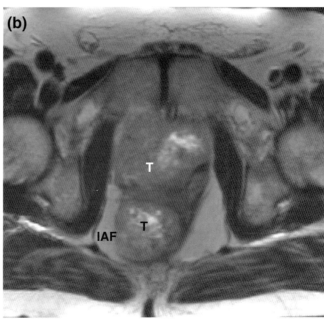

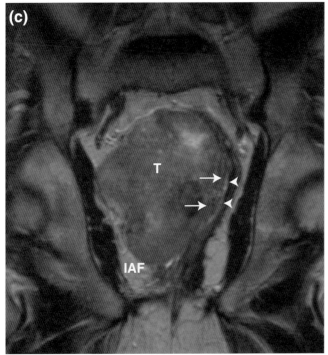

Figure 14.12. Tumour mass involving the bladder, seminal vesicles, rectum, and pelvic floor.

(a) and (b) Transaxial and (c) coronal T2WI in which a large soft tissue sarcoma tumour (T) can be seen to displace and infiltrate the rectum (arrows) with high signal oedema or haemorrhage of the rectal mucosa best seen on the coronal view (arrowheads). The tumour mass is displacing the lower rectum and anal canal, infiltrating the pelvic floor on the right side with extension into the right ischioanal fossa (IAF). The right seminal vesicle and the medial left seminal vesicle (SV) are totally engulfed by tumour which is also involving the right lateral bladder wall (open arrows in (a)). Extent of surgery required by MRI criteria: total pelvic clearance with resection of the pelvic floor.

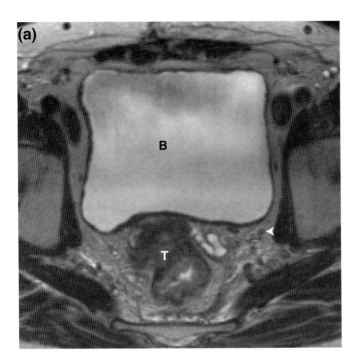

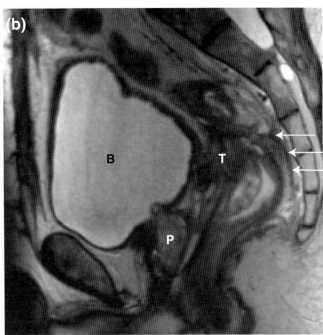

Figure 14.13. Tumour involving the seminal vesicles and pre-sacral fascia.

(a) Transaxial and **(b)** sagittal T2WI demonstrating a recurrent rectal tumour (T) involving the seminal vesicles and extending posteriorly to involve the pre-sacral fascia (arrows in (b)). One small left internal iliac node is seen (arrowhead in (a)) which is not significant by size criteria but whose signal intensity is similar to that of the tumour proper. Note that the sacrum is not involved and that the prostate (P) is also free from tumour infiltration. The tumour abuts the posterior wall of the bladder (B) to which it may be adherent but there is no evidence of tumour extension into or through the wall, with preservation of the normal low signal intensity of the bladder wall. Extent of the surgery required by MRI criteria: posterior exenteration, prostatectomy and possible cystectomy since the tumour may be adherent to the posterior bladder wall. Although the prostate is not involved, it has to be removed with the seminal vesicles.

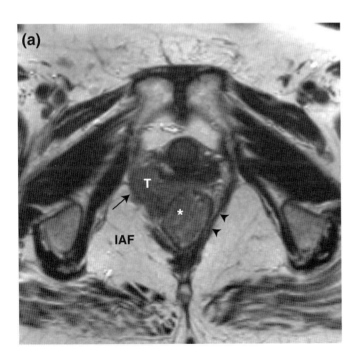

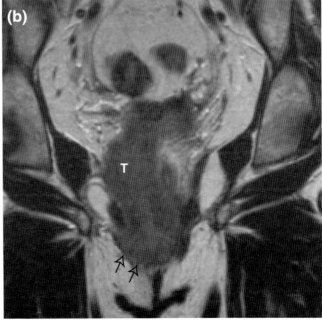

Figure 14.14. Tumour involving the pelvic floor.

(a) Transaxial and **(b)** coronal T2WI demonstrating a recurrent vaginal tumour (T) infiltrating the right anterior pubococcygeal portion of the levator ani muscle with extension of tumour into the anterior ischioanal fossa (IAF) (arrow) and infiltration of the anterior wall of the anal canal (asterisk). Note the normal signal intensity left pelvic floor (arrowheads). In (b) the craniocaudal extent of the tumour recurrence is appreciated and extension into the perineum (open arrows) can be identified. Extent of surgery required by MRI criteria: total pelvic clearance with resection of the pelvic floor.

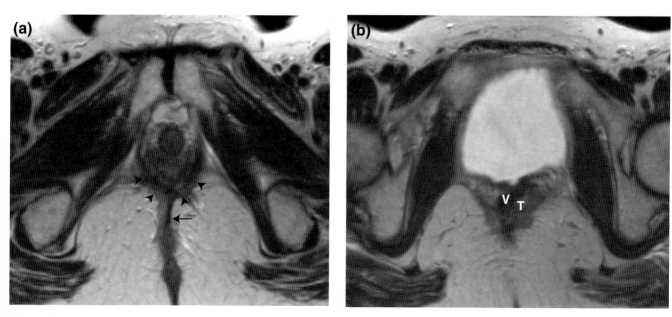

Figure 14.15. Recurrent rectal cancer involving the pelvic floor.

(a) Transaxial T2WI demonstrating the normal post-surgical appearances after abdomino-perineal resection when the perineal scar (arrow) becomes continuous with the oversewn inferior portion of the levator ani muscles (arrowheads). Note the low signal intensity of both the scar and the pelvic floor. (b) Transaxial T2WI at a more cranial level than (a) demonstrates a small lobular soft tissue recurrent tumour (T) which is of higher signal intensity than the levator and apex of the surgical scar. It is involving the vaginal vault (V) which is of low signal intensity due to post hysterectomy fibrosis. Extent of surgery required by MRI criteria: vaginectomy and resection of the pelvic floor.

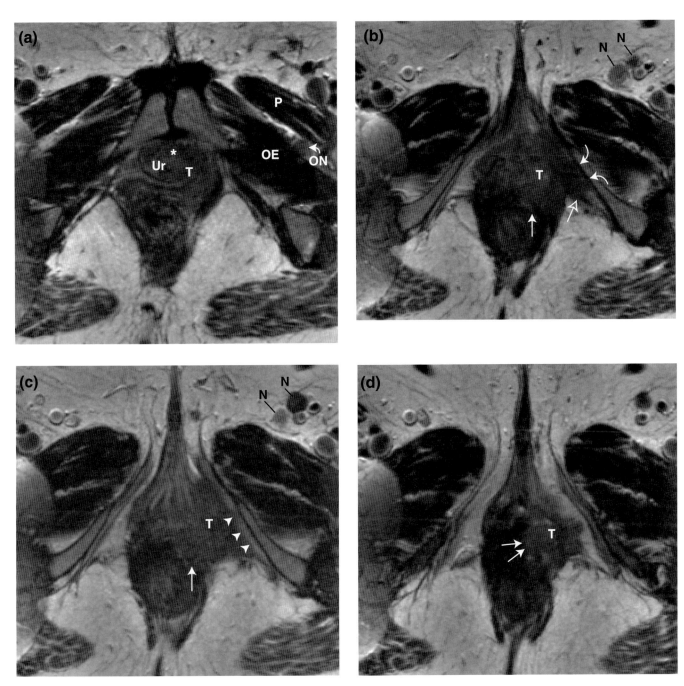

Figure 14.16. Perineal involvement by recurrent vaginal cancer.

(a) to (d) Transaxial T2WI demonstrating a recurrent vaginal tumour with the tumour mass (T) involving the urethra (Ur) in (a) where there is contiguous tumour extending from the left vagina to the left lateral margin of the urethra. Note the abnormal signal intensity of the urethra proper with intermediate to low signal intensity tumour within it (asterisk) and loss of its normal target appearance. In (b) and (c) the mass can be seen to have extended posteriorly to involve the anterior anal canal (small arrow), and anteriorly to involve the antero-inferior recess of the ischioanal fossa (open arrow in (b)). The mass abuts the left crus of the clitoris (arrowheads in (c)), and directly abuts the periosteum of the inferior pubic ramus (curved arrows in (b)). The tumour is involving the perineal body (short arrows in (d)). Also note the left inguinal nodes (N) in (b) and (c) which are not enlarged by size criteria but have a signal intensity similar to the signal intensity of the tumour. A similar signal, small left anatomical obturator node (ON) is seen between obturator externus (OE) and pectineus (P) on the left side in (a) (small curved arrow). Extent of surgery required by MRI criteria: total pelvic clearance, resection of the pelvic floor and perineum, local resection of the left inferior pubic ramus and insertion of a myocutaneous flap. A left inguinal lymph node dissection could be performed also but the left anatomical obturator lymph node would not be dissected routinely.

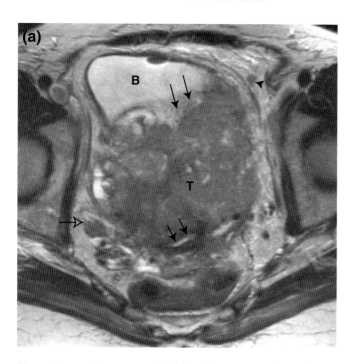

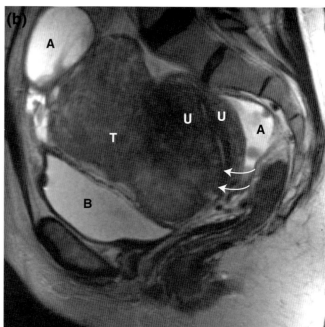

Figure 14.17. Pelvic sarcoma involving the uterus, cervix and bladder.

(a) Transaxial and (b) sagittal T2WI demonstrating a large central pelvic tumour (T) infiltrating into the uterus (U) with tumour extending through the anterior uterine body to infiltrate the inner junctional zone (small arrows in (a)). The tumour also infiltrates the cervix, best appreciated on the sagittal view (curved arrows). There is extensive tumour infiltration of the posterior wall of the bladder (arrows in (a)). Note a small but likely involved left paravesical lymph node (arrowhead in (a)) and an enlarged and likely metastatic right internal iliac lymph node (open arrow in (a)). A small air bubble is present in the anterior aspect of the bladder (B). This was due to recent cystoscopy. Ascites (A) is also present. Extent of surgery required by MRI criteria: anterior pelvic clearance. If there is malignant ascites, then the procedure becomes palliative.

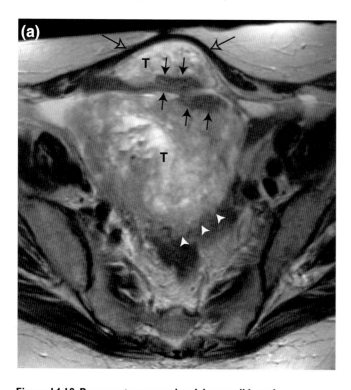

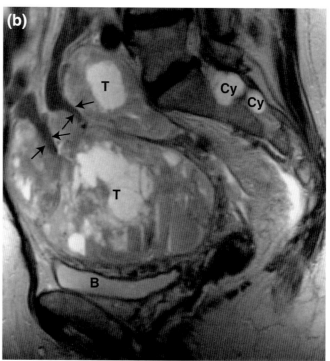

Figure 14.18. Recurrent sarcoma involving small bowel.

(a) Transaxial and (b) sagittal T2WI demonstrating a large central pelvic tumour (T) with fluid-fluid levels in the mass due to haemorrhage. The antero-superior surface of the mass is infiltrating around lower signal intensity small bowel loops (arrows in (a) and (b)). Posteriorly the tumour is also infiltrating into the recto-sigmoid (arrowheads in (a)). A component of the mass is displacing the rectus abdominis muscles anteriorly (open arrows in (a)) but there is no evidence of tumour infiltrating into the rectus abdominis muscles as their signal intensity is preserved. The bladder (B) is compressed but not involved by the mass. Note incidental arachnoid cysts (Cy) in the sacral spine in (b). Extent of surgery required by MRI criteria: local resection, recto-sigmoid colectomy and small bowel resection.

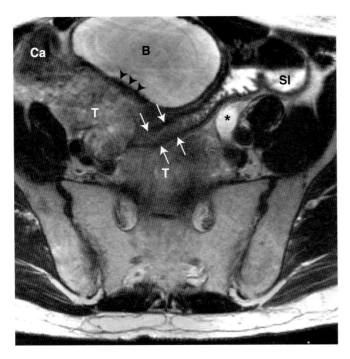

Figure 14.19. Tumour involvement of the caecum and small bowel.

Transaxial T2WI demonstrating a small bowel loop (arrows) being enveloped in the superior-most extent of a recurrent rectal tumour (T). The patient had subacute obstruction and a dilated loop of small bowel (SI) is seen in the left iliac fossa. The recurrent tumour mass is also extending antero-laterally to involve the caecum (Ca). Note the dilated left ureter (asterisk) due to entrapment at the pelvic brim. The tumour is also directly adjacent to the posterior wall of the bladder (B) which has altered high signal intensity of its outer muscle layer (arrowheads) indicating likely infiltration. Extent of surgery required by MRI criteria: total pelvic clearance with small bowel loop and caecal resection.

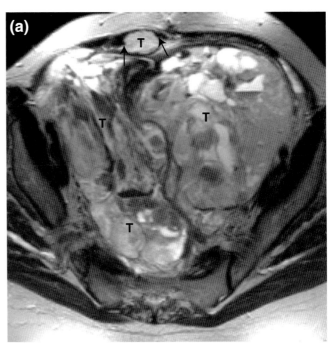

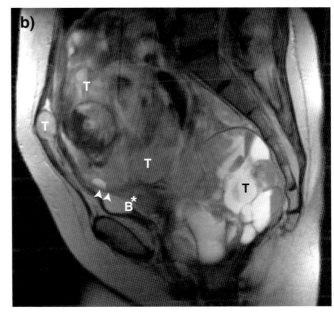

Figure 14.20. Anterior abdominal wall involvement by tumour.

(a) Transaxial and **(b)** sagittal T2WI demonstrating a recurrent pelvic leiomyosarcoma (T) with multiple fluid-fluid levels filling the pelvis and extending anteriorly into the right rectus abdominis muscle (arrows), with scalloping of the muscle:tumour interface. The tumour is compressing the bladder (B) and infiltrating the dome (arrowheads). There is some reactive oedema of the bladder mucosa (asterisk). Note the depression of the pelvic floor by the sheer size of the mass. Extent of surgery by MRI criteria: total pelvic clearance and localised abdominal wall resection.

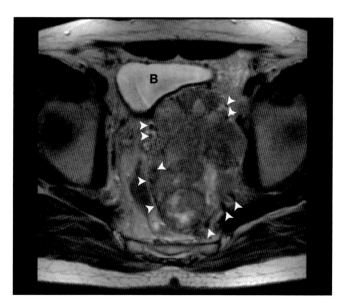

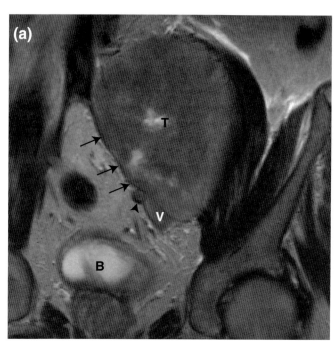

Figure 14.21. Vascular pelvic tumour.

Transaxial T2WI demonstrating a large pelvic tumour mass with multiple collateral vessels (arrowheads) identified as signal voids in and around the periphery of the mass. Note additional similar collateral vessels around the bladder (B). This finding should make the surgical team consider pre-operative angiography with a view to tumour embolisation. Intralesional signal voids can also be due to dystrophic calcification.

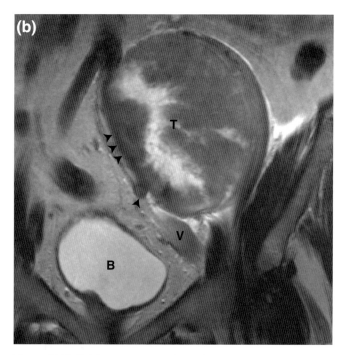

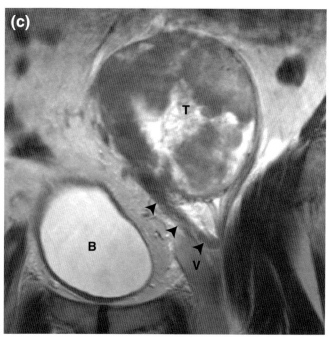

Figure 14.22. Pelvic tumour mass involving the external iliac vessels.

(a) to **(c)** Coronal T2WI demonstrating compression and displacement of the external iliac vein which is seen as a fine low signal intensity band at the margin of the large pelvic tumour (T) (arrows in (a)). Distal to the mass the vein demonstrates high signal intensity due to slow flow within its lumen (V in (a), (b) and (c)). The left common and external iliac artery are also markedly displaced and compressed by the tumour mass (arrowheads in (a) to (c)). Bladder (B). In these circumstances, it is often difficult to differentiate between adherence and involvement of the vessels. The pelvic surgeon should be warned that a vascular surgeon might be required to assist at the procedure.

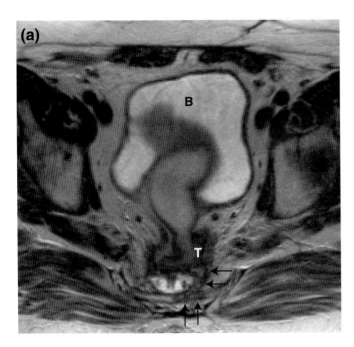

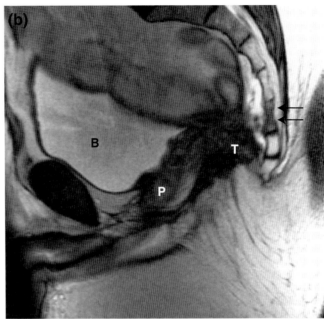

Figure 14.23. Tumour involvement of S5.

(a) Transaxial and (b) sagittal T2WI showing a small, recurrent rectal tumour (T) extending to involve S5 (arrows) and the bladder (B) and prostate (P). Extent of surgery required by MRI criteria: total pelvic clearance, resection of the pelvic floor and amputation of the sacrum below S3.

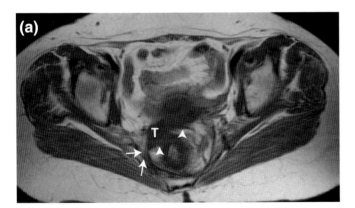

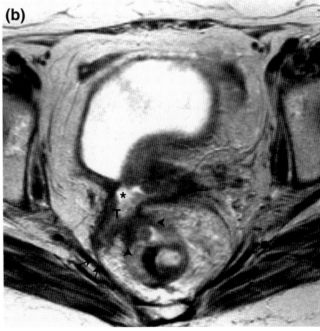

Figure 14.24. Tumour extension to the pelvic sidewall.

(a) Transaxial T1WI and (b) T2WI demonstrating a recurrent cervical tumour (T) extending to the right pelvic sidewall (arrows). The patient also has involvement of the rectum (arrowheads) and fluid in the vaginal vault (asterisk), which was due to a vesico-vaginal fistula. Pelvic sidewall disease is a contraindication to pelvic clearance.

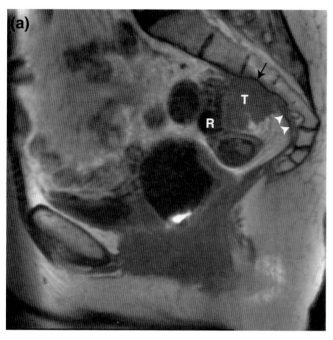

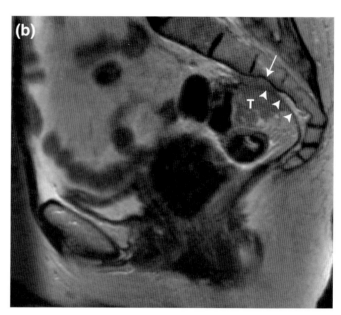

Figure 14.25. Extension of tumour into the sacrum.

(a) Sagittal T1WI and (b) sagittal T2WI demonstrating a recurrent ovarian tumour mass (T) involving the rectum (R) and extending through the pre-sacral fascia (arrowheads in (a) and (b)) to erode the periosteum of the sacrum at S2 and S3 levels (small arrows). This patient is ineligible for salvage surgery; she went on to have radiotherapy and is in remission after 5 years.

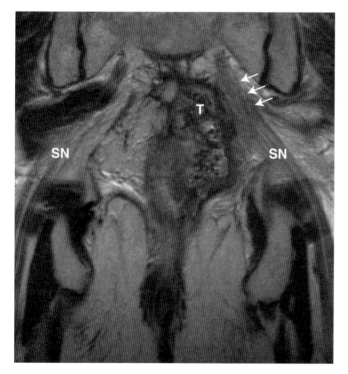

Figure 14.26. Involvement of sacral nerve roots by recurrent rectal tumour.

Coronal T2WI demonstrating a large partially necrotic posterior recurrent rectal tumour (T) which is adherent to the left exiting sacral nerve roots (arrows) down to the proximal-most portion of the sciatic nerve (SN). Note how the nerve roots are retracted towards the mass and the asymmetrical swelling of the sciatic nerve compared to the normal right side, indicating oedema or early infiltration. S1 or S2 nerve root involvement renders the patient ineligible for complete pelvic clearance.

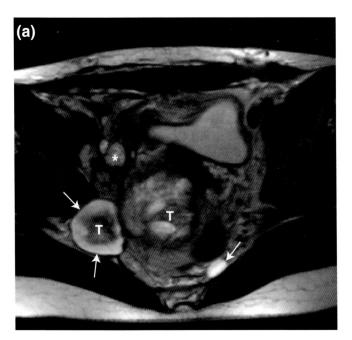

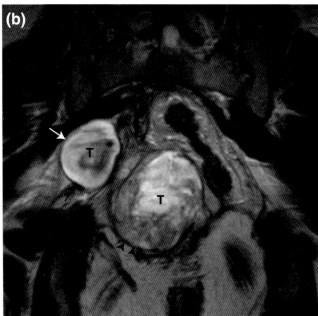

Figure 14.27. Tumour extension into the sciatic notch.

(a) Transaxial and **(b)** coronal T2WI in a patient with a multilobulated synovial sarcoma tumour (T) with a component extending into the sciatic notch (arrows in (a) and (b)). Another component of the mass is indenting the pelvic floor (arrowheads in (b)). Additional tumour locules are present within the pelvis, one adjacent to the right external iliac vessels (asterisk in (a)) and another situated on the left posterior pelvic sidewall adjacent to the sacrum (open arrow in (a)). This tumour is unsuitable for exenteration because of extension into the sciatic notch and involvement of the pelvic sidewall.

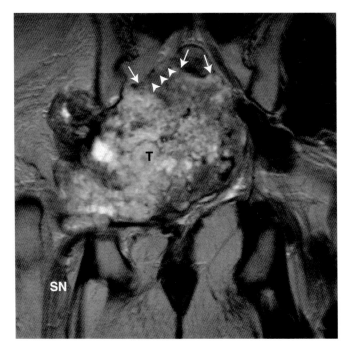

Figure 14.28. Involvement of the sacrum, sacral nerve roots, sciatic notch and sciatic nerve.

Coronal T2WI in a patient with a chondrosarcoma demonstrating a huge pelvic tumour (T), with signal voids within it indicating hypervascularity or calcifications, which is infiltrating the sacrum (arrows) with encroachment into the right S1 foramen (arrowheads). The tumour is extending through the sciatic notch and both the right sacral roots and the proximal sciatic nerve are completely engulfed. Note that the distal sciatic nerve (SN) appears normally positioned. The patient had severe neurological symptoms of pain and weakness and the gluteal muscles are shown to be completely wasted on the right side.

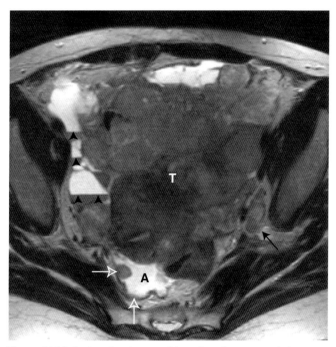

Figure 14.29. Ascites, implants and lymph node metastasis in a patient being evaluated for pelvic clearance.

Transaxial T2WI demonstrating a huge central pelvic tumour (T) with fluid-fluid levels (arrowheads) likely to indicate haemorrhage within the mass. In the posterior pelvis, there is a small volume of ascites (A) and peritoneal implants (open arrows). Note an enlarged left internal iliac lymph node (long arrow), which has a similar signal intensity to the tumour proper making it likely to be a metastatic node. This patient is ineligible for curative pelvic clearance.

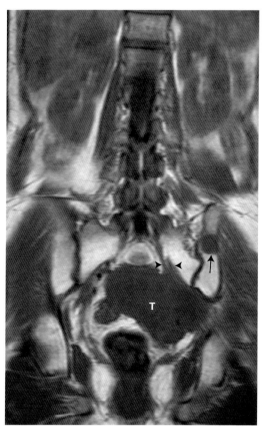

Figure 14.30. Bone metastases in a pelvic clearance candidate.

Coronal T1WI in a patient with a fibrosarcoma tumour (T) for which radiotherapy had already been administered. The tumour is infiltrating the left SI foramen (arrowheads). At the margin of the radiotherapy field there is high signal intensity within the marrow which has been irradiated and intermediate signal intensity in unradiated portions of the sacrum and iliac blades. A bone metastasis (arrow) has developed at the margin of the field.

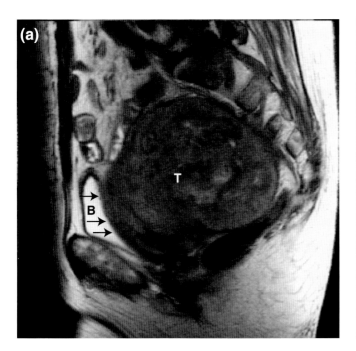
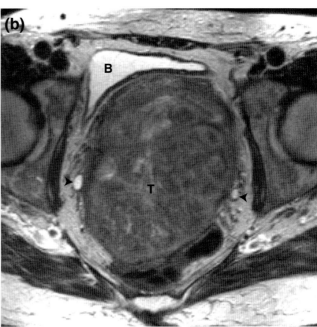

Figure 14.31. Large pelvic mass simulating visceral involvement.

(a) Sagittal and **(b)** transaxial T2WI in a patient with a large pelvic tumour (T) which is compressing both the rectum and the bladder (B). The posterior bladder wall demonstrates altered signal intensity on the sagittal images (arrows) but can be seen to be preserved on the transaxial image. This finding is explained by the plane of imaging, which is not perpendicular to the bladder wall on the sagittal sequence. On the transaxial image, the bladder wall is shown to be intact. Therefore, it is important to assess organ involvement in two planes. Note the bilateral hydroureter in (b) (arrowheads). This was not due to ureteric obstruction but to marked displacement of the ureters by the size of the central mass; they could be traced around the margins of the mass down to the vesico-ureteric junction.

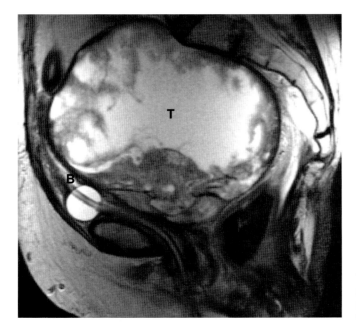

Figure 14.32. Tumour compressing pelvic organs.

Transaxial T2WI demonstrating a large recurrent ovarian tumour (T) compressing the bladder (B), which contains a urinary catheter. The mass is displacing the pelvic floor structures inferiorly. In these patients, it is often difficult to distinguish compression from adherence or infiltration.

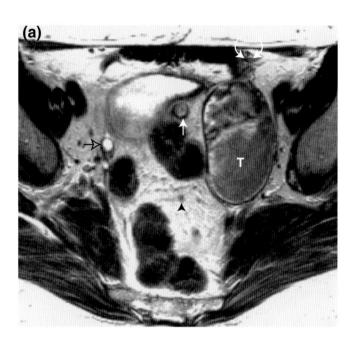

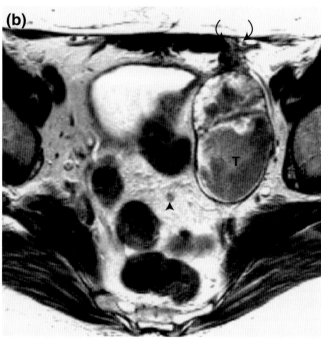

Figure 14.33. Small volume peritoneal disease.

(a) and **(b)** Transaxial T2WI in a patient with a recurrent ovarian tumour (T) which is adherent to the left abdominal wall (curved arrows). Additional small volume peritoneal deposits are seen adjacent to the bladder (arrow) and in the low pelvic peritoneum (arrowheads in (a) and (b)). Unusually, there is a retained right ovary (open arrow in (a)) with a small cyst within it.

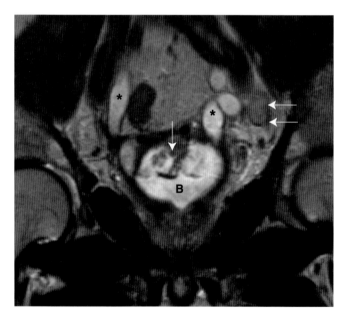

Figure 14.34. Hyperplastic lymph node.

Coronal T2WI in a patient with bladder cancer. There is a large left obturator node (arrows). The signal of the node does not match the signal intensity of the tumour (open arrow) which projects into the bladder lumen (B). At surgery, this node was shown to be reactive, probably due to inflammation and oedema induced at the time of biopsy. Note bilateral hydronephrosis (asterisks).

Index